Young Adult Drinking Styles

Dominic Conroy · Fiona Measham
Editors

Young Adult Drinking Styles

Current Perspectives on Research, Policy and Practice

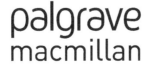

Editors
Dominic Conroy
School of Psychology
University of East London
London, UK

Fiona Measham
Department of Sociology
University of Liverpool
Liverpool, UK

ISBN 978-3-030-28609-5   ISBN 978-3-030-28607-1 (eBook)
https://doi.org/10.1007/978-3-030-28607-1

© The Editor(s) (if applicable) and The Author(s), under exclusive license to Springer Nature
Switzerland AG 2019
This work is subject to copyright. All rights are solely and exclusively licensed by the Publisher, whether
the whole or part of the material is concerned, specifically the rights of translation, reprinting, reuse
of illustrations, recitation, broadcasting, reproduction on microfilms or in any other physical way, and
transmission or information storage and retrieval, electronic adaptation, computer software, or by
similar or dissimilar methodology now known or hereafter developed.
The use of general descriptive names, registered names, trademarks, service marks, etc. in this
publication does not imply, even in the absence of a specific statement, that such names are exempt
from the relevant protective laws and regulations and therefore free for general use.
The publisher, the authors and the editors are safe to assume that the advice and information in this
book are believed to be true and accurate at the date of publication. Neither the publisher nor the
authors or the editors give a warranty, expressed or implied, with respect to the material contained
herein or for any errors or omissions that may have been made. The publisher remains neutral with
regard to jurisdictional claims in published maps and institutional affiliations.

Cover illustration: Brian Buckley/Alamy Stock Photo

This Palgrave Macmillan imprint is published by the registered company Springer Nature Switzerland AG
The registered company address is: Gewerbestrasse 11, 6330 Cham, Switzerland

Preface

The phrase 'young adult drinking' conjures up evocative images, at least until recently, of excess, anti-social behaviour and harm. More recently, the images of young adults on our screens have been of a more restrained, and indeed often strained, ilk, associated with a prioritisation of health and wellness in image and deed, plant-based diets (evident in the growing popularity of vegan products marketed at young adults) and concerns about their own future and the future of the planet, with movements like Extinction Rebellion reflecting a shift from a culture of consumption to a culture of restraint and sustainability.

At the close of the second decade of the twenty-first century, research and scholarly discussion concerning young adult alcohol use increasingly recognises the myriad ways in which alcohol can be understood and studied. Evidence now consistently points to broad demographic shifts in drinking behaviour among young adults. This is reflected in changes in expectations and stereotypes around drinking styles and behaviours among women and men and in the significant increase in the number of non-drinkers found among young adults in many developed countries. The rapid rise of social media use and mobile/smartphone technology also hold significant implications for future trends in alcohol, not just for drinkers but also for health promotion, and for alcohol industry manufacturing, marketing and retail practices.

Views on drinking behaviour and approaches to alcohol use practices among young adults continue to evolve. Accordingly, new research agendas and some evidence of movement away from a purely 'pathological' model for thinking about drinking behaviour among young adults have occurred. This new research climate is partly reflected in the great increase in qualitative and mixed methods research and a growth in multidisciplinary collaborations involving anthropologists, epidemiologists, psychologists, criminologists and sociologists, to name but a few. This diversification of topic focus and method application in the field of alcohol research is critically important from both clinical and policy perspectives. Progressive, successful modes of promoting more moderate drinking over the life course among young adults seem likely to benefit from the 'real world' emphasis of some contemporary alcohol research in which drinking experiences and drinking contexts are emphasised in empirical programmes.

Why should the drinking practices among individuals whom we are terming 'young adults' (those aged approximately 18–30 years old) warrant particular attention? Some authors consider that there are typical characteristics and decisions involved in this life stage—e.g. relating to living arrangements; acquiring secure/meaningful employment; initiation and experimentation with illicit drugs and altered states of intoxication; engaging with choices and meanings associated with identity and sexuality—that qualitatively distinguish young adulthood from earlier or later life stages. While early phases of experimentation may be behind them, many young adults are leaving the protective influences of family and local community for university, work and cohabiting with friends and partners, and beginning to lay down particular understandings about alcohol's role in their life which may form the basis for how alcohol is used (or not) for the remainder of that individual's life. Therefore, from their late teens onwards, young adults are, in many cases, presented with a relatively unfamiliar but considerable range of settings and occasions which demand decisions and action relating to alcohol use (and non-use).

How might 'drinking styles' provide a useful shift of focus? The lexicon for describing and understanding drinking behaviours and practices, and for identifying particular 'types' of drinkers is vast but is also culturally and historically situated. For example, we can think of drinking behaviour in terms of 'social drinking', 'moderate drinking', 'problem drinking', 'anti-social drinking', 'binge drinking', 'light drinking' and the list continues. Given the constructive power of the terminology surrounding alcohol consumption in the context of young adult drinking practices, questions are raised about possible alternatives that manage to navigate a route through these hard definitions to produce a more coherent appreciation of young adult drinking practices, cultural and policy change surrounding alcohol consumption, and new trends in research. The term 'drinking styles', which has appeared previously on occasions in the alcohol literature, helps guide the development of theory that accounts for fluidity and inconsistency in drinking practices over time. In terms of 'real world' advantages, the term 'drinking styles' provides a term that recognises that drinking behaviour is chosen and re-chosen between and within events involving the potential for alcohol consumption. Put another way, to discuss an individual's (or group's) drinking styles provides a way of acknowledging the multiple factors (and therefore multiple sites) for pursuing a health promotion agenda to promote safe, sustainable drinking practices among young adults.

While there is persistent coverage of alcohol-related issues in the media, academic, policy and broader cultural settings, what is much less clearly available is a space dedicated to a consideration of the trends, nuances and contexts for young adult drinking linked with life stage transitions and identity/identities in the post-Internet world. In exploring the complexities of drinking behaviour among young adults, the contributors to this collection avoid traditional understandings of young adult drinking that pathologise and generalise. We advocate instead for an inclusive approach evident in the wide range of disciplinary backgrounds, cultural perspectives and international settings represented in this book, in order to better understand the economic, cultural and pharmacological crossroads at which we now stand.

Never before has there been such a wide range of methods and approaches to considering drinking behaviour and practices among young adults. Our collection reflects this diversity with a range of methodological traditions which help expose nuance and difference in young adult drinking behaviour. Much of this is comprised of interview-based data, but this book also contains research based on focus groups, on studies of policy documents and on analyses of large scale survey data. We think this variety has helped to produce a more engaging and stimulating text but has also offered a collection that acknowledges the range of methodological lenses that can be applied to alcohol research focused on young adults and, as such, offers a more representative reflection of current field research.

We have structured the book into four short but distinct parts. Part I is organised around the theme of 'Trends in young adult drinking' reflecting both growing interest in what appears to be a decline in alcohol consumption among young people in recent years but also how drinking practices in young adulthood may transition to different drinking practices later in life. Part II is titled 'Young adult drinking in context' and presents a series of examples of how young adult drinking behaviour might be usefully framed in a contextualised sense involving specific places, time periods, online spaces or particular groups of people. Part III titled 'Recognizing the breadth of young adult drinking styles' turns to issues relating to identity. By definition, focusing on identity almost inevitably evokes an eclectic range of issues and topic areas for alcohol researchers and this diversity is reflected by the three contributions in this part. Chapter 11 in Part III attends to non-drinkers and non-drinking. As discussed elsewhere in this chapter, addressing the terminology used to understand and explore drinking practices among young adults can be instrumental in producing more coherent and accurate accounts of young adult drinking practices. Accordingly, the Part title—'Recognising the breadth of young adult drinking styles'—is a deliberate acknowledgement that drinking practices among young adults (or, indeed, anyone) can be usefully understood as *styles* and, as such, are situated, provisional modes of drinking practice that involve agency and context. Part IV ('Alcohol policy relating to young adult drinking practices') shifts attention to consider alcohol policy and does so with illustrations considering policy from different cultural perspectives and as applied to particular settings.

London, UK   Dominic Conroy
Liverpool, UK   Fiona Measham

Acknowledgements

Thank you to all our contributors and collaborators for their willingness to engage with this project initially. Without the generosity of spirit of our academic colleagues in the alcohol field in engaging with the process of feedback and discussion involved in developing chapter content, this collection would not have been possible.

We would also like to thank Palgrave Macmillan for their consistent support and patience throughout the production of this book. Particular thanks to Joanna O'Neill and Grace Jackson for steering the process of producing this book from initial discussions through to the final stages of production.

We have made every effort to trace all copyright holders in the production of this book. If, however, any have been overlooked, the publishers will be willing to make the required arrangements to address this at the earliest opportunity.

Contents

1 Book Introduction: Young Adult Drinking Styles 1
Dominic Conroy and Fiona Measham

Part I Trends in Young Adult Drinking

2 Have Recent Declines in Adolescent Drinking Continued into Young Adulthood? 21
Michael Livingston and Rakhi Vashishtha

3 Alcohol, Young Adults and the New Millennium: Changing Meanings in a Changing Social Climate 47
Gabriel Caluzzi and Amy Pennay

4 Life Transitions into Adulthood and the Drinking Trajectory 67
Marjana Martinic and Arlene Bigirimana

xii   Contents

Part II   Young Adult Drinking in Context

5   Into the Woods: Contextualising Atypical Intoxication
by Young Adults in Music Festivals and Nightlife
Tourist Resorts   87
Tim Turner and Fiona Measham

6   Drinking Norms and Alcohol Identities in the Context
of Social Media Interactions Among University
Students: An Overview of Relevant Literature   115
Brad Ridout

7   Social Media and Young Adults' Drinking Cultures:
Research Themes, Technological Developments
and Key Emerging Concepts   133
Ian Goodwin and Antonia Lyons

8   Friendship and Alcohol Use Among Young Adults:
A Cross-Disciplinary Literature Review   153
Dominic Conroy and Sarah MacLean

9   Gender in Young Adult's Discourses of Drinking
and Drunkenness   173
Alexandra Bogren

10   Alcohol Consumption Among Young People
in Marginalised Groups   191
Lana Ireland

**Part III   Recognizing the Breadth of Young
Adult Drinking Styles**

11   Non-drinkers and Non-drinking: A Review, a Critique
and Pathways to Policy   213
Emma Banister, Dominic Conroy and Maria Piacentini

Contents   xiii

12 Can't Dance Without Being Drunk? Exploring the Enjoyment and Acceptability of Conscious Clubbing in Young People   233
Emma Davies, Joanne Smith, Mattias Johansson, Kimberley Hill and Kyle Brown

13 Young People and Temporary Alcohol Abstinence During Dry January   253
Richard de Visser

Part IV Alcohol Policy Relating to Young Adult Drinking Practices

14 University Alcohol Policy: Findings from Mixed Methods Research and Implications for Students' Drinking Practices   275
Rose Leontini, Toni Schofield, Julie Hepworth and John Germov

15 Policies Addressing Alcohol-Related Violence Among Young People: A Gendered Analysis Based on Two Australian States   295
Aaron Hart and Claire Wilkinson

16 Making Sense of Alcohol Consumption Among Russian Young Adults in the Context of Post-2009 Policy Initiatives   313
Vadim Radaev

17 Evaluating the Recent 'Integrated Approach' to Alcohol Policy Designed to Promote Moderate Alcohol Consumption Among Dutch Young People   333
Rob Bovens and Dike van de Mheen

xiv   Contents

18   Conclusion and Reflections on Future Directions   351
Dominic Conroy and Fiona Measham

Index   359

Notes on Contributors

Emma Banister is a Senior Lecturer at the University of Manchester. Her research expertise is in transformative consumer research, informing policy outcomes and addressing inequalities and vulnerabilities in the marketplace. She is co-chair of the Academy of Marketing's 'Consumer Research with Social Impact' Special Interest Group. Her research mainly focuses around issues of identity, consumer culture and policy in relation to alcohol, motherhood, fatherhood and parental leave. Her work has been published in a range of journals including *Sociological Review, Sociology, Sociology of Health and Illness, Marketing Theory, Journal of Business Research, European Journal of Marketing* and *Consumption Markets and Culture*.

Arlene Bigirimana is a Science and Policy Research Associate at the International Alliance for Responsible Drinking in Washington, DC. Her research interests include alcohol policy topics related to youth and underage drinking, pricing practices, and screening and brief interventions. Previously, Arlene worked as a research assistant at the Baltimore arm of CDC's National HIV Behavioral Surveillance Study, BESURE. She graduated with honours from Johns Hopkins University a dual degree in Public Health and Spanish and obtained her masters in public health in Health Policy and Management from Johns Hopkins Bloomberg School of Public Health.

Alexandra Bogren is Associate Professor and Senior Lecturer in sociology at Södertörn University, Stockholm, Sweden. She has a long-standing interest in analysing gendered discourses on alcohol and other drugs and has published several articles on the topic, including a study comparing gendered media discourses on alcohol and psychotropics and a study on the Swedish media discourse of gender, alcohol and rape (with J. Bernhardsson).

Rob Bovens (1955) is Senior Researcher and Coordinator of the Academic Collaborated Center for Addiction of Tranzo. He studied Law and Criminology at the University of Nijmegen. He was a researcher for the Ministry of Justice where he was awarded his Ph.D. on research concerning 'Courses for alcohol traffic offenders, in and outside prison'. He worked on a national level as staff member and Managing Director in probation services for addicted offenders from 1990 to 2004, was campaign leader of the alcohol campaigns in the Netherlands until 2010, and was Professor at the University of Applied Sciences, Zwolle from 2010 to 2017.

Kyle Brown is an experimental psychologist with a research focus on alcohol-related cognitions and biases surrounding alcohol consumption. Specifically, his research examines the role of alcohol-related cues (e.g. brand labelling, advertisements and alcohol-related contexts) and value on both the choice and consumption of alcohol. His recent projects focus on the impact of alcohol warning messages on students' risk perceptions and alcohol-related discourses. He is also part of a collaboration examining the feasibility of alternatives to alcohol-related activities, with a view to reduce student alcohol consumption.

Gabriel Caluzzi is a Ph.D. student with CAPR at La Trobe University. His Ph.D. is a qualitative exploration of the factors contributing to declining youth drinking in Australia. Gabriel completed a Bachelor of Arts (Honours) in 2016, with a minor thesis examining at the role of conformity in heavy episodic drinking among university students. He has an interest in both the sociology and social psychology of alcohol use, and how different types of alcohol use demarcates different social groups.

Dominic Conroy is Lecturer in psychology at the University of East London. Dominic has published quantitative and qualitative research concerning health behaviour among young adults over the last decade. His qualitative, quantitative, and mixed methods research primarily concerns drinking practices including temporary abstinence initiative participation among young adults. He is interested in developing effective behavioural interventions designed to reduce excessive alcohol consumption among young adults. He is also interested in exploring young adult drinking practices that illuminate issues of intimacy and social bonding underpinning alcohol use and developing understanding of flexible drinking styles and agency involved in young adults' alcohol use.

Emma Davies is a Senior Lecturer in psychology at Oxford Brookes University. Her research expertise is in the field of health psychology and has a particular focus on behaviour change theories and developing interventions to improve young people's health and well-being. Recent key projects have explored the potential of using digital tools to reduce alcohol misuse in adolescents and students. She is also interesting in exploring the meanings attached with drinking (and non-drinking) practices and experiences within different groups.

Richard de Visser is a reader in psychology at the University of Sussex in the UK, where he teaches in the School of Psychology and the Brighton & Sussex Medical School. He is co-author of the textbook *Psychology for Medicine & Health Care*, the second edition of which was recently published. He uses quantitative, qualitative and mixed methods to explore social aspects of various health-related behaviours, with a particular focus on alcohol use.

John Germov is a Professor of Sociology, Pro-Vice-Chancellor (Academic) and Pro-Vice-Chancellor of the Faculty of Education and Arts at the University of Newcastle, Australia. His research interests span the social determinants of health, with a particular focus on food and alcohol consumption in the context of public health. His books include *Public Sociology: An Introduction to Australian Society* (with

Marilyn Poole), *A Sociology of Food and Nutrition: The Social Appetite* (with Lauren Williams), *Second Opinion: An Introduction to Health Sociology*, and *Histories of Australian Sociology* (with Tara McGee).

Ian Goodwin is a Senior Lecturer in the School of English and Media Studies, Massey University, Wellington. With a background in cultural studies, his research is wide-ranging and often interdisciplinary, yet focuses on understanding the societal changes associated with the rise of digital media technologies. His work explores intersections between contemporary media forms, youth culture, popular culture, activism, citizenship, media policy, consumption, and health and well-being.

Aaron Hart is a Research Fellow at the University of Melbourne and the Brotherhood of St Laurence, an Australian non-government organisation. His research uses qualitative sociological methods to investigate public health and social welfare policy issues. His interests include applied analyses of social issues, critical theory and science and technology studies, the capabilities approach and theories of justice, gender theory and political science. He has published in the alcohol and other drug fields, performed evaluations of social service programs and lectured in research methods at Victoria University. His current work investigates the health of older aged care workers.

Julie Hepworth is a health psychologist working in public health and primary health-care research. She has published extensively on young adults' mental health, including alcohol use and eating disorders, patients' experiences of health-care and chronic conditions, health-care professionals' perspectives on health-care delivery and health policy. She is Professor at the Queensland University of Technology, Brisbane, Australia, where she teaches healthy policy, health-related theory and methodology, and Honorary Professor at The University of Queensland, Australia.

Kimberley Hill is a Senior Lecturer in psychology at The University of Northampton. Her research expertise is in the area of health promotion and health risk prevention, with a particular interest in understanding the role of complex social contexts on the behaviour of young people. As well as exploring the meaning that alcohol-free spaces have for young people, some of Kimberley's most recent projects have focused on the functional significance of on- and off-premise alcogenic environments, with recommendations for preventing substance misuse and related harms, as well as creating new, on-campus contexts to safeguard students from sexual violence and related harms.

Lana Ireland is a Lecturer in psychology at Glasgow Caledonian University (GCU). Her research interests span social and forensic psychology and include substance use, domestic abuse, identity and including hard-to-reach and excluded populations in the research process. Recent research projects have involved working with victims of crime; prisoners; Gypsy, Roma, Traveller (GRT) groups; and LGBT groups. She is a member of the Substance Use and Misuse Research Group at GCU, is a Chartered Psychologist with the British Psychological Society (CPsychol, BPS) and a Senior Fellow with the Higher Education Academy (SFHEA).

Mattias Johansson is a Lecturer in sport and exercise psychology, at Örebro University, Sweden. His research focuses mainly on psychological effects and experiences of mind-body methods such as qigong, dance and mindfulness as well as other forms of physical activities. A recent research project of Mattias was a randomised controlled mixed methods free dance intervention in which the effects and experiences of dancing were explored on body esteem, objectification, body awareness, stress, mindfulness and psychological well-being.

Rose Leontini is a Lecturer in the School of Public Health and Community Medicine, UNSW Sydney. She has an interdisciplinary background in health sociology and health ethics, with research interests in youth and alcohol, the social and ethical dimensions of genetic testing, risk and harm minimisation, the sociology of health and illness, health and hygiene education, and illness narratives.

Michael Livingston is Senior Research Fellow with the Centre for Alcohol Policy Research (CAPR) at La Trobe University. Michael completed his Ph.D. on the effects of liquor licensing policy on alcohol-related harms in 2012 and has subsequently worked on a series of projects examining trends in drinking among young people. Michael has worked in alcohol epidemiology and policy research since 2006 and has a strong interest in understanding population-level changes in alcohol consumption.

Antonia Lyons is a Professor of Health Psychology at Victoria University of Wellington, New Zealand. Her research explores the social, cultural and mediated contexts of behaviours related to health, including the role that social media play in drinking cultures. She is currently co-editor of the *Journal Qualitative Research in Psychology* and serves as an Associate Editor for *Psychology and Health*. She also is co-editor (with Professor Kerry Chamberlain) of the Routledge book series *Critical Approaches to Health*.

Sarah MacLean uses practice theory and other sociological frameworks to understand cultures that frame alcohol and other drug use and gambling within specific social groups. Her research highlights how discrimination and disadvantage impact on, and are in turn produced by, substance use. Her Ph.D. explored the capacity of inhalant (volatile substance) use to offer socially excluded young people opportunities to enact desired selfhoods, after which she completed postdoctoral research investigating place-based differences in young adults' alcohol consumption. She is employed as Associate Professor in the Discipline of Social Work and Social Policy at La Trobe University in Melbourne, Australia, and has been appointed joint Editor-in-Chief of *Health Sociology Review* for the period 2019–2021.

Marjana Martinic has over two decades of experience in cross-cultural research on alcohol and the development of policy and interventions. Marjana established and led the scientific function at the global think tank International Center for Alcohol Policies and subsequently served as Deputy CEO at the International Alliance for Responsible Drinking. She received her degree in biology from Harvard University and her doctorate in neuroscience from Northwestern University and conducted basic research as a Fellow at the University of Virginia Medical School and the US National Institutes of Health. She has published extensively on alcohol issues, including the 2008 volume *Swimming with Crocodiles* examining extreme drinking among young people.

Fiona Measham was appointed Chair in Criminology at the University of Liverpool in 2019. She has conducted research for nearly three decades across a broad area of criminology and social policy, exploring changing trends in legal and illegal drugs; night time and festival economies and the sociocultural context to consumption; new psychoactive substances; and broader drug policy. She is an instructor and trainer with the Inside-Out Prison Exchange Programme that she introduced to the UK with Durham University colleagues in 2014. She is also co-founder and co-director of The Loop UK and The Loop AU non-profit harm reduction NGOs, best known for introducing Multi Agency Safety Testing to the UK in 2016.

Amy Pennay is Research Fellow with the Centre for Alcohol Policy Research (CAPR) at La Trobe University. She completed an ethnographic Ph.D. in 2012, which explored the social, cultural, economic and environmental influences of alcohol and party drug use among a group of young adults. She has worked in alcohol and drug research for more than 13 years, using a diverse range of methodologies, but has a particular interest in qualitative research. Her research has primarily focused on risky drinking, drug use and energy drink use in the night- time economy, but she also has an interest in cultures of drinking and stigma, relating to socio-economic status, ethnicity and sexual orientation.

Maria Piacentini is Professor of Consumer Research at Lancaster University Management School and Director of the Centre for Consumption Insights. Her research focuses on consumer vulnerability, and she has explored this theme in a number of contexts of public policy concern. Her work has been published in *Sociology, Sociology of Health & Illness, European Journal of Marketing, Journal of Business Research, Journal of Marketing Management and Marketing Theory*. She was co-editor of *Consumer Vulnerability: Conditions, contexts and characteristics*, published as part of the *Routledge Studies in Critical Marketing* series. She was a co-chair of the ESRC seminar series on Vulnerable Consumers (2012–2014). Along with Emma Banister and Kathy Hamilton, she is co-chair of the Academy of Marketing's 'Consumer Research with Social Impact' Special Interest Group.

Vadim Radaev is Professor, Head of the Laboratory for Studies in Economic Sociology and First Vice-Rector of the National Research University Higher School of Economics (Moscow, Russia). He is also Editor-in-Chief of *Journal of Economic Sociology* (https://ecsoc.hse.ru/en/). He received his Ph.D. from the Department of Economics, Moscow State University (1986) and Doctor Habilitat in Economics and Sociology from the Institute of Economics, Russian Academy of Sciences (1997). His research interests are economic sociology, legal and illegal markets, alcohol consumption. He has published articles in *Alcohol and Alcoholism, International Journal of Drug Policy, Addiction* and other journals.

Brad Ridout is a Research Fellow with the Faculty of Health Sciences, a PBA Registered Psychologist and member of the Australian Psychological Society. He completed his Ph.D. research at the University of Sydney and was the first in the world to demonstrate that Facebook can be used to facilitate social norm interventions to reduce problem drinking in young people. He is currently working with Kids Helpline to develop the world's first secure and anonymous social media platform for supporting the mental health of young people through online group counselling. He has published in *Current Opinion in Psychology* and *Australasian Drug & Alcohol Review* and is at the forefront of developing evidence-based best practice for the use of technology to support mental health. In his clinical work, he specialises in the treatment of anxiety and depression, with a special interest in using technology to support the psychological well-being of children and adolescents.

Associate Professor Toni Schofield is a researcher and writer based at the Universities of New England and Sydney. She is the author and co-author of more than 70 publications, including *A Sociological Approach to Health Determinants* (2015, Cambridge University Press) and reports for major Australian and international agencies such as the Department of Prime Minister and Cabinet, the Australian Human Rights Commission and the WHO. She is currently involved in a three-year ARC-funded study to investigate the impacts of an adult literacy campaign on Aboriginal communities in Western NSW.

Joanne Smith is a final-year Ph.D. candidate at Northumbria University exploring the positive social factors which underpin and maintain student drinking behaviour. During her Ph.D., Joanne has adopted both quantitative and qualitative approaches, and her final study used social network analysis to explore popularity and alcohol consumption among student athletes who participate in team sports. Joanne's work to date has provided an insight into the culture surrounding alcohol and sport at university, highlighting the complex role of alcohol in the social lives of student athletes and the impact of drinking choices on athlete mental health. As of January 2018, Joanne has taken up a research position in the NHS, where she is offering support and advice to health professionals who are conducting research and evaluating health initiatives.

Tim Turner is Senior Lecturer in criminology at Coventry University. He previously worked as a forensic mental health nurse and is the joint editor of Critical Issues in Mental Health (Palgrave). As a Registered Intermediary, he has worked extensively with vulnerable witnesses in the criminal justice system. His doctorate research, an ethnography of British youth in Ibiza, was conducted over three summers and examined the situated social meaning of poly-drug use in the context of tourism. His research interests are focused on the relationship between drug use, pleasure and space.

Dike van de Mheen is Full Professor and Director of Tranzo, Scientific Center for care and Wellbeing at Tilburg University. She studied Health Sciences at Maastricht University, the Netherlands, and is an epidemiologist. She worked as Researcher and Senior Advisor at the Rotterdam Area Health Authority, and as Researcher and Assistant Professor at Erasmus University Rotterdam. She was Director of IVO Addiction Research Institute Rotterdam from 2000 to 2017. From 2007 to 2017, she was Professor of Addiction Research at Erasmus University Rotterdam. From 2012 to 2017, she was also Professor (of Care and Prevention of Risky Behaviour and Addiction) at Maastricht University.

Rakhi Vashishtha is a Ph.D. student with CAPR at La Trobe University. Her current Ph.D. research involves quantitative investigation of the factors leading to the decline in adolescent drinking in

Australia. Rakhi completed her Masters in Public Health in 2016 with a research project that focused on examining the factors responsible for alcohol quitting among older population in Australia. Her research interests include statistical analysis of alcohol drinking behaviour in various subgroups and exploring the role of various drivers of alcohol drinking in bringing the changes in alcohol consumption.

Claire Wilkinson is a Research Fellow with the Social Policy Research Centre (SPRC) at UNSW and an Honorary Research Fellow at the Centre for Alcohol Policy Research (CAPR) at La Trobe University. She completed a comparative mixed methods Ph.D. in 2017, which examined approaches to restricting the physical availability of alcohol at a local level and assessed how and to what extent different approaches shaped local alcohol availability. She has conducted alcohol policy research for over a decade, exploring changing trends in public opinion and media coverage of alcohol policy issues; the association of alcohol outlet density with alcohol-related harms; the enforcement and implementation of alcohol outlet regulation; and the ways in which public health research and local/community opinion are considered in decisions to issue new liquor licenses in Australian liquor licensing laws and regulation.

List of Figures

Fig. 2.1	Average annual consumption by age and birth cohort, 2001–2016, National Drug Strategy Household Survey	26
Fig. 16.1	Alcohol consumers for the last 30 days, by age group (%, $n = 258,526$)	325
Fig. 16.2	Average volume of alcohol consumption during the last 30 days by age groups (grams of pure alcohol, $n = 80,839$)	326
Fig. 16.3	Excessive drinkers by age groups (%, $n = 80,839$)	327
Fig. 17.1	Trends in hospital admissions 2000–2005 due to intoxication by alcohol in the Netherlands (Valkenberg, Van der Lely, & Brugmans, 2007)	337

List of Tables

Table 2.1	Risky drinking trends among young adults	28
Table 2.2	Trends in other drinking measures among young adults	33
Table 12.1	Pearson correlations between AUDIT scores, social connectedness, life satisfaction, attitudes towards conscious clubbing and acceptability of policy to introduce conscious clubbing	242
Table 13.1	Reasons for taking part in Dry January	262
Table 13.2	Context of taking part in Dry January	263
Table 13.3	Multivariate predictors of successful completion of Dry January	265
Table 14.1	Patterns of drinking behaviour by living situation	280
Table 16.1	Excise tax rates on alcoholic beverages, RBL/L 2009–2017, and excise increase by 2009 (%)	320

1

Book Introduction: Young Adult Drinking Styles

Dominic Conroy and Fiona Measham

The phrase 'young adult drinking' conjures up evocative images, at least until recently, of excess, antisocial behaviour and harm. These images linking alcohol consumption by young adults with personal and social harms remain readily available in mass media depictions of archetypal leisure time activities involving drinking and drunkenness. The dangers posed to young adults by alcohol as a substance that too readily leads to over-indulgence, over-dependence and an array of other risks such as personal injury and potentially risky sexual encounters are often closely woven into the assumptions of empirical research in the social sciences. More recently, the images of young adults on our screens have been of a more restrained and, indeed, often strained, ilk, associated with a prioritisation of health

D. Conroy (✉)
School of Psychology, University of East London, London, UK
e-mail: D.Conroy@uel.ac.uk

F. Measham
Department of Sociology, University of Liverpool, Liverpool, UK
e-mail: f.measham@liverpool.ac.uk

© The Author(s) 2019
D. Conroy and F. Measham (eds.), *Young Adult Drinking Styles*,
https://doi.org/10.1007/978-3-030-28607-1_1

and wellness in image and deed, plant-based diets (evident in the growing popularity of vegan products marketed at young adults) and concerns about their own future and the future of the planet, with movements like Extinction Rebellion reflecting a shift from a culture of consumption to a culture of restraint and sustainability.

At the close of the second decade of the twenty-first century, research and scholarly discussion concerning young adult alcohol use increasingly recognises the myriad ways in which alcohol can be understood and studied. This more nuanced attitude towards alcohol research acknowledges alcohol's varied role within social rituals (such as preloading and drinking games) and permits scope for increased recognition of alcohol's valued role in initiating and maintaining friendships among young adults. Evidence now consistently points to broad demographic shifts in drinking behaviour among young adults. This is reflected in changes in expectations and stereotypes around drinking styles and behaviours among women and men and in the significant increase in the number of non-drinkers found among young adults in many developed countries. The rapid rise of social media use and mobile/smartphone technology also holds significant implications for future trends in alcohol, not just for drinkers but also for health promotion, and for alcohol industry manufacturing, marketing and retail practices. However, research on a possible association between the explosion in smartphone use, gaming and immediate, consistent internet access, and a reduction in young adult alcohol consumption is in its infancy. Such research needs to also consider how being online during drinking occasions might present new and different potential threats to young adult health and well-being.

Views on drinking behaviour and approaches to alcohol use practices among young adults continue to evolve. Accordingly, social scientists have recognised the importance of efforts to shift the emphasis of research agendas towards progressive and sometimes non-traditional models of young adult drinking behaviour. One notable characteristic of this shift is a conscious movement away from a purely 'pathological' model for thinking about drinking behaviour in which 'problem cognitions' (e.g. alcohol beliefs) or 'problem dispositions' (e.g. personality) are identified as key drivers of higher risk drinking among young adults. This new research climate is partly reflected in the great increase in qualitative and mixed methods research used to explore alcohol-related behaviour, experiences and practices. In addition, exploring alcohol use among young adults has been recognised as an ongoing multidisciplinary project with continued important contributions from anthropologists, epidemiologists, psychologists, criminologists and sociologists, to name but a few. This diversification of topic focus and method application in the field of alcohol research is critically important from both clinical and policy perspectives. Progressive, successful modes of promoting more moderate drinking over the life course among young adults seem likely to benefit from the 'real-world' emphasis of some contemporary alcohol research.

This empirical work and theoretical debate that we allude to above have helped generate greater awareness of alcohol use among young adults as something nuanced, complex, both pleasurable and problematic and, critically, tightly bound within broader social contexts and life relationships. We aim to present a sample of the breadth of this research in this collection and to explore where the emphases of progressive alcohol research concerning young adults may usefully go from here.

Who Are 'Young Adults'?

There is great variety in how young adults are referred to in the academic literature and in wider public discourse. We prefer the term 'young adults' and have chosen this term here to refer to individuals aged approximately 18–30 years of age. This is preferable to 'adolescents' that would span younger demographic groups, and 'youths' and 'young people' that are less clearly defined usually include early and mid-teenage groups and are associated with particular connotations and theoretical emphases. In approaching this book, we are mindful, however, that different terms will have particular currency in different international settings and within different disciplines.

We turn now to how the term 'young adults' was reached and how this works in relation to terminology used to describe the focal group of interest for our contributors. Accounting for the life stage (or life stages) following adolescence yet before later years of adulthood has attracted theoretical interest. Most prominent here is Arnett's (2000) theory of 'emerging adulthood' designed to articulate an understanding of the experiences of young adults aged roughly 18–25 years. Emerging adulthood, as a theory, helped to acknowledge changes in life stage circumstances in younger adult life that have taken place in industrialised societies needing to be accommodated to replace more traditional theories of life stage transition (e.g. Erikson, 1950). The advantages of emerging adulthood as a theoretical approach is that it *does* draw attention to important and distinctive features that may be experienced during this period of the lifespan characterised by uncertainty and identity exploration. However, we take the position that any strong categorisation of lifespan stages in this way runs the risk of impinging on understanding among a clearly heterogeneous group who will inevitably be situated in terms of their history and culture.

Research involving young adults, as preparation for this book has borne out time and again, is frequently conflated with research involving significantly younger individuals in a life stage more like middle adolescence (e.g. 15–17-year-olds) or even early adolescence (e.g. 11–14-year-olds). In focusing on 'young adults', we have a particular editorial view and definition which we believe helps narrow focus to a group of individuals who warrant particular attention and dedicated focus in the alcohol literature. The term 'young adults' helps narrow focus on individuals aged over eighteen and therefore adults, for at least some purposes, in a legal sense, in the UK and many other jurisdictions. Imposing an upper limit is more problematic of course, and this is acknowledged in long-standing theoretical discussion on emerging and established adulthood (Green, 2016; Levinson, 1986). In this edited collection, we chose to focus on 'young adults' as individuals aged approximately 18–30 years. Given that different terms mean different things to different people anyway (who may, quite reasonably, have little interest or investment in particular terms to describe the age range of the sample on whom their own research focuses), but also to promote the principle of academic freedom, we have adopted an inclusive approach and you will see variations in terminology and age ranges in this book including, predominantly, the terms 'young people' and 'young adults'.

What Is 'Drinking'?

As with the other elements of our title, pinning down what is meant by drinking presents similar difficulties. The alcohol literature contains a wide-ranging (and ever-increasing) vernacular for defining the focal activities of interest and relevance to this book and to this field. To illustrate, we could refer to these activities using the following expressions: 'drinking', 'drinking behaviour', 'drinking practices' and 'alcohol consumption'. A parallel range of terms exist to define and encapsulate the behaviour (and individuals) who do not drink alcohol (either as a lifestyle choice or within a particular time/place): 'non-drinking', 'abstinence', 'alcohol abstinence', 'sobriety', 'temporary sobriety' or 'social non-drinking'.

Each term brings its own point of emphasis, and its own advantages and caveats. The expression 'drinking behaviour' would be broadly accepted from a post-positivist psychology research perspective, where an understanding of alcohol use would typically prioritise an individual-level understanding of activity that can be understood in discrete and objectively definable 'behavioural' terms. Other social science research perspectives would be likely to problematise this starting point, noting that 'drinking behaviour' disaggregates an understanding of alcohol use (including, for example, an understanding of motivations to initiate alcohol consumption and to drink alcohol in large quantities) from the social and environmental context to which it is intimately tied. By contrast, there are advantages to referring to 'drinking practices', which blurs the individual and the social and does not imply clearly defined time frames for alcohol consumption, over more individually orientated terms such as 'drinking behaviour', and therefore, it is favoured in this book. No arrangement of terminology can attract or appease all audiences, however. We are aware here that, as an editorial team, we approach this book collection from our own disciplinary and sub-disciplinary perspectives. Like other decisions relating to terminology in this book, we have taken a loose, non-prescriptive approach both to our contributors' choice of vocabulary and to our own terms for defining alcohol use among young adults.

Why an Interest in Young Adult Drinking?

To this point, we have drawn attention to the changing landscape of alcohol-related research concerning young adults and note particularly that there seem to be new, invigorating opportunities and challenges ahead for research in this field. We have begun to consider the terminology that can or should be used to define the group of individuals who are the focus of our attention for this collection and, similarly, to define the activities relating to alcohol use that are to be focused on. Putting this together, we now turn to the question stated in the title of this subsection: Why should the drinking practices among individuals whom we are terming 'young adults' (those aged approximately 18–30 years old) warrant particular attention? Different perspectives are helpful in addressing this question.

One might draw on Arnett's (2000) account of emerging adulthood again here to consider what have been presented as typical characteristics of this life stage that have a bearing on considering alcohol use during this period of life. Indeed, this has been the focus of specific discussion and research in the emerging adulthood literature (e.g. Arnett, 2005; Maynard, Salas-Wright, & Vaughn, 2015). These might include pivotal decisions relating to living arrangements and lifestyle choices; embarking on higher education; acquiring secure/meaningful employment; accessing licensed leisure in adult nightlife and festival economies; initiation and experimentation with illicit drugs and altered states of intoxication; identifying whether and what relationship circumstances suit an individual; and similar issues relating to choices and meanings associated with identity and sexuality. These important considerations mark 'young adults' as a group for whom alcohol use is one in a constellation of factors to consider from a research and policy perspective.

Another perspective might draw greater attention to the particular pressures faced by young adults in the closing quarter of the twenty-first century to work with (whether to adhere to or resist) cultural understandings of what becoming and 'being' a young adult could or should entail. The visibility and importance of alcohol use as features of 'being young' are something that are recognised and capitalised on by the alcohol, hospitality, events and festival industries when considering their own marketing strategies (Hastings et al., 2010). Alcohol branding and sponsorship have a near-omniscient presence in much young adult leisure from the naming of entertainment arenas and live music stadia to festival bars, particularly with growing restrictions on sponsorship of sporting events and of alcohol marketing more generally in many developed countries (Rowley & Williams, 2008).

A pragmatic approach to health promotion offers a further perspective to help explain why focusing on alcohol use among young adults might attract research attention. Whilst secondary school (i.e. schools for children aged 11–16 years) has traditionally provided an important opportunity for formal educational input on health education and life skills, the expansion of higher education to cover nearly half of young adults in many developed countries results in young adults representing an additional and under-recognised demographic group to target with age and life stage appropriate health promotion, education and prevention campaigns. Whilst reviews have identified the most effective prevention programmes for secondary school youth being those that focus on normative education and enhancing social and social resistance skills relating to substance use, more consideration is needed regarding their efficacy with young adults (Botvin & Griffin, 2007). For whilst the earliest phase of experimentation may be behind them, many young adults are leaving the protective influences of family and local community for university, work and cohabiting with friends and partners, and beginning to lay down particular understandings about alcohol's role in their life which may form the basis for how alcohol is used (or not) for the remainder of that individual's life. Therefore, from their late teens onwards, young adults are, in many cases, presented with a relatively unfamiliar but considerable range of settings and occasions which demand decisions and action relating to alcohol use (and non-use).

Why Drinking 'Styles'?

Terminology, as discussed above, is central to understanding. The lexicon for describing and understanding drinking behaviours and practices, and for identifying particular 'types' of drinkers is vast but is also culturally and historically situated. For example, we can think of drinking behaviour in terms of 'social drinking', 'moderate drinking', 'problem drinking', 'antisocial drinking', 'binge drinking', 'light drinking' and the list continues. We might also think about 'risky drinking', 'harmful drinking', 'immoderate drinking' and, increasingly visibly, the terminology of 'responsible drinking' in the USA and other international settings (e.g. International Alliance of Responsible Drinking, 2019). These terms set down the parameters through which we might think about drinking behaviour, and drinking behaviour among young adults particularly, as morally acceptable/unacceptable, as harmful/beneficial to the self and as harmful/beneficial to others in our immediate and wider vicinity. Moreover, these terms set down yardsticks by which research questions are framed, by which research projects are designed and implemented, by which research evidence informs and governs the development and delivery of alcohol policy, and by which evidence also informs the justification, choice and delivery of interventions and clinical practice relevant to alcohol consumption.

Discussion here is intended partly to draw attention to the constructive power of the terminology surrounding alcohol consumption in the context of young adult drinking practices, and the theoretical and practical difficulties that hard definitions can produce for understanding behaviour that is inherently complex and multifaceted. For example, contemporary use of the term 'binge drinker' would serve to produce an understanding of an individual's approach to alcohol consumption as excessive and harmful regardless of the company and environment in which the individual finds themselves in, the cultural and sub-cultural norms pertinent to that individual, surrounding life circumstances and demands, and how drinking practices can be understood from the perspective of life narrative including transition between particular life stages. Historically, the term might have been associated with a prolonged and intense drinking session or 'bender' (Herring, Berridge, & Thom, 2008). Therefore, drinker categories like 'binge drinker', useful as they may be as shorthand in academic and everyday language, can create a persistently decontextualised understanding of young adult drinking practices.

1 Book Introduction: Young Adult Drinking Styles   9

This raises questions about possible alternatives that manage to navigate a route through these hard definitions to produce a more coherent appreciation of young adult drinking practices, cultural and policy change surrounding alcohol consumption, and new trends in research. The term 'drinking styles' has theoretical and 'real-world' advantages. In theoretical terms, 'drinking styles' shifts emphasis of young adult drinking behaviour to take account for fluidity and inconsistency in drinking practices over the course of a social event, a week, a month, a life stage or a lifespan. This shifts the research agenda towards an emphasis on contradictory and counter-intuitive features of drinking practices which may fluctuate in association with contextual considerations. In practical terms, 'drinking styles' provides a term that recognises that drinking behaviour is chosen and re-chosen between and within events involving the potential for alcohol consumption. As a term, drinking styles also provides a rhetorical way of acknowledging that a given young adult has possibilities open to them in terms of how they understand the role of alcohol, its subjective effects, its social role and its community and cultural understandings. Put another way, to discuss individual (or group) drinking styles provides a way of acknowledging the multiple factors (and therefore multiple sites) for pursuing a health promotion agenda to promote safe, sustainable drinking practices among young adults.

The notion of 'styles' appears rarely in the context of health behaviour or health practices. This is perhaps surprising given the appearance of this term among, for example, educationalists, where theories of differing 'learning styles' have proven influential (e.g. Messick, 1984; Peterson, Rayner, & Armstrong, 2009) and, from the perspective of some educational commentators, controversial (Kirschner, 2017; Willingham, Hughes, & Dobolyi, 2015). Researchers with an interest in health behaviours do not conventionally refer to 'eating styles', 'styles of sexual practice', 'physical activity styles' or 'drinking styles'. Drinking styles is not a new term, however. It has appeared in discussion of patterns of drinking behaviour among individuals with a diagnosis of alcoholism and the children of alcoholics (e.g. Johnson, Leonard, & Jacob, 1989; Olenick & Chalmers, 1991). However, deployment of the term in a way that aligns with our suggested use—to recognise variations in drinking behaviour and the context-dependent nature of drinking practices—is present in the work of Betsy Thom and colleagues who, for example, have documented the nuances in motivations to drink and drinking practices among young men (Harnett, Thom, Herring, & Kelly, 2000). These nuances are also evident in work on 'peer attachment styles' (Bartholomew & Horowitz, 1991) and 'romantic attachment styles' (Hazan & Shaver, 1987) in young adulthood.

What Is the Purpose of This Book?

Whilst there is persistent coverage of alcohol-related issues in the media, academic, policy and broader cultural settings what is much less clearly available is a space dedicated to a consideration of the trends, nuances and contexts for young adult drinking linked with life stage transitions and identity/identities in the post-Internet world. Studies are just turning their focus to consider the sociocultural context to drinking in a world shifting from cultures of consumption to cultures of austerity, alongside the growing impact of online, digital and virtual worlds. We have seen the ebbs and flows of both alcohol consumption and licensed leisure more broadly, with a rise in binge drinking across developed countries in the late 1990s and early 2000s associated with growing disposable income and notions of extended adolescence delaying life stage milestones like marriage, mortgage and parenthood. Then, in the post-millennial decade, there has been an apparent downturn in alcohol and in consumption more generally, associated with economic recession and associated austerity measures leading to growing economic restrictions on licensed leisure and a turn against conspicuous consumption.

In exploring the complexities of drinking behaviour among young adults, the contributors to this collection take a deliberate discursive turn away from traditional understandings of young adult drinking that pathologise and generalise. We advocate instead for an inclusive approach evident in the wide range of disciplinary backgrounds, cultural perspectives and international settings represented in this book, in order to better understand the economic, cultural and pharmacological crossroads at which we now stand.

Never before has there been such a wide range of methods and approaches to considering drinking behaviour and practices among young adults. A prominent strand of alcohol research involves discursive methods which have guided understanding of how individual rhetoric and interactions are involved in shoring up credentials as a particular kind of drinker (e.g. non-drinkers, Nairn, Higgins, Thompson, Anderson, & Fu, 2006; Conroy & de Visser, 2014) or in positioning particular drinking styles in pejorative terms (e.g. Conroy & de Visser, 2013). The book also reflects different methodological traditions in exposing subtleties and difference in young adult drinking behaviour. Much of this is comprised of interview-based data, but this book also contains research based on focus groups, on studies of policy documents and on analyses of large-scale survey data. Several analytic methods are described across the book including thematic analysis (Leontini et al., Chapter 14), discourse analysis (Banister, Conroy & Piacentini, Chapter 11) and content analysis (Davies, Brown, Hill, Johansson, & Smith, Chapter 12). We think this variety has helped to produce a more engaging and stimulating text but has also offered a collection that acknowledges the range of methodological lenses that can be applied to alcohol research focused on young adults and, as such, offers a more representative reflection of current field research.

Overview of the Book

We have structured the book into four short but distinct sections. Part I is organised around the theme of 'Trends in young adult drinking' reflecting both growing interest in what appears to be a decline in alcohol consumption among young people in recent years and also how drinking practices in young adulthood may transition to different drinking practices later in life. Changing trends in alcohol consumption have been well documented over the past decade but are difficult to decipher. In Chapter 2, Michael Livingston and Rakhi Vashishtha provide an authoritative overview of this international phenomenon, comparing and contrasting a number of European and English-speaking countries in turn, and illustrating the progression from adolescent to adult trends in each case. The authors also discuss the complexity involved in presenting a standardised picture of drinking behaviour trends across different countries. Given this change in drinking trends, the clear question arises: 'why have drinking trends changed' and more specifically to the purposes of this book 'why are young adults around the world, living in different countries, socio-cultural and policy contexts, drinking less than previously?'. There are no easy answers to this question and Chapter 3 written by Gabriel Caluzzi and Amy Pennay is a critical consideration of a range of theoretical perspectives that link these changes in alcohol consumption to the changing nature of family, leisure, identities, digital technologies and both physical and mental health considerations. Caluzzi and Pennay contextualise decreased young adult drinking in a wider decline in 'risky' practices traditionally associated with young adulthood and a shift from associating alcohol with sociability and social well-being, to associations with negative mental health outcomes, and warn that this in itself might have detrimental consequences for well-being. Then, in Chapter 4, Marjana Martinic and Arlene Bigirimana discuss how drinking patterns can be understood as in a state of flux and how drinking trajectories involve multiple, interweaving factors including socio-economic and cultural factors alongside family dynamics and the changing experience of employment, parenthood and gender in contemporary adult lives. Such changes challenge us not only to revisit the evidence on the development of young adult drinking patterns but also to reconsider our preconceptions about the traditional life transitions that have been considered the markers of adulthood.

Part II is titled 'Young adult drinking in context' and presents a series of examples of how young adult drinking behaviour might be usefully framed in a contextualised sense involving specific places, time periods, online spaces or particular groups of people. Chapter 5 begins this section with a contribution prepared by Tim Turner and Fiona Measham that sets the scene for young adult drinking in contemporary leisure through their consideration of 'atypical intoxication' as a central feature of the literal and symbolic journeys through the weekend in music festivals and nightlife tourist resorts. Using the three-phase monomyth of separation, immersion and return, Turner and Measham explore the tensions of transgressive leisure and intoxication within these commodified play spaces. It is the increasingly atypical intoxication that results in additional risk but also

1 Book Introduction: Young Adult Drinking Styles

additional opportunity for engagement in festival and club-goers' health, safety and well-being. Next, Chapter 6 presents Brad Ridout's discussion of how contemporary young adult identity construction takes place in the context of social media platforms, with a particular focus on students, exposing how online drink-related content may hold important implications for how drinking norms are embedded in young people's lives and therefore for how health promotion strategies should be pursued. Chapter 7 by Ian Goodwin and Antonia Lyons explores an emergent area of alcohol research—the relationship between social media, online drinking cultures and young adult identities—and the wider implications of this for a health promotion agenda. Alcohol brands no longer simply tailor their marketing to consumer groups but utilise social media to embed their brands in the identity work, social lives and social practices of young adults, thereby blurring the lines between user-generated and commercial content. In this new world of multiple, dynamic and differentiated social network sites (SNSs), Goodwin and Lyons highlight the creation of a 'cybernetic sociality' for 'perpetually connected' young adults who increasingly interact in real-time loops with social media during their leisure time drinking and nightlife. Their work highlights how ripe this field is for future research exploring the holistic ecology of SNS—visual and aural as well as textual—and the social dynamics and synchronisation of these new forms of communication and representation with young adult drinking cultures. In Chapter 8, Dominic Conroy and Sarah MacLean consider how young adult drinking influences friendships and how young adult friendships influence drinking, in a critical review that incorporates both social cognitive literature and qualitative research to explore what appear to be sometimes dynamic and reciprocal relationships between different features of what can be understood by friendship and drinking practices in this emerging area of alcohol research. The section continues with Chapter 9 which presents a contribution from Alexandra Bogren who discusses four strands of gendered discourse relating to young adult drinking practices as evident from studies of everyday talk and media presentations of alcohol consumption among young adults. Young adult drinking in Swedish popular and policy discourse is represented as risky, as pleasurable or as problematic, and these discourses also varied in relation to cultural understandings of femininity and masculinity. Chapter 10 concludes this section with Lana Ireland's discussion of drinking patterns and associated problems among marginalised groups of young people in Scotland, focusing on drinking and violence as experienced by disadvantaged young men, LGBT groups and domestic abuse survivors, concluding that we should not presume a 'one-size-fits-all' approach to alcohol interventions and instead tailor such approaches with input from peers.

Part III ('Recognising the breath of young adult drinking styles') turns attention to non-drinkers and non-drinking. As discussed elsewhere in this chapter, addressing the terminology used to understand and explore drinking practices among young adults can be instrumental in producing more coherent and accurate accounts of young adult drinking practices. Accordingly, the section title—'Recognising the breadth of young adult drinking styles'—is a deliberate acknowledgement that drinking practices among young adults (or, indeed, anyone) can be usefully understood as *styles* and, as such, are situated, provisional modes of drinking practice underpinned by issues of agency and context. Chapter 11 opens this section with a contribution by Emma Banister, Dominic Conroy, and Maria Piacentini that provides an overview of recent research concerning experiences and perceptions of non-drinkers and non-drinking, before problematising relevant terminology and outlining considerations for future research, policy and practice. These authors highlight a concern that many previous studies on this subject have framed non-drinkers as a culturally homogeneous and problematised 'outgroup', having as their starting point that drinking is a normalised leisure activity among young adults. Next, Chapter 12 written by Emma Davies, Kyle Brown, Kimberley Hill, Mattias Johansson, and Joanne Smith provides a discussion of experiences of alcohol-free events among young adults, drawing on recent mixed methods research on the conscious clubbing phenomenon. By highlighting the value of dancing and togetherness at nightclubs without alcoholic beverages available, they suggest that focusing on the wider social context to alcohol consumption rather than simply individual behaviour change could be more effective in reducing the problems associated with young adult drinking and drunkenness. In Chapter 13, Richard de Visser explores engagement with the UK-based 'Dry January' campaign and adults' motives and outcomes after participating in the non-drinking challenge, highlighting the differential

1 Book Introduction: Young Adult Drinking Styles

roles of financial, health and charity motives between younger and older adults.

Our fourth and final book section (Part IV: 'Alcohol policy relating to young adult drinking practices') shifts attention to consider alcohol policy and does so with illustrations considering policy from different cultural perspectives and as applied to particular settings. Chapter 14 starts this section in a contribution from Rose Leontini, Toni Schofield, John Germov, and Julie Hepworth discussing the limitations of current policies aimed at targeting university students' alcohol use in Australia, including valuable data addressing not just student but also university staff perspectives on student drinking and university regulation. The authors conclude with five recommendations for the higher education sector to reduce alcohol-related harms. Again focusing on Australia, Aaron Hart and Claire Wilkinson provide an analysis of the contrasting policy trajectories regarding alcohol-related violence and the recent 'lock-out laws' in Sydney and Melbourne in Chapter 15. They highlight how social and gender norms, and indeed the gendering of the conceptualisation of alcohol problems and the problematisation of the conceptualisation of alcohol-related violence, are important yet neglected factors in creating effective and progressive alcohol and nightlife policies. The section then presents accounts and discussion of alcohol-related policy relevant to young adults in two further national settings. Chapter 16 by Vadim Radaev discusses the impact of a new alcohol policy introduced in Russia in 2009 which combined with broader economic turbulence to result in a reduction in the affordability of alcohol and consequently a reduction in young adult drinking practices and preferences. Chapter 17 is a contribution from Rob Bovens and Dike van de Mheen who present a review of post-2017 alcohol policy in The Netherlands and discuss how the ambitions and goals of this policy may translate in future drinking practices among Dutch young adults.

References

Arnett, J. J. (2000). Emerging adulthood: A theory of development from the late teens through the twenties. *American Psychologist, 55*(5), 469-480.

Arnett, J. J. (2005). The developmental context of substance use in emerging adulthood. *Journal of Drug Issues, 35*(2), 235–254.

Bartholomew, K., & Horowitz, L. M. (1991). Attachment styles among young adults: A test of a four-category model. *Journal of Personality and Social Psychology, 61*(2), 226–244.

Botvin, G. J., & Griffin, K. W. (2007). School-based programmes to prevent alcohol, tobacco and other drug use. *International Review of Psychiatry, 19*(6), 607–615.

Conroy, D., & de Visser, R. O. (2013). 'Man up!': Discursive constructions of non-drinkers among UK undergraduates. *Journal of Health Psychology, 18*(11), 1432–1444.

Conroy, D., & de Visser, R. O. (2014). Being a non-drinking student: An interpretative phenomenological analysis. *Psychology & Health, 29*(5), 536–551.

Erikson, E. (1950). *Childhood and society.* New York: Norton.

Green, L. (2016). *Understanding the life course: Sociological and psychological perspectives.* Cambridge: Polity Press.

Harnett, R., Thom, B., Herring, R., & Kelly, M. (2000). Alcohol in transition: Towards a model of young men's drinking styles. *Journal of Youth Studies, 3*(1), 61–77.

Hastings, G., Brooks, O., Stead, M., Angus, K., Anker, T. & Farrell, T. (2010, January 23). Alcohol advertising: The last chance saloon. *BMJ, 340,* 184–186.

Hazan, C., & Shaver, P. (1987). Romantic love conceptualized as an attachment process. *Journal of Personality and Social Psychology, 52*(3), 511–524.

Herring, R., Berridge, V., & Thom, B. (2008). Binge drinking: An exploration of a confused concept. *Journal of Epidemiology and Community Health, 62,* 476–479.

International Alliance of Responsible Drinking. (2019). *Mission statement.* http://www.responsibledrinking.org/. Accessed 17 June 2019.

Johnson, S., Leonard, K. E., & Jacob, T. (1989). Drinking, drinking styles and drug use in children of alcoholics, depressives and controls. *Journal of Studies on Alcohol, 50*(5), 427–431.

Kirschner, P. A. (2017). Stop propagating the learning styles myth. *Computers & Education, 106,* 166–171.

Levinson, D. J. (1986). A conception of adult development. *American Psychologist, 41*(1), 3–13.

Maynard, B. R., Salas-Wright, C. P., & Vaughn, M. G. (2015). High school dropouts in emerging adulthood: Substance use, mental health problems, and crime. *Community Mental Health Journal, 51*(3), 289–299.

Messick, S. (1984). The nature of cognitive styles: Problems and promise in educational practice. *Educational Psychologist, 19,* 59–74.

Nairn, K., Higgins, J., Thompson, B., Anderson, M., & Fu, N. (2006). 'It's just like the teenage stereotype, you go out and drink and stuff': Hearing from young people who don't drink. *Journal of Youth Studies, 9*(3), 287–304.

Olenick, N. L., & Chalmers, D. K. (1991). Gender-specific drinking styles in alcoholics and nonalcoholics. *Journal of Studies on Alcohol, 52*(4), 325–330.

Peterson, E. R., Rayner, S. G., & Armstrong, S. J. (2009). Researching the psychology of cognitive style and learning style: Is there really a future? *Learning and Individual Differences, 19,* 518–523.

Rowley, J., & Williams, C. (2008). The impact of brand sponsorship of music festivals. *Marketing Intelligence & Planning, 26*(7), 781–792.

Willingham, D. T., Hughes, E. M., & Dobolyi, D. G. (2015). The scientific status of learning styles theories. *Teaching of Psychology, 42*(3), 266–271.

Part I
Trends in Young Adult Drinking

2

Have Recent Declines in Adolescent Drinking Continued into Young Adulthood?

Michael Livingston and Rakhi Vashishtha

Introduction

Studies from around the world highlight that alcohol consumption typically peaks in early adulthood, at least in intoxication-oriented drinking cultures. For example, in Britton, Ben-Shlomo, Benzeval, Kuh, and Bell (2015) combination of nine UK cohort studies, men aged 25 were estimated to consume around 23 units of alcohol per week, while those in their 50s consumed less than 15. Similar patterns are evident in studies from the USA (Kerr, Greenfield, Bond, Ye, & Rehm, 2009), Sweden (Kraus et al., 2015), the UK (Meng, Holmes, Hill-McManus, Brennan, & Meier, 2014) and Australia (Livingston et al., 2016). These patterns are

---

M. Livingston (✉) · R. Vashishtha
Centre for Alcohol Policy Research, La Trobe University,
Melbourne, VIC, Australia
e-mail: M.Livingston@latrobe.edu.au

M. Livingston
Department of Clinical Neuroscience, Karolinska Institutet,
Stockholm, Sweden

© The Author(s) 2019
D. Conroy and F. Measham (eds.), *Young Adult Drinking Styles*,
https://doi.org/10.1007/978-3-030-28607-1_2

reflected in alcohol-related harms. Alcohol is the number one risk factor for injury and disease globally for people aged between 15 and 44 (Institute for Health Metrics, 2016). It is a particularly important risk factor for adolescents and young adults, contributing to around 8% of the total disease burden in this population (and substantially more than this in high-income countries) (Institute for Health Metrics, 2016).

Understanding changes in how young adults drink is therefore critical to understanding the public health implications of alcohol consumption in a society. Governments and other public health actors spend considerable resources in trying to reduce drinking in this age group, with public campaigns, health promotion interventions and policies often targeted at their drinking. Historically, however, monitoring of drinking patterns in this age group has been inconsistent and often entirely lacking. Researchers and governments have long wanted to understand trends in alcohol consumption within populations, and a tradition of regular population surveys measuring alcohol consumption (and often the use of other substances) was developed through the latter part of the twentieth century. Despite this, changes to questionnaire design, survey methodologies and inconsistent funding have meant that consistent long-term trends in survey-related measures of drinking are often lacking. While there are some exceptions where long-term survey data are available (e.g. Harkonen, Savonen, Virtala, & Makela, 2017; Meng et al., 2014), sub-analyses for young adults remain rare.

This is in stark contrast to adolescent drinking, where regular and comparable data collection provides detailed and consistent trend data. This is largely driven by two major cross-national studies that have been conducted since at least the 1990s. These two studies—the European School Survey Project on Alcohol and Other Drugs (ESPAD) and the Health Behaviour in School Children Study (HBSC)—both provide multi-country trends on adolescent alcohol use and have been running for more than twenty years. Furthermore, countries not included in these studies often have their own long-running (and broadly comparable) school surveys—for example, Australia's School Student Alcohol and Drug Survey (ASSAD) has been running since 1984 (White & Williams, 2016). Thus, our knowledge of trends in adolescent drinking is much more comprehensive than it is for trends in drinking among young adults.

Adolescent Drinking Trends

A series of research studies from across Europe, North America and Australasia have identified sharp declines in alcohol consumption for adolescents since the early 2000s (de Looze et al., 2015; Kraus et al., 2018; Livingston, 2014). For example, de Looze et al. (2015) examined data on teenagers between 11 and 15 years of age from the Health Behaviour in School Children (HBSC) survey between 2002 and 2010, finding sharp declines in past-week alcohol use in 20 of 28 countries examined. Similarly, Pape (Pape, Rossow, & Brunborg, 2018) presents data from the ESPAD from 26 countries, finding significant declines in past-month drinking between 2003 and 2015 for 22. These trends appear to have affected multiple drinking behaviours, with marked increases in abstention, delayed onset of drinking and reduced rates of heavy episodic drinking. There remain debates about the implications of these trends for these cohorts as they age into adulthood. Will their consumption levels remain lower than they were for previous cohorts in early adulthood or will they simply 'catch up' once they age out of adolescence, where particular factors (e.g. parenting practices, legal supply issues) may be holding them back.

There is a substantial body of evidence demonstrating strong associations between alcohol consumption in adolescence and heavy drinking in adulthood (Englund, Egeland, Oliva, & Collins, 2008; Grant & Dawson, 1997; Wechsler, Dowdall, Davenport, & Castillo, 1995). Similarly, studies have repeatedly shown that earlier age of onset of drinking is associated with higher rates of alcohol use disorders and other problems in adulthood. With this in mind, we would expect the decline in adolescent drinking described here to flow through into lower rates of heavy drinking and reduced alcohol-related harm among young adults. Given that the adolescent trends appear to have established in many countries by the early 2000s, there has been sufficient time to observe the initial impacts of the decline in youth drinking on adult consumption, but we could find no comprehensive attempt to do so. A number of Australian studies have shown falls in young adult alcohol consumption in recent years (Livingston, Callinan, Raninen, Pennay, & Dietze, 2018; Livingston & Dietze, 2016), while a Finnish study provides some counter-evidence, with marked differences between cohorts in adolescent drinking disappearing by the age of 18 (Lintonen, Härkönen, Raitasalo, Härkänen, & Mäkelä, 2016).

Methods

We have compiled data from 12 countries on recent trends in drinking for young adults. The lack of the systematic multi-country surveys that are run within schools (e.g. ESPAD, HBSC, GSHS) makes this a more challenging task. For this reason, the data here are likely to be incomplete. Systematic online searches were conducted to identify either peer-reviewed publications outlining trends in young adult drinking for particular jurisdictions or, more commonly, grey literature summarising survey data within countries. We limited searches to high-income countries with a strong tradition of alcohol research likely to have conducted regular high-quality population surveys—thus, our data come from predominantly Anglo countries and Western Europe. References in media reports and other publications were used to identify data sources for some countries. We also used our network of contacts in alcohol research groups around the world where published data for specific countries could not be located (e.g. for Norway). The main audience for population monitoring surveys on alcohol and drugs is generally the government and population of the jurisdiction in question, so many survey reports were written in languages other than English. Where necessary, Google Translate was used to extract key data from survey reports. Gender breakdowns are provided where they were readily available in published reports.

We have not attempted to produce comparable measures across countries. Reporting practices vary markedly—different countries use different measures of standard drinks (Kalinowski & Humphreys, 2016) and different thresholds for risky drinking (National Health and Medical Research Council, 2009), meaning standard reports in surveys are inconsistent between countries. Instead, we group the results in two sets—firstly, any measure of *risky* drinking, however it is defined, and secondly, any other drinking measure not specifically focussed on risk (frequency, abstinence vs past-year drinking, etc.). Similarly, there are no standardised age groups for report age-specific drinking trends, so we have relied on the specific age breakdowns provided in published reports. In some countries, this includes some respondents below the legal purchase age of alcohol (e.g. 15- to 24-year-olds in Canada), but generally data span the late teens and early twenties. The time periods for which data are available are also inconsistent—we attempted to collate data from the early 2000s onwards to provide a similar time frame to that used in previous work on adolescent drinking declines. These variations in reporting practices across countries thus make it almost impossible to compare drinking patterns *between* countries. Fortunately, we are mainly interested here in understanding whether changes in drinking *within* countries look similar around the world.

Results

Before presenting country-by-country trend data, we conduct some specific analyses of Australian survey data to assess whether the declines in drinking among recent cohorts of adolescents have continued as they have aged into adulthood. We use repeated cross-sectional data between 2001 and 2016 from the National Drug Strategy Household Survey (NDSHS), a major national survey of alcohol and drug use that is conducted every three years (e.g. Australian Institute of Health and Welfare, 2017). The repeated cross sections allow us to conduct quasi-cohorts—samples of people born in the same period in each survey wave who should be broadly representative of the population born in that period. Thus, for example, we take the cohort of people born between 1985 and 1987 as representative of all 14- to 16-year-olds in 2001 and of all 29- to 31-year-olds in 2016. This provides us with snapshots of the life-course drinking patterns of a series of different birth cohorts across the study period. Of course, we do not have full data for every cohort—for respondents born in 1979–1981, the earliest data available (2001) is for the ages 20–22, while for the most recent birth cohort (1997–1999), we only have data up to the ages of 17–19.

We used data on annual drinking volume sourced from standard graduated quantity-frequency questions (Bhattacharya, 2016). Respondents who had never consumed alcohol or did not drink in the past 12 months were assigned a drinking volume of 0. The average annual consumption of alcohol (in 10 g standard drinks) is presented for each cohort at each age group in Fig. 2.1.

The data in Fig. 2.1 clearly illustrate significant cohort differences in young adulthood. For almost all cohorts, drinking peaks in the early 20s, but there are substantial differences. For example, between the ages of 20 and 22, young people born in between 1991 and 1996 (in 2013 and 2016) were drinking nearly 200 standard drinks per year less than those born in between 1979 and 1981 (in 2001).

These findings provide good evidence that the decline in adolescent drinking continues into adulthood, at least in Australia. Similar analyses should be conducted in other countries that have seen marked falls in youth drinking to provide more comprehensive evidence that drinking over the life course has been affected by the recent shifts in youth drinking. Ideally, studies of actual cohorts at different ages would provide even more concrete evidence, rather than relying on these quasi-cohorts constructed

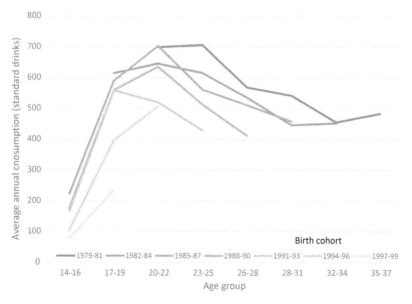

Fig. 2.1 Average annual consumption by age and birth cohort, 2001–2016, National Drug Strategy Household Survey

from repeated cross sections. The remainder of this chapter will present descriptive data on key countries to assess these trends.

Australia

Data on risky drinking for Australia come from the NDSHS. Table 2.1 includes the trends in two measures of risky drinking for 18- to 24-year-olds between 2007 and 2016, extracted from the most recent survey report (Australian Institute of Health and Welfare, 2017). Rates of both measures of risky drinking have declined sharply for both men and women over the past decade, with long-term risky drinking nearly halving (e.g. falling from 39% for men in 2007 to 23% in 2016).

England and the United Kingdom

Similar to Australia, England has seen marked reductions in adolescent drinking since the early 2000s (Bhattacharya, 2016). Data on long-term risky drinking and risky single-occasion drinking were available in two different surveys. The Health Survey for England collects data on the proportion of the population drinking an average of more than 2 UK units per day (16 g of pure alcohol per day), while the Opinion and Lifestyle Survey collects data on past-week heavy drinking (>32 g in a session for men, >24 g for women). Trends in both measures are presented in Table 2.1 for 16- to 24-year-olds.

Both measures showed substantial declines for both men and women in recent years. The data for risky single-occasion drinking provide a longer time-series and suggest that the decline in drinking was concentrated around 2008–2010 for both men and women. In fact, on this measure, drinking rates have been relatively stable in the past five survey waves. In contrast, the long-term risky drinking data point towards declines between 2011 and 2016, with some fluctuations (potentially due to small sample sizes when age-group-specific data are examined).

A recent overview using data from a range of sources suggests that these declines have been driven by both an increase in abstention among young

Table 2.1 Risky drinking trends among young adults

			2001	2004	2005	2006	2007	2008	2009	2010	2011	2012	2013	2014	2015	2016	2017
	Australia						2007			2010			2013			2016	
18–24	Long-term risky drinking[a]	Men					39%			39%			28%			23%	
		Women					20%			22%			23%			13%	
	Risky single-occasion drinking[b]	Men					61%			60%			53%			46%	
		Women					46%			47%			40%			37%	
	England				2005	2006	2007	2008	2009	2010	2011	2012	2013	2014	2015	2016	2017
16–24	Long-term risky drinking[c]	Men									27%	31%	28%	24%	24%	21%	
		Women									20%	17%	14%	17%	14%	14%	
	Risky single-occasion drinking[d]	Men			45%	41%	44%	43%	35%	32%	32%	31%	27%	31%	36%	28%	30%
		Women			41%	40%	40%	38%	37%	31%	30%	29%	29%	31%	32%	27%	31%
	USA				2005	2006	2007	2008	2009	2010	2011	2012	2013	2014	2015		
19–20	Heavy episodic drinking[e]	Both			33%	28%	25%	26%	24%	19%	25%	28%	18%	21%	12%		
21–22		Both			33%	31%	40%	30%	36%	35%	31%	34%	27%	29%	32%		
23–24		Both			39%	35%	36%	36%	34%	31%	36%	29%	28%	27%	26%		
25–26		Both			39%	31%	34%	28%	29%	33%	36%	31%	39%	28%	31%		
	Sweden				Change between 2004-2010						Change between 2010-2017						
17–29	Intensive drinking (past month)[f]	Both			-28%						7%						
	Germany		2001	2004	2005		2008			2010	2011	2012		2014	2015	2016	

Age	Indicator	Sex													
18–25	Long-term risky drinking[g]	Men	22%	23%	24%	24%		20%	22%	19%			17%	16%	15%	
		Women	13%	16%	14%	12%		11%	15%	13%			14%	12%	11%	
	Heavy episodic drinking[h]	Men	n.a.	57%	53%	53%		49%	54%	53%			44%	45%	42%	
		Women	n.a.	30%	25%	28%		26%	29%	n.a.			26%	25%	23%	
Norway											2012	2013	2014	2015	2016	2017
16–24	Risky drinking[i]	Both									27%	24%	23%	19%	18%	20%
Denmark													2014	2015	2016	2017
15–25	Frequent risky drinking[j]	Both											48%	39%	34%	35%
New Zealand					2006/07						2011/12	2012/13	2013/14	2014/15	2015/16	
18–24	Hazardous drinking[k]	Both			43%						30%	32%	33%	34%	33%	
	Monthly 6 + drinking[l]	Both			44%						36%	42%	35%	37%	35%	
Canada				2004		2008	2009	2010	2011	2012	2013		2015			2017
15–24	Drinking above acute guidelines[m]	Both		14%		18%	17%	15%	13%	13%	15%		14%			14%
	Drinking above chronic guidelines[n]	Both		19%		23%	20%	18%	15%	17%	19%		17%			18%
Spain			1997	1999	2001	2003	2005	2007	2009	2011	2013		2015			

(continued)

Table 2.1 (continued)

15–34	Prevalence of past-year intoxication	Men	39%	38%	36%	41%	40%	39%	44%	41%	43%	38%
		Women	19%	20%	18%	21%	21%	23%	26%	24%	26%	23%
	France				2005			2010				
20–25	Risky drinking	Both			11%			18%				

[a]Long-term risky drinking involves consuming at least 20 g of pure alcohol per day (on average) over the past 12 months, National Drug Strategy Household Survey

[b]Risky single-occasion drinking involves consuming more than 40 g of alcohol in a single occasion at least 12 times in the past 12 months, National Drug Strategy Household Survey

[c]Average of >2 units per day (16 g of pure alcohol), Health Survey for England

[d]At least one occasion of >32 g (men) or >24 g (women) of pure alcohol in the past week, Opinion and Lifestyle Survey, England

[e]At least one occasion of >70 g alcohol in the past fortnight, Monitoring the Future Survey

[f]>80 g of pure alcohol in a session, CAN (Centralförbundet för Alkohol- och Narkotikaupplysning) Survey

[g]>24 g/12 g of pure alcohol per day for men/women, Federal Centre for Health Education Surveys

[h]>60 g of pure alcohol in a given day, Federal Centre for Health Education Surveys

[i]>180 g pure alcohol per week for men, >120 g pure alcohol per week for women, Alkoholbruk i den voksne befolkningen Survey

[j]At least 2 occasions of >60 g of pure alcohol in the past month, Full of Life Survey

[k] AUDIT score of 8 or higher (Svensson & Dan-Erik, 2016), New Zealand Health Survey

[l]60 g of pure alcohol at least once per month, New Zealand Health Survey

[m]>41 grams of pure alcohol (women)/ >54 grams of pure alcohol on any one day in the past week, CAS, CADUMS and CTADS Surveys

[n]>136 grams of pure alcohol (women)/ >204 grams of alcohol (men) in the past 7 days, CAS, CADUMS and CTADS Surveys

people and a reduction in the amount of alcohol consumed by drinkers (Oldham, Holmes, Whitaker, Fairbrother, & Curtis, 2018).

United States of America

The USA has a quite different context to most other countries discussed in this chapter. The minimum legal purchase age for alcohol is 21, the highest in the world (World Health Organisation, 2014), and in recent years has markedly relaxed regulations around cannabis, with as yet unclear effects on drinking patterns (Hall & Lynskey, 2016). The declining trend in adolescent drinking in the USA predates most other countries with rates of drinking falling since the 1990s (Jang, Patrick, Keyes, Hamilton, & Schulenberg, 2017; Johnston, O'Malley, Bachman, & Schulenberg, 2006a, 2006b; Patrick et al., 2017)

The USA also has some of the most comprehensive data sources on alcohol consumption in the world, with multiple sources available to assess recent trends. In Table 2.1, we present data on heavy episodic drinking from Monitoring the Future, a long-running study of youth substance use, as published in Patrick et al. (2017). These data point to declines in drinking, although the declines are much steeper for those under the legal drinking age, with prevalence dropping by more than half between 2005 and 2015 for 19- to 20-year-olds compared with much smaller declines in the older age groups.

In contrast, Grucza et al. (2018) found no significant recent trends for heavy drinking among 18- to 29-year-olds when they compiled data from six other national surveys. It is worth noting that US data on adolescent drinking show substantial declines between 1991 and 2013 (Johnston et al., 2006b) but, while some sources of data have identified recent declines in drinking for young adults, the overall picture appears to be one of stability.

Sweden

Sweden is another country that has seen a marked decline in adolescent drinking since the early 2000s (Hallgren, Leifman, & Andreasson, 2012;

Larm, Raninen, Åslund, Svensson, & Nilsson, 2018; Norström & Svensson, 2014; Svensson & Dan-Erik, 2016). In general, Sweden has a relatively restrictive approach to alcohol policy, with a government monopoly on retail sales, relatively high taxes and restrictions on advertising and opening hours of outlets. The 'Europeanisation' of alcohol policy in Sweden to comply with European Union regulations has led to some relaxation of these policies (Cisneros, 2009) and gradual increases in per capita consumption since the early 2000s (even while youth drinking declined sharply) (Norström & Ramstedt, 2018).

We present here data on young adult drinking come from a monthly monitoring survey conducted by CAN (Centralförbundet för Alkohol- och Narkotikaupplysning). The most recent report (Jang et al., 2017) provides a series of different measures of alcohol consumption for 17- to 29-year-olds. These data are summarised in Tables 2.1 and 2.2.

On most measures, alcohol consumption for young adults in Sweden has declined, but that decline was concentrated between 2004 and 2010—in subsequent years, drinking has been relatively stable and, for some measures, increased. Thus, for example, the average volume of alcohol consumed by 17- to 29-year-olds in the past month fell by 23% between 2004 and 2010, while the prevalence of risky single-occasion drinking fell by 28%. Between 2010 and 2017, however, average volume fell by only 3%, while risky drinking prevalence increased by 7%.

Germany

Overall, alcohol consumption in Germany has been steadily declining from its peak of nearly 14 litres of pure alcohol per person in the late 1970s down to less than 10 litres per person in the most recent data available (Anderson & Pinilla, 2017). The most recent data on adolescent drinking come from the 2014 HBSC report (World Health Organisation, 2018), which finds that weekly drinking had roughly halved for both boys and girls between 2002 and 2014.

The most reliable German data on young adult drinking patterns come from a series of surveys run by the Federal Centre for Health Education. These surveys have been run irregularly between 2001 and 2016, with

Table 2.2 Trends in other drinking measures among young adults

	Sweden		Change between 2004–2010					Change between 2010–2017					
17–29	Any drinking (past month)[a]	Both	−12%					5%					
	Number of drinking days in the past month[a]	Both	−20%					21%					
	Volume of alcohol (past month)[a]	Both	−23%					−3%					
	Germany		2001	2004	2005	2008		2010	2011	2012	2014	2015	2016
18–25	Weekly drinking[b]	Men	52%	59%	55%	53%		48%	55%	52%	47%	46%	41%
		Women	27%	28%	25%	20%		20%	24%	24%	23%	20%	19%
	Finland		1968	1976	1984	1992	2000	2008	2016				
15–19	Median volume of pure alcohol consumed in the past year[c]	Men	0.2	1.6	0.6	1.9	1.9	0.8	0.5				

(continued)

Table 2.2 (continued)

		Women	0.1	0.6	0.2		1.0	1.1	0.8	0.3						
20–29	Median	Men	2.0	3.3	2.1		3.3	3.7	3.7	1.8						
	volume of pure alcohol consumed in the past year[c]	Women	0.2	0.7	0.4		1.0	1.0	1.0	0.9						
	Norway										2012	2013	2014	2015	2016	2017
16–24	Past-year drinking[d]	Both									87%	86%	82%	80%	80%	80%
	Denmark												2014	2015	2016	2017
15–25	Lifetime abstainer[e]	Both											11%	12%	18%	19%
	New Zealand					2006/07					2011/12	2012/13	2013/14	2014/15	2015/16	
18–24	Past-year drinking[f]	Both				89%					85%	86%	84%	86%	84%	
	Canada				2004		2008	2009	2010	2011	2012	2013		2015		2017
15–24	Past 12 month use[g]	Both			83%		78%	76%	72%	71%	70%	73%		72%		71%

[a]CAN (Centralförbundet för Alkohol- och Narkotikaupplysning) Survey
[b]Federal Centre for Health Education Surveys Denmark
[c]Drinking Habits Survey, Finland
[d]Alkoholbruk i den voksne befolkningen
[e]Full of Life Survey, Norway
[f]New Zealand Health Survey
[g]CAS, CADUMS and CTADS Surveys

some changes to specific measures meaning certain data are not available (e.g. heavy episodic drinking was not measured in 2001). Three different measures of drinking for 18- to 25-year-olds are presented in Tables 2.1 and 2.2.

These data show declines for all measures of drinking, especially for men. For example, between 2004 and 2016, the prevalence of heavy episodic drinking for men fell from 57 to 42%, while the decline for women was from 30 to 23%. In contrast to Sweden, the declines in Germany mostly occurred in recent years (i.e. after 2012).

Finland

Finland has seen some major alcohol policy changes in recent years, with spirits and beer taxes cut by around one-third in 2004 before increasing by 10% in 2009. Per capita consumption moved as expected following these tax changes, increasing between 2003 and 2008 and then declining after the tax increase in 2009 (Anderson & Pinilla, 2017). In contrast, adolescent drinking fell across the period, seemingly unaffected by tax policy changes (Raitasalo, Simonen, Tigerstedt, Mäkelä, & Tapanainen, 2018).

Finnish data for young adults come from their long-running Drinking Habits Survey that has been collecting detailed and comparable data on Finnish drinking every eight years since the late 1960s (Grucza et al., 2018). Because of the idiosyncratic nature of the questions used, the clearest measure of change over time is the median volume of pure alcohol reported by respondents. Trends for men and women among older teenagers (Grant & Dawson, 1997; Kalinowski & Humphreys, 2016; Lintonen et al., 2016; Livingston & Dietze, 2016; Livingston et al., 2018) and younger adults (Australian Institute of Health and Welfare, 2017; Bhattacharya, 2016; Hall & Lynskey, 2016; Jang et al., 2017; Johnston et al., 2006a, 2006b; National Health and Medical Research Council, 2009; Oldham et al., 2018; Patrick et al., 2005; World Health Organisation, 2014) are presented in Table 2.2.

These data show a significant decline between 2000 and 2016, especially for men. Median drinking for older teenagers fell sharply for both men and women between 2000 and 2016 (dropping by more than half), while for 20- to 29-year-olds there was a sharp drop for men between 2008 and 2016, but little change for women.

Norway

Norway is another country with broadly restrictive alcohol policies. Per capita consumption steadily increased by nearly 50% between 1993 and 2008 but has since been in decline. Drinking for 15-year-olds in the HBSC survey has fallen to almost non-existent levels, with fewer than 5% of boys and girls reporting weekly drinking in 2014, from nearly 20% in 2002.

Consistently recorded data on Norwegian drinking are available only from 2012 onwards, via the Alkoholbruk i den voksne befolkningen (alcohol consumption in the adult population) survey (Larm et al., 2018). Data on past-year drinking and past-year risky drinking are available across the period and are presented in Tables 2.1 and 2.2.

There have been small but significant declines in both measures for Norwegian young adults (aged 16–24) over the six years of survey data available.

Denmark

Denmark has the most liberal alcohol policy of the Nordic countries, with widespread alcohol availability and relatively relaxed drinking age laws. Per capita consumption there has historically been high, although it has fallen by 20% since a peak of 10.1 litres of pure alcohol per person in 1996 (Anderson & Pinilla, 2017). These declines come during a period when adolescent drinking was a key policy focus, with a minimum purchase age of 16 implemented in 2004, even as taxes were cut in 2003. Danish adolescents have historically been among the heaviest drinking adolescents in Europe, but there have been steep declines as in many other countries since 2002 (Andersen, Rasmussen, Bendtsen, Due, & Holstein, 2014).

Consistently collected, long-term data on drinking by Danish young adults could not be located. Instead, we rely on recent surveys conducted as part of the 'Full of Life' campaign conducted between 2014 and 2017

(Hallgren et al., 2012). The most consistent alcohol use measures were (1) abstinence from alcohol and (2) the frequency of binge drinking (more than 5 drinks (60 g pure alcohol) on a single occasion) in the past month for 15- to 25-year-olds. Trends for these measures are presented in Tables 2.1 and 2.2.

Young adults are increasingly choosing not to drink at all, with the proportion reporting no alcohol consumption at all increasing from 11% in 2014 to 19% in 2017. Risky drinking rates have fallen sharply, from 48 to 35% over the same four-year period.

New Zealand

Per capita consumption in New Zealand has been relatively stable since the early 2000s, while adolescent consumption has declined sharply (Clark et al., 2013).

Data for New Zealand come from the New Zealand Health Survey (NZHS). The NZHS was conducted in 2006/2007 and then annually from 2011/2012. The drinking questions were changed in 2016/2017, so only data up to 2015/2016 are presented here (New Zealand Ministry of Health, 2017). There are three measures collected consistently over the period: hazardous drinking as measured by the AUDIT score, regular drinking occasions of 6 + standard drinks (60 g or more of pure alcohol) and any past-year drinking.

There have been some declines in all measures of drinking for 18- to 24-year-olds in New Zealand, although these shifts predominantly occurred between 2006/2007 and 2011/2012. All measures have been relatively stable since 2011/2012. For example, monthly 6 + drinking rates decreased from 44% in 2005 to 36% in 2012 and have been stable subsequently.

Canada

Per capita consumption in Canada increased slightly through the early part of the 2000s and has been stable since about 2008. Adolescent alcohol consumption has also fallen substantially in Canada (de Looze et al., 2015).

Canadian alcohol consumption data for young adults come from three sources: the Canadian Addiction Survey (CAS, 2004), the Canadian Alcohol Drug Use Monitoring Survey (CADUMS, 2008–2012) and the Canadian Tobacco Alcohol and Drugs Survey (CTADS, 2013–2017). These three surveys are closely related and, while the methodologies have changed across waves, key alcohol questions are consistent across time allowing for some tentative comparisons. We have relied on published estimates for 15- to 24-year-olds from the CAS and CADUMS (Health Canada, 2012) but had to manually combine estimates for 15- to 19-year-olds and 20- to 24-year-olds (based on population estimates provided in the results) from the CTADS (Health Canada, 2018) due to changes in reporting practices. Risky drinking prevalence trends are presented in Table 2.1 (for both acute and chronic risks), while trends in any alcohol consumption are presented in Table 2.2.

The data presented show a decline in past 12-month use, especially between 2004 and 2010. In contrast, risky drinking rates were stable across the study period.

Spain

Alcohol research has been a much lower priority in Southern European countries than in the Anglo and Northern European countries discussed above. Per capita consumption in Spain has historically been markedly higher than most of the countries discussed thus far, but drinking patterns have tended to be less intoxication oriented and the risks of alcohol consumption have been less of an emphasis in research and public policy (Room & Mäkelä, 2000). Despite the substantially different context, adolescent drinking in Spain appears to show the same trends as many of the other countries discussed in this chapter, with weekly drinking declining by more than half between 2002 and 2014 (World Health Organisation, 2018).

Data on alcohol consumption trends for young adults in Spain come from the Encuesta sobre Alcohol y Drogas en España (EDADES—Survey on Alcohol and Drugs in Spain), reported in a major compendium of alcohol and drug data for the period 1995–2015 (Observatorio Espanol de las Dragas y las Addiciones, 2017). Age-specific trend data were only reported for the past-year prevalence of intoxication (self-reported), which is largely subjective and potentially influenced by changing norms around what 'intoxication' might mean. Trends are presented in Table 2.1 for men and women aged 15–34.

Self-reported rates of intoxication were stable for men and slightly increasing for women between 1997 and 2015.

France

Per capita consumption has declined in France since the 1950s, falling by more than half from nearly 20 litres of pure alcohol per person to around 9 (Anderson & Pinilla, 2017). Adolescent drinking in France has declined, but not as steeply as it has in many other European countries (World Health Organisation, 2018).

We could not locate consistently reported data on drinking for young adults in France. We did, however, identify data from France's public health barometer series that suggests rates of risky drinking for young adults have *increased* there in recent years. Between 2005 and 2010, the proportion of 20- to 25-year-olds who drank 50 g of pure alcohol or more in a session at least monthly increased from 11 to 18% (Beck & Richard, 2011). For subsequent years, data were presented using different age groups, making comparisons difficult, but small reported increases in monthly risky drinking for 15- to 24-year-olds and 25- to 34-year-olds (Richard et al., 2015) suggest that risky drinking rates for French young adults continue to rise.

Discussion

The data presented here highlight substantial reductions in alcohol consumption for young adults from across a range of high-income countries. The time periods, measures and age groups for which data are available vary markedly, which makes drawing the data together into a simple summary difficult. It is clear, however, that some countries have seen marked declines in drinking among young adults. In Australia and the UK, measures of risky drinking have fallen by at least a quarter since 2007, while Denmark has seen a similar sized drop in just the past five years. In general, where sex-specific data were available, trends for men and women have been similar, with the notable exception of Finland, where the median amount of pure alcohol consumed by men aged 20–29 fell from 3.7 l in 2000 to 1.8 l in 2016, while for women of the same age consumption fell from 1.0 l to 0.9 l.

There were also countries where a significant decline in young adult drinking was not identified—notably traditional wine cultures, France and Spain. A number of other countries had seen declines in drinking, but not in recent years. Thus, for example, all measures of drinking for Swedish young people (aged 17–29) fell between 2004 and 2010, but there has been stability or increases in subsequent years. Similar patterns were evident in Canada and New Zealand. Thus, while the overall picture is one of declining young adult drinking, there remains significant variation to consider. These variations raise fascinating questions. Why, for example, do we see no decline in young adult drinking in Spain despite dramatic reductions in adolescent drinking? Why do Swedish and Australian trends for young adults look so different when adolescent drinking statistics for the two countries are markedly similar? These questions require much more in-depth research data than that which can be attained using monitoring surveys. We have not included here any analysis of key socio-demographic factors likely to influence the experience of being young adults across these countries—for instance, employment prospects for young adults are likely to vary considerably. Cultural practices around alcohol and young adulthood are similarly unlikely to be consistent around the world, and research from a range of theoretical and methodological traditions is necessary to provide a more nuanced understanding of the drivers of the trends reported here.

Of course, the data presented here are limited in numerous ways—age-specific alcohol consumption data rely inherently on self-report surveys which are prone to a wide range of biases that have the potential to change over time (Gmel & Rehm, 2004). These issues are magnified by the marked changes in survey methodologies that have occurred in many of the series we report on, not to mention the diversity of measures we have relied on due to the vast variation in survey practices between countries. These limitations contrast with the general consistency of methods and approach in the two major cross-national studies of adolescent drinking (HBSC and ESPAD) and raise the question as to whether a similar standardisation of approach is necessary to ensure we better understand the changing patterns of alcohol consumption in young adulthood, a period where the risk of alcohol-related harm is substantial.

On the whole though, these results are encouraging from a purely public health point of view—in many countries risky drinking among young adults has fallen significantly in the past 10–15 years. Young adulthood is a life stage in which alcohol represents one of the major contributors to morbidity and mortality, but there are an array of non-health harms associated with heavy drinking as well (Laslett et al., 2011). Of course, alcohol also plays a positive role in the lives of the many millions of people who drink it and intoxication is a key way of experiencing pleasure for many young adults (e.g. Measham, 2004). The shifts reported here represent a fascinating shift in behaviour (at least in some jurisdictions) that requires urgent examination. While some researchers have begun exploring the reasons for the decline in teenage drinking (Pennay, Livingston, & MacLean, 2015), there has been little work exploring how and why these declines continue into adulthood. The potential reasons for the declines discussed here will be the subject of the following chapter.

References

Andersen, A., Rasmussen, M., Bendtsen, P., Due, P., & Holstein, B. E. (2014). Secular trends in alcohol drinking among Danish 15-year-olds: Comparable representative samples from 1988 to 2010. *Journal of Research on Adolescence, 24*(4), 748–756.

Anderson, K. & Pinilla, V. (2017). *Annual database of global wine markets, 1835 to 2016.* Adelaide: Wine Economics Research Centre, University of Adelaide.

Australian Institute of Health and Welfare. (2017). *National Drug Strategy Household Survey—Detailed report 2016.* Canberra: AIHW.

Beck, F., & Richard, J.-B. (2011). *Les Comportements de Santé des Jeunes—Analyses du Baromètre santé 2010* [Youth health behaviours—Analysis of the 2010 health barometer]. Paris, France: Sante Publique France.

Bhattacharya A. (2016). *Youthful Abandon: Why are young people drinking less?* London: Institute for Alcohol Studies.

Britton, A., Ben-Shlomo, Y., Benzeval, M., Kuh, D., & Bell, S. (2015). Life course trajectories of alcohol consumption in the United Kingdom using longitudinal data from nine cohort studies. *BMC Medicine, 13*(1), 47.

Cisneros Örnberg, J. (2009). *The Europeanization of Swedish alcohol policy.* Stockholm: Statsvetenskapliga institutionen.

Clark, T. C., Fleming, T., Bullen, P., Denny, S., Crengle, S., Dyson, B., ... & Utter, J. (2013). *Youth'12 overview: The health and wellbeing of New Zealand secondary school students in 2012.* Auckland, New Zealand: The University of Auckland.

de Looze, M., Raaijmakers, Q., ter Bogt, T., Bendtsen, P., Farhat, T., Ferreira, M., ... & Simons-Morton, B. (2015). Decreases in adolescent weekly alcohol use in Europe and North America: Evidence from 28 countries from 2002 to 2010. *The European Journal of Public Health, 25*(Suppl. 2), 69–72.

Englund, M. M., Egeland, B., Oliva, E. M., & Collins, W. A. (2008). Childhood and adolescent predictors of heavy drinking and alcohol use disorders in early adulthood: A longitudinal developmental analysis. *Addiction, 103*(Suppl. 1), 23–35.

Gmel, G., & Rehm, J. (2004). Measuring alcohol consumption. *Contemporary Drug Problems., 31,* 467–540.

Grant, B. F., & Dawson, D. A. (1997). Age at onset of alcohol use and its association with DSM-IV alcohol abuse and dependence: Results from the national longitudinal alcohol epidemiologic survey. *Journal of Substance Abuse, 9,* 103–110.

Grucza, R. A, Sher, K. J., Kerr, W. C., Krauss, M. J., Lui, C. K., McDowell, Y. E., ... Bierut, L. (2018). Trends in adult alcohol use and binge drinking in the early 21st-century United States: A meta-analysis of 6 national survey series. *Alcoholism: Clinical and Experimental Research, 42*(10), 1939–1950.

Hall, W., & Lynskey, M. (2016). Why it is probably too soon to assess the public health effects of legalisation of recreational cannabis use in the USA. *The Lancet Psychiatry, 3*(9), 900–906.

Hallgren, M., Leifman, H., & Andreasson, S., (2012). Drinking less but greater harm: Could polarized drinking habits explain the divergence between alcohol consumption and harms among youth? *Alcohol and Alcoholism, 47*(5), 581–590.

Härkönen, J., Savonen, J., Virtala, E., & Mäkelä, P. (2017). *Suomalaisten alkoholinkäyttötavat 1968—2016* [Finnish drinking habits, 1968–2016]. Helsinki, Finland: Terveyden Ja Hyvinvionnin Laitos.

Health Canada. (2012). *Canadian Alcohol and Drug Use Monitoring Survey— Survey tables* November 14, 2018. Available from: https://www.canada.ca/en/health-canada/services/health-concerns/drug-prevention-treatment/drug-alcohol-use-statistics/canadian-alcohol-drug-use-monitoring-survey-tables-2011.html.

Health Canada. (2018). *Canadian Tobacco, Alcohol and Drugs Survey* November 14, 2018. Available from: https://www.canada.ca/en/health-canada/services/canadian-tobacco-alcohol-drugs-survey.html.

Institute for Health Metrics. (2016). *GBD Compare Data Visualization.* Seattle WA: IHME, University of Washington. Available from: http://vizhub.healthdata.org/gbd-compare.

Jang, J. B., Patrick, M. E., Keyes, K. M., Hamilton, A. D., & Schulenberg, J. E. (2017). Frequent binge drinking among US adolescents, 1991 to 2015. *Pediatrics, 139*(6), e20164023.

Johnston, L., O'Malley, P., Bachman, J., & Schulenberg, J. (2006a). *Monitoring the future national survey results on drug use, 1975–2005. Volume I: Secondary school students* (NIH Publication No. 06-5883).

Johnston, L., O'Malley, P., Bachman, J., & Schulenberg, J. (2006b). *Monitoring the future national survey results on drug use, 1975–2005. Volume II: College students and adults ages 19–45.*

Kalinowski, A., & Humphreys, K. (2016). Governmental standard drink definitions and low-risk alcohol consumption guidelines in 37 countries. *Addiction, 111*(7), 1293–1298.

Kerr, W. C., Greenfield, T. K., Bond, J., Ye, Y., & Rehm, J. (2009). Age–period–cohort modelling of alcohol volume and heavy drinking days in the US National Alcohol Surveys: Divergence in younger and older adult trends. *Addiction, 104*(1), 27–37.

Kraus, L., Seitz, N. N., Piontek, D., Molinaro, S., Siciliano, V., Guttormsson, U., … Hibell, B. (2018). 'Are the times A-changin'? trends in adolescent substance use in Europe. *Addiction, 113*(7), 1317–1332.

Kraus, L., Tinghög, M. E., Lindell, A., Pabst, A., Piontek, D., & Room, R. (2015). Age, period and cohort effects on time trends in alcohol consumption in the Swedish adult population 1979–2011. *Alcohol and Alcoholism, 50*(3), 319–327.

Larm, P., Raninen, J., Åslund, C., Svensson, J., & Nilsson, K. W. (2018). The increased trend of non-drinking alcohol among adolescents: What role do internet activities have? *European Journal of Public Health, 29*(1), 27–32.

Laslett, A. M., Room, R., Ferris, J., Wilkinson, C., Livingston, M., & Mugavin, J. (2011). Surveying the range and magnitude of alcohol's harm to others in Australia. *Addiction, 106*(9), 1603–1611.

Lintonen, T., Härkönen, J., Raitasalo, K., Härkänen, T., & Mäkelä, P. (2016). Decreasing adolescent drinking: Is there evidence of a continuation into future adult cohorts? APC analysis of adolescent drinking in Finland, 1983–2013. *Scandinavian Journal of Public Health, 44*(7), 654–662.

Livingston, M. (2014). Trends in non-drinking among Australian adolescents. *Addiction, 109*(6), 922–929.

Livingston, M., Callinan, S., Raninen, J., Pennay, A., & Dietze, P. M. (2018). Alcohol consumption trends in Australia: Comparing surveys and sales-based measures. *Drug and Alcohol Review, 37*, S9–S14.

Livingston, M., & Dietze, P. (2016). National survey data can be used to measure trends in population alcohol consumption in Australia. *Australian and New Zealand Journal of Public Health, 40*(3), 233–235.

Livingston, M., Raninen, J., Slade, T., Swift, W., Lloyd, B., & Dietze, P. (2016). Understanding trends in Australian alcohol consumption—An age, period, cohort model. *Addiction, 111*(7), 1203–1213.

Measham, F. (2004). The decline of ecstasy, the rise of 'binge' drinking and the persistence of pleasure. *Probation Journal, 51*(4), 309–326.

Meng, Y., Holmes, J., Hill-McManus, D., Brennan, A., & Meier, P. S. (2014). Trend analysis and modelling of gender-specific age, period and birth cohort effects on alcohol abstention and consumption level for drinkers in Great Britain using the general lifestyle survey 1984–2009. *Addiction, 109*(2), 206–215.

National Health and Medical Research Council. (2009). *Australian guidelines to reduce health risks from drinking alcohol.* Canberra: NHMRC.

New Zealand Ministry of Health. (2017). *Annual Data Explorer 2016/2017: New Zealand Health Survey* November 13, 2018. Available from: https://minhealthnz.shinyapps.io/nz-health-survey-2016-17-annual-update/.

Norström, T., & Ramstedt, M. (2018). The link between per capita alcohol consumption and Alcohol-related harm in Sweden, 1987–2015. *Journal of Studies on Alcohol and Drugs, 79*(4), 578–584.

Norström, T., & Svensson, J. (2014). The declining trend in Swedish youth drinking: Collectivity or polarization? *Addiction, 109*(9), 1437–1446.

Observatorio Espanol de las Dragas y las Addiciones. (2017). *Estadisticas. 2017—Alcohol, tabaco y drogas ilegales in Espana: Encuesta Sobre Alcohol y Drogas en Espana, 1995–2015* [Statistics 2017—Alcohol, tobacco and illicit drugs in Spain: Survey on alcohol and drugs in Spain, 1995–2015]. Madrid, Spain: Observatorio Español de las Drogas y las Adicciones (OEDA).

Oldham, M., Holmes, J., Whitaker, V., Fairbrother, H., & Curtis, P. (2018). *Youth drinking in decline.* Sheffield, UK: The University of Sheffield.

Pape, H., Rossow, I., & Brunborg, G. S. (2018). Adolescents drink less: How, who and why? A review of the recent research literature. *Drug and Alcohol Review, 37,* S98–S114.

Patrick, M. E., Terry-McElrath, Y. M., Miech, R. A., Schulenberg, J. E., O'Malley, P. M., & Johnston, L. D. (2017). Age-specific prevalence of binge and high-intensity drinking among U.S. young adults: Changes from 2005 to 2015. *Alcoholism: Clinical and Experimental Research, 41*(7), 1319–1328.

Pennay, A., Livingston, M., & MacLean, S. (2015). Young people are drinking less: It is time to find out why. *Drug and Alcohol Review, 34*(2), 115–118.

Raitasalo, K., Simonen, J., Tigerstedt, C., Mäkelä, P., & Tapanainen, H. (2018). What is going on in underage drinking? Reflections on Finnish European School Survey Project on Alcohol and Other Drugs Data 1999–2015. *Drug and Alcohol Review, 37*(S1), S76–S84.

Richard, J.-B., Palle, C., Guignard, R., Nguyen-Thanh, V., Beck, F., & Arwidson, P. (2015). *La consommation d'alcool en France en 2014* [The Consumption of Alcohol in France in 2014]. Paris, France: Institut National de Prévention et d'Education Pour la Santé.

Room, R., & Mäkelä, K. (2000). Typologies of the cultural position of drinking. *Journal of Studies on Alcohol, 61*(3), 475–483.

Svensson, J. A., & Dan-Erik. (2016). What role do changes in the demographic composition play in the declining trends in alcohol consumption and the increase of non-drinkers among Swedish youth? A time-series analysis of trends in non-drinking and region of origin 1971–2012. *Alcohol and Alcoholism, 51*(2), 172–176.

Wechsler, H., Dowdall, G. W., Davenport, A., & Castillo, S. (1995). Correlates of college student binge drinking. *American Journal of Public Health, 85*(7), 921–926.

White, V., & Williams, T. (2016). *Australian secondary school students' use of tobacco, alcohol, and over-the-counter and illicit substances in 2014.* Melbourne, VIC: Cancer Council Victoria.

World Health Organisation. (2014). *Global status report on alcohol and health* (2014th ed.). Geneva, Switzerland: WHO.

World Health Organisation. (2018). *Adolescent alcohol-related behaviours: Trends and inequalities in the WHO European Region, 2002–2014.* Copenhagen, Denmark: WHO Regional Office for Europe.

3

Alcohol, Young Adults and the New Millennium: Changing Meanings in a Changing Social Climate

Gabriel Caluzzi and Amy Pennay

Since the turn of the millennium, significant declines in drinking have been observed among young adults (a term covering the transitional period from adolescence to adulthood) in many developed countries. Population shifts in drinking patterns often reflect broader changes in alcohol's position within society. Thus, examining periods of change in consumption is important for providing insight into broader social change. In this chapter, we argue for the importance of examining young adults' current drinking practices within the context of unique post-millennial developments.

Around the turn of the millennium, drinking rates among young people peaked across many developed countries as market conditions and the acceptability of drinking and drunkenness enabled 'cultures of intoxication' (Measham & Brain, 2005). The identity work, choice and self-expression that were provided through alcohol consumption have been well documented by researchers (e.g. Measham, 1996; Parker, Measham,

---

G. Caluzzi (✉) · A. Pennay
Centre for Alcohol Policy Research, La Trobe University,
Melbourne, VIC, Australia
e-mail: G.Caluzzi@latrobe.edu.au

© The Author(s) 2019
D. Conroy and F. Measham (eds.), *Young Adult Drinking Styles*,
https://doi.org/10.1007/978-3-030-28607-1_3

& Aldridge, 1998). Around the same time, neoliberal discourses concerning 'safe alcohol consumption' placed responsibility back on the individual consumer, and public health concerns grew over young adults' heavy drinking styles. This created conditions that both promoted and punished excessive consumption (see Bauman, 1988). Since the peaks of the early 2000s, there has been a widespread decline in drinking among young adults (refer to Chapter 2 of this book). Emerging research has focused on isolated policy, parenting and recreational changes as triggers (Bhattacharya, 2016; Pape, Rossow, & Brunborg, 2018). However, it is important to recognise that declines have occurred amidst broader social changes such as growing economic precarity, the Internet boom, increasingly globalised communities and heightened anxiety over young adult behaviour in public discourse (Measham, 2008; Törrönen, Roumeliotis, Samuelsson, Kraus, & Room, 2019). Simultaneously, public health efforts have nudged young adults towards a drinking culture based on health, safety and 'sensibility' (Fry, 2010). In this chapter, we suggest that moderation and abstinence are becoming more mainstream as a consequence of new meanings ascribed to alcohol use, new salience of short- and long-term harms and more credible lifestyles and leisure activities for young adults to pursue without alcohol.

Understanding the Current Generation of Young Adults: A Social Generations Perspective

We understand young adulthood as a fluid concept constructed by a range of biological, psychological, cultural and social discourses. Young adults exist within socio-historical conditions that actively shape and are shaped, creating generations of shared experiences and social conditions (see Mannheim, 1952 [1927]). For example, today's adolescents are developing in a time where traditional transitions into work, family formation and home ownership have become protracted over a longer period, now commonly occurring anywhere from the late teens well into the thirties. Whilst young adults face contemporary conditions that affect all other age groups, the way in which they manage transitions into new roles of independence and responsibility makes them more susceptible to social change and more likely to experiment with different ways of living as a response (Woodman & Wyn, 2014).

Sociologists have suggested young adults today are experiencing a number of unique conditions: precarious labour markets marked by job competitiveness, higher education levels, ubiquity of digital communications, greater pursuit of satisfying careers, difficulty building and maintaining intimate relationships, delayed family formation and a diversification of lifestyles (Furlong & Cartmel, 2006; Woodman, 2016). In particular, familiarity and incorporation of technology into the everyday lives of young adults has reshaped social worlds (e.g. the ability communicate and network) and economic worlds (e.g. the push for 'knowledge-based' economies based on digitally technical jobs).

Shared commonalities and experiences shape values and actions, in turn leading to new methods of self-expression and social movements among generations (Mannheim, 1952 [1927]). The concept of social generations is not without criticism though. In treating generations as a collective, intra-generational divisions (such as class, gender and ethnicity) and intergenerational interactions (such as familial support and social networks) can be under-valued. Thus, generation should be recognised as only one element of social location. Indeed, whilst social generations provide shared sites of experience and meaning, individuals within a generation can still have opposing reactions to shared social conditions. The divergence between light and heavy drinking young adults for example (see Caluzzi, 2018) highlights how social conditions are not deterministic of clear collective actions.

By accepting that generational patterns are not linear, universal or deterministic, social generations theory is useful for thinking about the diversity of lifestyles young adults can now lead and their shared experiences of fragmentation and social change. This approach is particularly relevant as globalisation and communications technology have forged a 'post-traditional cosmopolitan world' (Beck, 2000: 211) for young adults since the new millennium. From here, we will explore in more detail the generational changes that may be shifting the position of alcohol for young adults, including the changing nature of family, leisure, digital technology and mental health.

Parental Influence on Young Adults' Drinking

One of the more consistent findings in research on declines in young adult drinking has demonstrated the importance of parents in monitoring, setting norms and building closer relationships with their children (see Pape et al., 2018). Parental permissiveness or strictness around alcohol is now recognised as key to the development and shaping of drinking norms and practices in later life (Raitasalo & Holmila, 2017; Yap, Cheong, Zaravinos-Tsakos, Lubman, & Jorm, 2017). Moreover, longer periods of economic constraint and delayed independence suggest that the role of intergenerational familial relationships has become increasingly important, even as children transition into young adulthood. Findings from the Australian Life Patterns Study and the Canadian Paths on Life's Way study indicate that since the late 2000s, family relationships have been the most significant influence on the lives of young participants (Wyn, 2011). Since traditional markers of independence (such as moving out) are also associated with increased autonomy, it stands to reason that delays in such transitions would also delay, or limit, consumption practices; for example, hedonistic consumption practices might become structurally bound by family, limiting in a practical sense the time and space young adults have to 'let loose' (e.g. Measham, 1996; Parker et al., 1998). Since alcohol use for many young adults remains opportunistic, it may be that longer periods of dependence and increased familial supervision might act as inhibitors.

The advent of social learning has also increased awareness of the role parents play in setting norms and expectations around alcohol use. Parental modelling is likely to influence age of alcohol initiation, and this has been suggested to influence children's drinking habits into adulthood (Pennay, Livingston, & MacLean, 2015). Thus, efforts have been made to delay initiation and increase parental awareness of how they set drinking norms through both formal policy (e.g. secondary supply laws and education campaigns) and informal depictions of the 'good' and 'bad' parent (Assarsson & Aarsand, 2011). In addition, public health responses aimed at reducing consumption might be making parents more confident (or obliged) to develop stricter alcohol rules and expectations with their children (Hagell & Witherspoon, 2012). Family formation is progressively happening later in life, and parents are raising less children; this has been suggested to result in greater parental investment (Bugental, Corpuz, & Beaulieu, 2014). The amount of time parents spend with their children has increased and been linked to a number of positive social outcomes (Sani & Treas, 2016). Spending more time with their children, and encouraging engagement in sport, music and other activities, may be working as protective factors against heavy consumption. Indeed, it has been suggested that improved family cohesion, parent–child relationships, monitoring and discipline have potentially contributed to declining alcohol use (Bhattacharya, 2016; Pape et al., 2018).

Decreasing Risky Activities and Increasing Safe Alternatives?

There is good evidence to suggest that drinking is not the only young adult practice that has declined. Age of learning to drive, socialising independent of parents, attending parties, dating and having sex for the first time have also declined for young adults across gender, socio-economic status and ethnicities (Kann et al., 2015; Twenge, 2017). These have paralleled declines in drug use and 'delinquent behaviours' such as truancy, violence and crime (Farrell, Tilley, & Tseloni, 2014; Vaughn et al., 2018). Twenge and Park (2017) theorise that because more contemporary young adults live in contexts with access to resources and parental support, they are more carefully planning out their lives, whilst avoiding risk and delaying 'adult' activities. Indeed, young abstainers tend to be characterised by greater academic engagement, parental cohesion, less propensity for risk and having fewer substance-using peers (Vaughn et al., 2018). However, whilst Twenge and Park suggest young people are delaying the transition to adulthood, it should be noted that they are exposed to more adult information and imagery through digital media at a younger age than their generational predecessors and are demonstrating more forward planning at a younger age (Wyn, 2016). Thus, it might not be that young people are transitioning more slowly into adulthood, but are choosing different lifestyles and pathways to perform adulthood. Indeed, it may be that many activities previously thought of as 'adult' (e.g. alcohol use, drug use and other 'risk' practices) have lost their connection to young adulthood.

The decline of not only drinking, but also other 'risky' behaviours suggests that risk-taking and experimentation are no longer key to young adults' achievement of independence, identity and maturity, and there may now be alternative avenues for developing identity and independence. In particular, digital media has been suggested to have profoundly shaped the way young people interact, process information and explore social identities (Prensky, 2001). The growth of online immersive entertainment through the Internet, smartphones, videogames, streaming services, mobile apps and social media has changed the communication landscape, providing new methods of socialisation and competing forms of immersion. Access to a wealth of global information also means this digital discourse empowers young adults to challenge the norms and agendas of older generations (Itō et al., 2010). It has even been suggested that the ubiquity of digital and social media has crossed traditional divides based on wealth, ethnicity and geographic location (Tilleczek & Srigley, 2016).

This cultural digitisation has complex impacts on communication. It offers new leisure activities that may be pursued at the expense of peer interactions and potentially drinking with peers, whilst simultaneously encouraging young people to connect with their social networks. The ability to socialise digitally can be done remotely and often at home, where parents can monitor behaviour. With the Internet increasingly being used to initiate and maintain social relationships, both romantic and otherwise (Tyler, 2002), the use of alcohol as a social lubricant may also be less necessary, and the imperative to find potential partners in licensed venues may have weakened. Social media sites in particular have become central to practices of performance, identity work and socialising (Goodwin & Griffin, 2017). Social media has been argued to encourage alcohol use by aiding event planning, enhancing sociability and setting positive alcohol norms through the sharing of photos and narratives (Supski, Lindsay, & Tanner, 2017), and there is some evidence to suggest a link between increased social media use and drinking (Larm, Raninen, Åslund, Svensson, & Nilsson, 2018; Pape et al., 2018). Social media sites also regularly expose their users to alcohol advertising, thus actively shaping discourses around alcohol normalisation and brand engagement, and raising questions about the 'intoxigenic' nature of digital spaces (Griffiths & Casswell, 2010). However, the link between alcohol and social media is likely to be mediated by social networks, as well as how individuals wish to portray themselves. Young adults may be increasingly aware of the 'pedagogy of regret' that can accompany a night out (Brown & Gregg, 2012), with the idea that anyone (including parents, future employers, romantic interests and friends) can survey social media content. This encourages curated presentations of health, style and discipline, making social media's effect on alcohol consumption complicated.

In contrast to music, dancing, parties and other social activities where substance use acts a complement (Lee et al., 2018), alcohol-free leisure activities have also become more popular. Digital gaming, and the accessibility of TV shows and movies, now provides young people with alternatives to the night-time economy, a substitution that is arguably safer, more controlled and cheaper. There is some evidence to suggest that gaming is linked with less alcohol use in young people (Pape et al., 2018) particularly among those who play more over weekends (Twenge, 2017). Online gaming and increased access to networked media like Netflix and YouTube have become a meaningful, accessible and pleasurable source of social engagement in the modern age. As credible pastimes, these leisure activities are also sites for identity construction and communication, thus providing legitimate consumption alternatives that may be replacing or at least supplementing the role of alcohol.

The Link Between Mental Health and Alcohol

Despite general improvements to health, living conditions, life expectancy and population-level affluence, psychological concerns continue to impact on the well-being of many young adults. A systematic review by Bor, Dean, Najman and Hayatbakhsh (2014) showed that for young adults in the twenty-first century, internalising problems such as stress, anxiety and depression had reportedly risen, particularly among females. Another review by Collishaw (2015) showed that these trends were part of longer-term increases in affective and emotional problems, beginning in a number of countries from the 1970s and 1980s. Despite previously identified associations between heavy alcohol use and worse mental health, increasing mental health symptoms have occurred at the same time as decreasing alcohol use among young adults. It could be that mental health problems are better reported and recorded. However, there is suggestive evidence that mental health symptoms are increasing among young adults at a population level (Collishaw, 2015; Mojtabai, Olfson, & Han, 2016). Because the relationship between alcohol and mental health is complex and often bi-directional (Hagell et al., 2012), it is important to explore the changing issues around mental health and its relationship with alcohol for young adults.

Whilst objective quality of life measures has improved, many other culturally specific goals continue to shape perceptions of happiness. For example, stresses around body image, academic performance, career success, unstable employment conditions and economic independence are all associated with psychological distress for young adults (West, 2016; Wyn, Cuervo, & Landstedt, 2015). And whilst more young adults receive education for longer, they are less rewarded for their efforts in a highly competitive job market. For some, such as sexual minorities, life satisfaction seems to have increased in countries where structural stigma has weakened (Bränström, 2017). But young adults remain part of a generation intuitively concerned about global political issues, including human rights issues and climate change (Williams & Page, 2011). Worries about precarious and uncertain futures, for both themselves and the world, mean that stress and anxiety are features of the lives of young adults.

The intersection between digital technologies and mental health is another important consideration. Elevated use of electronic devices has been associated with worse psychological health (Wang, Li, Kim, Lee, & Seo, 2019), where time spent on digital technology may come at the cost of key factors associated with mental health, such as reduced sleep and exercise. Digital technology has also been linked to loneliness, anxiety, social withdrawal and isolation (Li & Wong, 2015; Odacı & Kalkan, 2010), and problematic use is now being recognised through Internet and gaming addictions (Faust & Prochaska, 2018; Young, 2004). Whilst quantity and quality of interactions with real-world friends is associated with better mental health, increased Facebook engagement risks the development of meaningful relationships and interactions and has been associated with poorer mental health and life satisfaction (Kross et al., 2013; Shakya & Christakis, 2017). Social media has become intertwined with new experiences of bullying and aggression and propagates standards of health, beauty and self-improvement that heighten anxieties around body image and self-presentation (Fardouly & Vartanian, 2016; Livingstone & Smith, 2014). Despite these negatives, however, digital technology has also created more accessible spaces for interaction, meaningful leisure pursuits, and has provided new interfaces to support mental health. How technology influences mental health, and how that might then mediate alcohol use, thus remains a complicated issue.

Given the self-medicating properties of alcohol and its relationship with poorer mental health (Pedersen & von Soest, 2015), it might be expected that young adults would increase drinking due to the stresses of social change. On the other hand, alcohol use might be avoided given its potential for disrupting productivity and diminishing mental health. A recent Australian survey found that young adults considered mental health and alcohol and drugs the two most important societal issues (Bullot, Cave, Fildes, Hall, & Plummer, 2017). In this sense, young adults' relationship with alcohol is complex: whilst it can provide positive benefits to well-being by enhancing confidence, sociability and sense of belonging, it is also linked with a number of well-known negative mental health outcomes including depression, stress, anxiety and relationship breakdown (Newbury-Birch et al., 2009). The mounting evidence linking alcohol and mental health problems may be a connection that young adults are increasingly wary of. Now with new ways of socialising and immersion without alcohol, and greater emphasis on mental health awareness and self-care strategies, alcohol's previously established association with sociability and, by extension, social well-being may be changing. Thus, we may be witnessing a generation of young adults whose response to stress is to be more risk-averse, and more attuned with their own mental health needs.

Changing Lives, Changing Drinking Cultures

Whilst we should not assume it has been denormalised, alcohol, like other goods, is a cultural commodity tied to social status, individualism, choice and identity. Evaluative judgements of good and bad taste reflect popular attitudes towards consumption, and performing a non- or light-drinking identity can also be considered a form of status. For example, young adults spend more time and money on dining out than previous generations (Zan & Fan, 2010), and recent subcultures of drinking alcohol based on taste, knowledge and food-pairing have emerged (Martinez, Hammond, Harrington, & Wiersma-Mosley, 2017), challenging traditional notions of youthful drinking as intoxication-fuelled or excessive.

As 'global citizens' of an increasingly multicultural and informed generation, young adults have also been characterised as being respectful of ethnic and cultural diversity and as having greater social awareness (Williams & Page, 2011). Heavy migration from lower drinking countries in Asia, Africa and Latin America has created culturally integrated and diverse communities. In the United States and Australia, immigrant groups from collectivist regions such as Asian and African countries report lower rates of excessive and recent drinking (Chan et al., 2016; Szaflarski, Cubbins, & Ying, 2011). Indirectly, it is hypothesised this may potentially diffuse out into young adults' drinking behaviour at the population level through acculturation and adaption to social networks (Amundsen, 2005). Although this is still speculative, not drinking for cultural reasons is seen as a credible alternative (Fry, 2010) and may be symptomatic of an acceptance of diversity, including choices around alcohol.

It is also important to remember that drinking status is not necessarily static. A recent Australian study showed over the past fifteen years more young adults tried to reduce or cease drinking—largely for health, lifestyle, financial and taste/enjoyment reasons (Pennay et al., 2018). The authors suggest that heavy and frequent drinking has become less acceptable. Alcohol can produce both positive and negatives outcomes, and being aware and ambivalent towards the negative effects of alcohol is not uncommon for both abstainers and heavy drinkers (de Visser & Smith, 2007). Young adults seem to demonstrate greater ambivalence towards losing control and greater stigmatisation of drunkenness (MacLean, Pennay, & Room,

2018). Thus, the changing boundaries of socially acceptable behaviour may have influenced the current decline in alcohol consumption just as it did with increases in the 1990s; just as social controls have shifted to reflect growing concerns over young adult behaviour, so too has the meaning of alcohol within their lives and the search for other alternatives.

What Does This Mean for Future Alcohol Consumption Trends?

There are two broad perspectives we might consider when thinking about recent changes in young adult alcohol consumption and what it might mean for future consumption. The first is that changes in drinking rates are a continuation of historical peaks and troughs of consumption (see Mäkelä, Walsh, Sulkunen, Single, & Room, 1981). The second is that the current reduction in consumption represents a unique historical and social phenomenon.

The first perspective sees drinking rates change over time through processes of normalisation (marked by the relaxing of formal and informal controls) and problematisation (marked by the tightening of alcohol policies and increased stigma). Thus, declines occur as a societal reaction to the excesses of previous generations, and increases occur through 'generational forgetting' (Johnston et al., 2018). In this respect, high rates of drinking in the late 1990s and the subsequent 'demonising' of young adult drinking might be seen as a precipitant to the current decline. The excesses of the 1990s saw an intersection of several public health concerns, including youth, drugs, crime and danger (Parker et al., 1998), allowing young adults to be pathologised and 'othered' as a risky subgroup. Focused sanctions and regulatory approaches that included taxes on pre-mixed drinks, lockout laws (i.e. legal restrictions on how late licensed premises can serve alcohol), secondary supply laws, minimum drinking ages and targeted education campaigns all highlight efforts to address 'moral panics' around young adult drinking (Cohen, 2011). However, formal policy and legislative responses tend to lag behind informal social responses (such as collective pressures by communities and the media) (Room, Osterberg, Ramstedt, & Rehm, 2009), and public health initiatives are as much symptoms of change as they are precipitators. Therefore, the problematisation of young adult alcohol use in popular media that occurred in the early 2000s may have encouraged a change in drinking styles and destabilised its normalised status, as it did with smoking in the late twentieth century (see Chapman, 2008). In this perspective, it stands to reason that young adult drinking will increase again when informal and formal controls relax in response to diminished public health concern. Whilst the rhetoric around risky young adult drinking is likely to have played a role in declining drinking rates, an apparent divergence between the drinking of younger drinkers and older populations (Livingston et al., 2016) suggests changes in young adults' consumption practices cannot simply be explained as a consequence of a historical trough. Deciphering whether and how alcohol regulations have contributed to young adult drinking is difficult. For example, from a UK perspective the Licensing Act 2003 (Mandatory Licensing Conditions) Order could be understood to have curbed the worst excesses of drinks promotions that characterised the preceding years (UK Government, 2010). However, assessing the global impact of alcohol regulations on young adult drinking practices, and whether there is impact in different cultural contexts, is difficult to meaningfully quantify.

The second perspective, that the current reduction in consumption represents a unique historical and social phenomenon, is therefore worthy of consideration. Declines might be part of a broader change in the way young adults are 'doing' or 'performing' young adulthood, and this may lead to a more sustained change. As we have argued, structural shifts in education and labour markets have forced young people to adapt to insecure and flexible labour, longer time in education, declining tradition, individualisation, growing diversity of information and choice and an expanding and globalised media. Young adults' struggle for autonomy may have restricted opportunities for consumption, including economic factors (i.e. purchasing power) and spatial restrictions (e.g. through spending more time in the family home). We note here that shifting circumstances for young adults make certainty with these arguments difficult; for example, the 'extended adolescence' thesis (e.g. Arnett's [2000] 'emerging adulthood' theory) would emphasise that extended time in the family home frees up young adults' disposable income resulting in delayed adult responsibilities (e.g. parenthood, independent living) for socialising. The practice of being a young adult (and indirectly, the meanings attributed to alcohol) is distinct from previous generations. Because of the tangled and rapid nature of these social changes, what they mean for the future of alcohol consumption is unclear. Whether this constitutes a continuation of historical drinking trends or a turning point for the place of alcohol in the lives of young adults requires further investigation. To add to this complexity, there is some evidence of a growingly polarised drinking culture between heavy and light drinkers, rather than collective declines (Caluzzi, 2018). Thus, any theories raised are likely to be provisional at best and should remain open to new ideas, explanations and conceptual ways of thinking.

Conclusion

Alcohol has been historically (and for many continues to be) a means of experiencing pleasure, time-out, enhancement and excitement, whilst also providing a sense of belonging, celebration and adulthood (Beccaria & Sande, 2003). However, with competing discourses of commodification and risk, young adults are required to negotiate ambiguous cultural messages that endorse both excess and restraint. Today's generation of young adults more than ever have to adapt to neoliberal conditions that emphasise individual responsibility and restraint (Babor, 2010). Policy, regulation and media problematisation of alcohol use have coincided with a boom in new digital forms of consumption and alternative lifestyles, which is likely to have had a synergistic effect and reinforced changes in alcohol use. Whilst recent declines in consumption represent a positive public health development, alcohol use has long been tied to social benefits, so we should remain wary of the indirect effects on young adults. Declines in alcohol use and other behaviours deemed risky may be part of a shift towards actively meeting institutional requirements (e.g. school, university, unpaid work and flexible employment) at the cost of leisure times and a potential decline in social well-being. Neoliberal discourses seem to have created an environment that opposes 'letting loose' and drunken comportment in favour of alternative lifestyles, new forms of consumption and entertainment and new ways to achieve status and identity. Future research should investigate how young adults reflexively build identities based on (non-)consumption, how activities and rituals may have changed and provided new ways of achieving adult identities, and the role of alcohol for young adults in the context of a globalised world of increasing precarity and pressure.

References

Amundsen, E. J. (2005). Drinking pattern among adolescents with immigrant and Norwegian backgrounds: A two-way influence? *Addiction, 100*(10), 1453–1463.

Arnett, J. J. (2000). Emerging adulthood: A theory of development from the late teens through the twenties. *American Psychologist, 55*(5), 469.

Assarsson, L., & Aarsand, P. (2011). "How to be good": Media representations of parenting. *Studies in the Education of Adults, 43*(1), 78–92.

Babor, T. (2010). *Alcohol: No ordinary commodity—Research and public policy* (2nd ed.). Oxford: Oxford University Press.

Bauman, Z. (1988). *Freedom.* Minnesota: University of Minnesota Press.

Beccaria, F., & Sande, A. (2003). Drinking games and rite of life projects: A social comparison of the meaning and functions of young people's use of alcohol during the rite of passage to adulthood in Italy and Norway. *Young, 11*(2), 99–119.

Beck, U. (2000). *The brave new world of work.* Malden, MA: Polity Press.

Bhattacharya, A. (2016). *Youthful abandon—Why are young people drinking less* [Institute of Alcohol Studies report]. Retrieved 1 November 2019 from http://www.ias.org.uk/uploads/pdf/IAS%20reports/rp22072016.pdf.

Bor, W., Dean, A. J., Najman, J., & Hayatbakhsh, R. (2014). Are child and adolescent mental health problems increasing in the 21st century? A systematic review. *Australian and New Zealand* Journal *of Psychiatry, 48*, 606–616.

Bränström, R. (2017). Hidden from happiness: Structural stigma, sexual orientation concealment, and life satisfaction among sexual minorities across 28 European countries—Richard Bränström. *European Journal of Public Health, 27*(suppl. 3).

Brown, R., & Gregg, M. (2012). The pedagogy of regret: Facebook, binge drinking and young women. *Continuum, 26*(3), 357–369.

Bugental, D. B., Corpuz, R., & Beaulieu, D. A. (2014). An evolutionary approach to socialization. In P. D. Hastings & J. E. Grusec (Eds.), *Handbook of socialization: Theory and research* (2nd ed., pp. 325–346). New York: The Guilford Press.

Bullot, A., Cave, L., Fildes, J., Hall, S., & Plummer, J. (2017). *Mission Australia's 2017 youth survey report.* Retrieved 1 November 2019 from https://www.missionaustralia.com.au/publications/youth-survey/746-youth-survey-2017-report/file.

Caluzzi, G. (2018). Changing but resistant: The importance of integrating heavier young drinkers within a declining drinking culture. *Drugs: Education, Prevention and Policy,* 1–5.

Chan, G. C., Kelly, A. B., Connor, J. P., Hall, W., Young, R. M., & Williams, J. W. (2016). Does parental monitoring and disapproval explain variations in alcohol use among adolescents from different countries of birth? *Drug and Alcohol Review, 35,* 741–749.

Chapman, S. (2008). *Public health advocacy and tobacco control: Making smoking history.* Hoboken, UK: Wiley.

Cohen, S. (2011). *Folk devils and moral panics: The creation of the mods and rockers.* London and New York: Taylor & Francis.

Collishaw, S. (2015). Annual research review: Secular trends in child and adolescent mental health. *Child Adolescent Psychology Psychiatry, 56*(3), 370–393.

de Visser, R. O., & Smith, J. A. (2007). Young men's ambivalence toward alcohol. *Social Science and Medicine, 64*(2), 350–362.

Fardouly, J., & Vartanian, L. R. (2016). Social media and body image concerns: Current research and future directions. *Current Opinion in Psychology, 9,* 1–5.

Farrell, G., Tilley, N., & Tseloni, A. (2014). Why the crime drop? *Crime and Justice, 43*(1), 421–490.

Faust, K. A., & Prochaska, J. J. (2018). Internet gaming disorder: A sign of the times, or time for our attention? *Addictive Behaviors, 77,* 272–274.

Fry, M.-L. (2010). Countering consumption in a culture of intoxication. *Journal of Marketing Management, 26*(13–14), 1279–1294.

Furlong, A., & Cartmel, F. (2006). *Young people and social change.* Buckingham, VA: McGraw-Hill Education.

Goodwin, I., & Griffin, C. (2017). Neoliberalism, alcohol and identity: A symptomatic reading of young people's drinking cultures in a digital world. In A. Lyons, T. McCreanor, I. Goodwin, & H. M. Barnes (Eds.), *Youth drinking cultures in a digital world: Alcohol, social media and cultures of intoxication* (pp. 16–30). Abingdon Oxon, UK: Routledge.

Griffiths, R., & Casswell, S. (2010). Intoxigenic digital spaces? Youth, social networking sites and alcohol marketing. *Drug and Alcohol Review, 29*(5), 525.

Hagell, A., Aldridge, J., Meier, P., Millar, T., Symonds, J., & Donmall, M. (2012). Trends in adolescent substance use and their implications for understanding trends in mental health. In A. Hagell & M. Rutter (Eds.), *Changing adolescence: Social trends and mental health* (pp. 117–150). Bristol, UK: Policy Press.

Hagell, A., & Witherspoon, S. (2012). Reflections and Implications. In A. Hagell & M. Rutter (Eds.), *Changing adolescence: Social trends and mental health* (pp. 165–178). Bristol, UK: Policy Press.

Itō, M., Baumer, S., Bittanti, M., Boyd, D., Cody, R., Herr-Stephenson, B., ... Tripp, L. (2010). *Hanging out, messing around, and geeking out: Kids living and learning with new media.* Cambridge: MIT Press.

Johnston, L. D., Miech, R. A., O'Malley, P. M., Bachman, J. G., Schulenberg, J. E., & Patrick, M. E. (2018). *Monitoring the future national survey results on drug use, 1975–2017: Overview, key findings on adolescent drug use* [data report]. Retrieved 1 November 2019 from https://eric.ed.gov/?id=ED578534.

Kann, L., McManus, T., Harris, W., Shanklin, S., Flint, K., Hawkins, J., ... Zaza, S. (2015). Youth risk behavior surveillance—United States, 2015. *Surveillance Summaries, 65*(6), 1–174. Retrieved 1 November 2019 from https://www.cdc.gov/mmwr/volumes/65/ss/pdfs/ss6506.pdf.

Kross, E., Verduyn, P., Demiralp, E., Park, J., Lee, D. S., Lin, N., ... Ybarra, O. (2013). Facebook use predicts declines in subjective well-being in young adults. *PLoS ONE, 8*(8), e69841.

Larm, P., Raninen, J., Åslund, C., Svensson, J., & Nilsson, K. W. (2018). The increased trend of non-drinking alcohol among adolescents: What role do internet activities have? *European Journal of Public Health, 29*(1), 27–32.

Lee, J. O., Cho, J., Yoon, Y., Bello, M. S., Khoddam, R., & Leventhal, A. M. (2018). Developmental pathways from parental socioeconomic status to adolescent substance use: Alternative and complementary reinforcement. *Journal of Youth and Adolescence, 47*(2), 334–348.

Li, T. M. H., & Wong, P. W. C. (2015). Youth social withdrawal behavior (hikikomori): A systematic review of qualitative and quantitative studies. *Australian and New Zealand Journal of Psychiatry, 49*(7), 595–609.

Livingston, M., Raninen, J., Slade, T., Swift, W., Lloyd, B., & Dietze, P. (2016). Understanding trends in Australian alcohol consumption-an age-period-cohort model. *Addiction, 111*(9), 1590–1598.

Livingstone, S., & Smith, P. K. (2014). Annual research review: Harms experienced by child users of online and mobile technologies—The nature, prevalence and management of sexual and aggressive risks in the digital age. *Journal of Child Psychology* and *Psychiatry, 55*, 635–654.

MacLean, S., Pennay, A., & Room, R. (2018). 'You're repulsive': Limits to acceptable drunken comportment for young adults. *International Journal of Drug Policy, 53*, 106–112.

Mäkelä, K., Walsh, B., Sulkunen, P., Single, E., & Room, R. (1981). *Alcohol, society, and the state: I. A comparative study of alcohol control.* Toronto, ON: Addiction Research Foundation.

Mannheim, K. (1952 [1927]). The problem of generations. In *Essays on the sociology of knowledge* (pp. 276–322). London: Routledge.

Martinez, D. C., Hammond, R. K., Harrington, R. J., & Wiersma-Mosley, J. D. (2017). Young adults' and industry experts' subjective and objective knowledge of beer and food pairings. *Journal of Culinary Science & Technology, 15*(4), 285–305.

Measham, F. (1996). The 'big bang' approach to sessional drinking: Changing patterns of alcohol consumption amongst young people in North West England. *Addiction Research, 4*(3), 283–299.

Measham, F. (2008). The turning tides of intoxication: Young people's drinking in Britain in the 2000s. *Health Education, 108*(3), 207–222.

Measham, F., & Brain, K. (2005). 'Binge' drinking, British alcohol policy and the new culture of intoxication. *Crime, Media, Culture: An International Journal, 1*(3), 262–283.

Mojtabai, R., Olfson, M., & Han, B. (2016). National trends in the prevalence and treatment of depression in adolescents and young adults (Report). *Pediatrics, 138*(6).

Newbury-Birch, D., Walker, J., Avery, L., Beyer, F., Brown, N., Jackson, K., … Gilvarry, E. (2009). *Impact of alcohol consumption on young people: A systematic review of published reviews* [research report]. Retrieved 1 November 2019 from https://dera.ioe.ac.uk/11355/1/DCSF-RR067.pdf.

Odacı, H., & Kalkan, M. (2010). Problematic internet use, loneliness and dating anxiety among young adult university students. *Computers & Education, 55*(3), 1091–1097.

Pape, H., Rossow, I., & Brunborg, G. S. (2018). Adolescents drink less: How, who and why? A review of the recent research literature. *Drug and Alcohol Review, 37*(S1), S98–S114.

Parker, H. J., Measham, F., & Aldridge, J. (1998). *Illegal leisure: The normalization of adolescent recreational drug use.* London and New York: Routledge.

Pedersen, W., & von Soest, T. (2015). Adolescent alcohol use and binge drinking: An 18-year trend study of prevalence and correlates. *Alcohol and Alcoholism, 50*(2), 219–225.

Pennay, A., Callinan, S., Livingston, M., Lubman, D. I., Holmes, J., MacLean, S., ... Dietze, P. (2018). Patterns in reduction or cessation of drinking in Australia (2001–2013) and motivation for change. *Alcohol and Alcoholism, 54*(1), 79–86.

Pennay, A., Livingston, M., & MacLean, S. (2015). Young people are drinking less: It is time to find out why. *Drug and Alcohol Review, 34*(2), 115–118.

Prensky, M. (2001). Digital natives, digital immigrants part 1. *On the Horizon, 9*(5), 1–6.

Raitasalo, K., & Holmila, M. (2017). Practices in alcohol education among Finnish parents: Have there been changes between 2006 and 2012? *Drugs: Education Prevention and Policy, 24*(5), 392–399.

Room, R., Osterberg, E. S. A., Ramstedt, M., & Rehm, J. (2009). Explaining change and stasis in alcohol consumption. *Addiction Research & Theory, 17*(6), 562–576.

Sani, G., & Treas, J. (2016). Educational gradients in parents' child-care time across countries, 1965–2012. *Journal of Marriage and Family, 78*(4), 1083–1096..

Shakya, H. B., & Christakis, N. A. (2017). Association of facebook use with compromised well-being: A longitudinal study. *American Journal of Epidemiology, 185*(3), 203–211.

Supski, S., Lindsay, J., & Tanner, C. (2017). University students' drinking as a social practice and the challenge for public health. *Critical Public Health, 27*(2), 228–237.

Szaflarski, M., Cubbins, L., & Ying, J. (2011). Epidemiology of alcohol abuse among US immigrant populations. *Journal of Immigrant and Minority Health, 13*(4), 647–658.

Tilleczek, K., & Srigley, R. (2016). Young cyborgs? Youth and the digital age. In A. Furlong (Ed.), *Routledge handbook of youth and young adulthood* (pp. 273–284). London, UK: Routledge.

Törrönen, J., Roumeliotis, F., Samuelsson, E., Kraus, L., & Room, R. (2019). Why are young people drinking less than earlier? Identifying and specifying social mechanisms with a pragmatist approach. *International Journal of Drug Policy, 64,* 13–20.

Twenge, J. M. (2017). *IGen: Why today's super-connected kids are growing up less rebellious, more tolerant, less happy—And completely unprepared for adulthood (and what this means for the rest of us).* New York, NY: Atria Books.

Twenge, J. M., & Park, H. (2017). The decline in adult activities among U.S. adolescents, 1976–2016. *Child Development*, 1–17.

Tyler, T. R. (2002). Is the internet changing social life? It seems the more things change, the more they stay the same. *Journal of Social Issues, 58*(1), 195.

UK Government. (2010). *The Licensing Act 2003 (Mandatory Licensing Conditions) Order 2010*. Accessed 6 June 2019 from http://www.legislation.gov.uk/uksi/2010/860/pdfs/uksi_20100860_en.pdf.

Vaughn, M. G., Nelson, E. J., Oh, S., Salas-Wright, C. P., DeLisi, M., & Holzer, K. J. (2018). Abstention from drug use and delinquency increasing among youth in the United States, 2002–2014. *Substance Use & Misuse*, 1–14.

Wang, C., Li, K., Kim, M., Lee, S., & Seo, D.-C. (2019). Association between psychological distress and elevated use of electronic devices among U.S. adolescents: Results from the youth risk behavior surveillance 2009–2017. *Addictive Behaviors, 90,* 112–118.

West, P. (2016). Health in youth: Changing times and changing influences. In A. Furlong (Ed.), *Routledge handbook of youth and young adulthood* (pp. 327–338). London: Routledge.

Williams, K. C., & Page, R. A. (2011). Marketing to the generations. *Journal of Behavioral Studies in Business, 3*(1), 37–53.

Woodman, D. (2016). The sociology of youth and generations. In A. Furlong (Ed.), *Routledge handbook of youth and young adulthood* (pp. 20–26). London, UK: Routledge.

Woodman, D., & Wyn, J. (2014). *Youth and generation: Rethinking change and inequality in the lives of young people*. London, UK: Sage.

Wyn, J. (2011). The sociology of youth: A reflection on its contribution to the field and future directions. *Youth Studies Australia, 30*(3), 34–39.

Wyn, J. (2016). Educating for late modernity. In A. Furlong (Ed.), *Routledge handbook of youth and young adulthood* (pp. 91–98). London, UK: Routledge.

Wyn, J., Cuervo, H., & Landstedt, E. (2015). The limits of wellbeing. In K. Wright & J. McLeod (Eds.), *Rethinking youth wellbeing: Critical perspectives* (pp. 55–70). Singapore: Springer.

Yap, M., Cheong, T., Zaravinos-Tsakos, F., Lubman, D. I., & Jorm, A. (2017). Modifiable parenting factors associated with adolescent alcohol misuse: A systematic review and meta-analysis of longitudinal studies. *Addiction, 112*(7), 1142–1162.

Young, K. S. (2004). Internet addiction: A new clinical phenomenon and its consequences. *American Behavioral Scientist, 48*(4), 402.

Zan, H., & Fan, J. X. (2010). Cohort effects of household expenditures on food away from home. *Journal of Consumer Affairs, 44*(1), 213.

4

Life Transitions into Adulthood and the Drinking Trajectory

Marjana Martinic and Arlene Bigirimana

The transition from adolescence into adulthood is assumed to be defined by certain life events that bring with them new roles and responsibilities and societal expectations around stage-appropriate and normative behavior. Leaving the parental home in pursuit of higher education or a job, full-time employment, marriage and domestic partnership, and parenthood are all defining stages of adult life, independence, and self-sufficiency. It is generally assumed that life stages are well delineated and defined, and that transitioning into them will occur in a particular and predictable sequence. In reality, life transitions are fluid and constantly evolving, as is the definition of when adolescence ends and adulthood begins. Boundaries have shifted, as have assumptions about timing and order of particular life events, like marriage, parenthood, or a career.

M. Martinic (✉)
MM Science and Policy Advisors, LLC, Washington, DC, USA
e-mail: mmartinic@mm-spa.com

A. Bigirimana
International Alliance for Responsible Drinking (IARD),
Washington, DC, USA

© The Author(s) 2019
D. Conroy and F. Measham (eds.), *Young Adult Drinking Styles*,
https://doi.org/10.1007/978-3-030-28607-1_4

As boundaries between life stages have shifted, so have gender- and age-bound definitions of particular social roles and of the behaviors we expect will accompany them. The consumption of alcohol in those societies where it is permitted and accepted is one such behavior. Particular drinking patterns, whether heavy or light, are expected to occur during particular life stages, and to be incompatible with others. In particular, drinking patterns during the transition from adolescence into early adulthood, with its many life-defining events, are expected to evolve along a predetermined trajectory—from initiation to experimentation and possibly excess, before finally stabilizing into a pattern that will persist well into adulthood. Yet, like life transitions, drinking patterns are dynamic. They change over time and reflect evolving social norms, expectations, and cultural shifts.

This chapter offers an overview of available research on the relationship between life transitions and the development of the drinking trajectory as adolescence becomes adulthood. Yet in light of the shifting timing, definition, and significance of particular life events, it may be time to revisit the evidence and to challenge what we know and, more importantly, what we expect, with regard to both life transitions and the development of drinking patterns.

Life Transitions, Social Roles, and Drinking Patterns

Across cultures, the first introduction to alcohol beverages typically occurs in adolescence or even childhood, frequently within the context of family celebrations and social occasions (Brunborg, Norstrom, & Storvoll, 2018; Ostergaard, Jarvinen, & Andreasen, 2018). Once the family fold and its social controls are left behind, drinking often becomes heavier, more frequent, and a way of testing limits (Martinic & Measham, 2008). The influence of peers grows and drinking may become a means for achieving social cohesion, shared experiences, and group bonding (Guo, Li, Owen, Wang, & Duncan, 2015; Pocuca et al., 2018). For many young people,

4 Life Transitions into Adulthood and the Drinking Trajectory 69

drinking is a central leisure-time activity and important for social interaction (reviewed in Leigh & Lee, 2008; Nelson & Taberrer, 2017; Windle & Windle, 2018).

As adolescents become adults, these experimental drinking patterns 'mature out' and are replaced by new ones compatible with adult roles and responsibilities. The frequency of drinking declines, as do binge and heavy drinking (Lee & Sher, 2018), and a more stable stage emerges along the drinking trajectory, mirroring the transition into full adulthood and the increasing importance of employment, stable relationships, family life, and parenthood (Lee & Sher, 2018).

Independence and the Testing of Boundaries

For many young people, the transition from adolescence to adulthood begins when they enter higher education. It marks the first foray into relative independence and, across different countries and cultures, has been associated with more frequent and heavier drinking (Staff et al., 2010). Evidence from various countries suggests that permissive social attitudes and enabling peer groups, as well as the central role of drinking in social interactions in student life, are closely linked to the development of heavy drinking patterns (Kypri, Paschall, Maclennan, & Langley, 2007; Paschall & Saltz, 2007), which may facilitate peer bonding and the establishment of group identity. Much research in the US has focused on the so-called Greek system of sororities and fraternities on many college campuses (McCabe, Veliz, & Schulenberg, 2018; Scott-Sheldon, Carey, Elliott, Garey, & Carey, 2014). Belonging to these groups is generally associated with more frequent and heavy drinking, reflecting permissive social norms around risk-taking behavior.

It has been argued that these drinking patterns are a symptom of deferred adulthood and extended adolescence (Staff et al., 2010). By moving into higher education, young people may be simply trading one sheltered environment for another, with few responsibilities other than academic and without the constraints of parental rules and supervision. Others have suggested that risk-taking, including in drinking, may be projections about

Employment as a Milestone to Adulthood

Within the context of 'maturing out,' steady employment might be expected to go hand in hand with reduced drinking and patterns compatible with adult roles. Yet, surprisingly, employment does not appear to be a consistent predictor of stable drinking patterns. The relationship is strongly influenced by gender, cultural context, personality, and individual-level factors (Geisner et al., 2018). Some studies have shown lower rates of drinking and less heavy drinking among individuals who are employed, compared to those who are unemployed; this correlation appears to be especially strong for women (Ahlström, Bloomfield, & Knibbe, 2001; Staff, Greene, Maggs, & Schoon, 2014). Other studies suggest that full-time employment (especially among men) is likely to be correlated with *higher* odds of being a current drinker, more frequent binge drinking (Greene, Eitle, & Eitle, 2014), and little reduction in heavy drinking (Staff et al., 2010). There is also evidence that men and women in professional jobs are likely to drink more frequently than those in non-professional jobs (Staff et al., 2014). Cross-cultural dimensions of the relationship have not been well studied, but what evidence there is supports a rather inconsistent picture. While some studies report employment as a predictor of lighter drinking, others report an increased likelihood of drinking, generally, and of heavier drinking (Kinjo et al., 2018; Qian, Newman, Yuen, Shell, & Xu, 2018; Taylor et al., 2017). It has been suggested that increased, or simply sustained, heavy drinking with full-time employment may actually be a reflection of greater disposable income. This relationship has been reported for both men and women across different cultures (Grittner, Nemeth, Kuntsche, Gaertner, & Bloomfield, 2015) and appears to be stronger in middle-income than in low-income countries.

Interruptions in stable employment (e.g., getting fired or being unemployed for extended periods) also affect the 'normal' trajectory of drinking.

There is evidence of an association between unemployment and both overall drinking and heavy episodic drinking., specifically (Aseltine & Gore, 2005), which may be influenced by gender. While women are more likely to reduce their drinking following unemployment, men appear more likely to increase their consumption and to become heavier drinkers.

Family Role Transitions: Domestic Partnerships, Marriage, and Parenthood

Of the various life transitions examined, shifts in family roles are most consistently associated with changes in drinking patterns. Stable intimate relationships (whether marriage, domestic partnership, or cohabitation) tend to be associated with a decline in alcohol consumption among both men and women (Dinescu et al., 2016; Kuntsche, Astudillo, & Gmel, 2016; Olson, Hummer, & Harris, 2017; Staff et al., 2014), and to the protective effect of family roles. There is also evidence suggesting that the effect may be greater for men than women (Duncan, Wilkerson, & England, 2006).

The 'shared lifestyle' of intimate relationships and marriage may account for some of this effect, which also translates into other health behaviors among spouses and life partners (Birditt, Cranford, Manalel, & Antonucci, 2018). Across cultures, the effect of spouses' and partners' drinking appears to be stronger for women than men (Ahlström et al., 2001; Kendler, Lonn, Salvatore, Sundquist, & Sundquist, 2016). Shared peer and social groups also play a role in shaping drinking by life partners (Polenick, Birditt, & Blow, 2018). Conversely, transitioning out of domestic partnerships has been associated with increased drinking (Keenan, Ploubidis, Silverwood, & Grundy, 2017; Liang & Chikritzhs, 2012), a higher likelihood of having an alcohol use disorder, and generally engaging in risky behaviors (Salvatore et al., 2017). Some studies have found this effect to be particularly strong in men (Ahlström et al., 2001; Kretsch & Harden, 2014). For those coping with the loss of a partner, increased drinking may be a way of coping (Eng, Kawachi, Fitzmaurice, & Rimm, 2005), but the loss of a partner may also represent the loss of a drinking companion and result in reduced levels and frequency. This transition to lighter drinking is observed particularly among women (Liew, 2012).

The centrality of marriage as an adult role has also been identified as an influence on the drinking trajectory. Based on research conducted in the United States, individuals who placed greater emphasis on marriage than on a career or even parenthood as a central life event were less likely to engage in risky behaviors, including problematic drinking patterns (Willoughby, Hall, & Goff, 2015). The meaning of this finding is unclear, but it may point to the influence of social and cultural pressure to adhere to the expected norms and behaviors associated with married life. The consistency of the relationship between marriage and drinking across cultures and its role as a stabilizing and protective factor has not been well studied, but there is evidence from studies using ethnicity as a proxy for culture that changes in drinking frequency and problem drinking after marriage may in part be culturally determined (Taylor et al., 2017; Qian et al., 2018; Wainberg et al., 2018).

Of all life transitions, parenthood appears to be the most significant influence on drinking and the most consistent predictor of drinking patterns. Becoming a parent is closely related to a decline in drinking, even among young adults whose drinking patterns are relatively heavy (Ahlström et al., 2001; Bowden, Delfabbro, Room, Miller, & Wilson, 2018; Little, Handley, Leuthe, & Chassin, 2009). It is observed in both men and women and across different cultures (Grittner et al., 2015). These findings suggest that the increased responsibilities of being a parent and the structure of parental life are reflected in changes in drinking and may make it difficult to devote time and resources to drinking.

There are some notable gender differences in the impact of parenthood on drinking patterns. Among women, a transition into more moderate drinking patterns or even abstention generally starts in pregnancy. Drinking is likely to resume after childbirth (Chapman & Wu, 2013; Levy, Le Strat, Hoertel, Ancelet, & Dubertret, 2018; Liu & Mumford, 2017), but generally at reduced levels (Matusiewicz, Ilgen, & Bohnert, 2016). Studies have also reported a so-called motherhood advantage, protective against risky drinking (Balan et al., 2014; Kendler, Lonn, Salvatore, Sundquist, & Sundquist, 2018) and particularly strong when women are living with younger children (Bowden et al., 2018; Kendler et al., 2018). However, these associations are not hard and fast. Socioeconomic status, deprivation, and educational level all play a role in the evolution of drinking patterns in motherhood (Liu & Mumford, 2017; Watt et al., 2014).

Possibly one of the strongest cultural influences on the drinking trajectory is the degree to which drinking is integrated into the social fabric of everyday life. In typical 'Mediterranean' or 'wet' drinking cultures, the impact of parenthood on changing drinking patterns appears to be less pronounced than in those where drinking is an isolated activity, as in 'Nordic' or 'dry' cultures (Ahlström et al., 2001). Culture also determines the contexts where drinking takes place, which, in turn, may determine changes in drinking patterns among parents (Paradis, Demers, Nadeau, & Picard, 2015). For example, men and women who are parents may be less likely to frequent bars and restaurants after having children. As a result, in cultures where most drinking occurs outside the home, parents may reduce their overall drinking (Paradis, 2011).

The Times, They Are a' Changing: Gender Roles and Drinking Trajectories

Over recent decades observable shifts in certain life transitions have had a disruptive effect on the expected and normative evolution of the drinking trajectory. Broader social and economic conditions, such as financial crises and instability, may disrupt the expected order of life stages, delay the timing of particular events, and redefine gender roles. All of these, in turn, are likely to contribute to shifting societal expectancies regarding drinking behavior.

Life Transitions, Drinking Patterns, and the Closing Gender Gap

For both men and women, gender roles are steadily evolving. The delineation between feminine and masculine roles and professions has blurred, along with expectations around the timing and nature of particular life transitions, and the 'appropriate' behaviors that might accompany them.

While there is still an undeniable gender differential between men and women in virtually every aspect of life, important strides have been made in the education and employment of women in many countries. The convergence of opportunity and equality, particularly in developed countries, is mirrored in some important shifts in life transitions and also in an observable convergence in alcohol consumption by men and women. While the number of male drinkers still exceeds the number of female drinkers globally, the gap has narrowed (Breslow, Castle, Chen, & Graubard, 2017). More women are drinking, even where previously not condoned, and some women are also drinking more than in previous generations, emulating typically 'male' drinking patterns. A clear convergence in the drinking patterns can already been seen among adolescent boys and girls (Currie et al., 2012; The ESPAD Group, 2016).

In spite of these significant shifts in drinking patterns, perspectives on normative drinking behaviors have not kept up with the rate of change. Some researchers have offered the view that rising rates of drinking among women 'constitute a public health crisis' (Grant et al., 2017). This view has resonated in media headlines and public perception. Headlines such as, 'For women, heavy drinking has been normalized. That's dangerous' (Kindy & Keating, 2016), and 'Young women become biggest binge drinkers as boys call time' (Hurst, 2017) reflect society's response to a changing trend.

There is good reason to be concerned about heavy drinking among women. As a function of the sheer increase in the number of drinking women, a rise in the prevalence of alcohol problems has been reported in various countries. There is also good reason to recommend lower consumption levels to women than to men. Physiological differences mean that women process alcohol differently than men and are likely to experience harms at lower levels of drinking. Recent evidence has also flagged a slightly increased risk of breast cancer, even at moderate drinking levels, and advice against drinking during pregnancy has been a staple of consumer information for some time. However, the tone of the public outcry suggests that it is colored not only by health concerns, but by a reaction to women engaging in what was long considered a 'masculine' behavior. Content analyses of media coverage of women's drinking suggest that depictions are rife with moralistic overtones and stereotypes of 'loose' women (Patterson, Emslie, Mason, Fergie, & Hilton, 2016; Rolando, Taddeo, & Beccaria, 2016). These stereotypes are at odds with the reality of educated, employed, and professional women for whom drinking is a lifestyle choice, and likely very compatible with other social roles. A paternalistic view of how women should drink, framed around potential health and social concerns, may well be misplaced in light of greater freedom, autonomy, and choice available to women today than ever before.

The new reality of the relationship between life transitions and drinking patterns described here has not yet been studied in a scientific and systematic way, but supports the notion that women who have children later in life, and also a career, are more likely to drink alcohol than those who have children earlier (Ahlström et al., 2001). Women who transition early into motherhood are also more likely to reduce their previous levels of drinking than those who first move into a career and later into motherhood (Amato & Kane, 2011). The pressures associated with the transition into employment and a career are an important consideration. Work stressors have been identified as one of the main drivers of drinking among the actively employed. A review of alcohol use and work has shown that those who work long hours are likely to drink more than those with a shorter workday; the relationship appears to be particularly strong in women (Virtanen et al., 2015). Externalizing pressure is often socially acceptable for men, but not always for women, and drinking to relieve workplace stress and general pressures is less socially accepted (Frone, 2016).

The 'work-family conflict' offers a particular challenge (Wolff, Rospenda, Richman, Liu, & Milner, 2013). Whereas professional and family roles have long been accepted as compatible for men, they are less so for women, who have traditionally been under pressure to choose one or the other. Yet transitioning into motherhood no longer marks the end of professional life for many women, who now have the option and the economic power to do both. In some countries, access to childcare and other work-life benefits enable women to combine the two roles. In many Western societies, men are also increasingly sharing in parenting and family roles once seen as the traditional domain of women.

While a dual role for women may be increasingly accepted, there is still significant social disapproval in many cultures, and women, whether or not they have a career, often continue to be expected to carry the major burden of parenting. Research into drinking patterns among individuals who engage in multiple social roles show that while men who have concurrent roles as parents, domestic partners, and members of the workforce are less likely to be heavy drinkers (Kuntsche, Knibbe, & Gmel, 2009; Kuntsche, Knibbe, & Gmel, 2010), this is not always the case for women. Women who either have a larger number of children or were employed in addition to having maternal duties were likely to drink *more* than those with fewer roles to juggle (Kuntsche, Knibbe, & Gmel, 2012). The disproportionate burden of family roles shouldered by women, regardless of occupational status, likely plays a major contributing role. The pressure of motherhood seems especially strong during the first years after childbirth, presumably reflecting the responsibilities of having a younger child (Alstveit, Severinsson, & Karlsen, 2011).

The timing of the transition into motherhood also plays a role in the evolving drinking trajectory (De Genna, Goldschmidt, Marshal, Day, & Cornelius, 2017). There is evidence to suggest that older women are more likely to drink during pregnancy than younger women (Kitsantas, Gaffney, Wu, & Kastello, 2014; Meschke, Holl, & Messelt, 2013) and to take up drinking again after birth. This is of particular significance given that more women are opting to have children at a later age than in prior generations. A similar relationship with drinking is seen with increasing level of education (Rossen et al., 2018), with more educated women more likely to drink than those with lower educational attainment.

Social disapproval of women who drink as they juggle motherhood and other social roles has also been reflected in media coverage. The so-called mummy drinking culture and the wine o'clock notion of having a drink outside of strictly prescribed times and occasions is increasingly a feature in media coverage and the reflection of society's discomfort with changing social roles and drinking patterns. The subtext is that there must surely be a problem with women who are mothers and drink, whether to relieve stress, or simply for enjoyment, and that these behaviors are still at odds with traditional expectations of 'feminine' roles. There remains a long way to go in dispelling ingrained notions of the appropriate role of women in society. Women are increasingly taking on traditionally 'male' roles in most of life's domains, and it stands to reason that a more egalitarian approach to drinking is part of the equation.

Conclusions

This chapter has attempted to offer an overview of the known associations between life transitions and the trajectory of drinking patterns, particularly during the transition into adulthood. As the survey of evidence shows, the available literature is neither extensive nor consistent and there are significant gaps, particularly relating to the evolution of drinking trajectories across cultures. The relationship with drinking in many lower- and middle-income countries looks quite different than it does in the developed world. It reflects a disparity in social roles and pressures at different stages of life and between genders, as well as perspectives on drinking, its place in society, and its appropriateness.

Further research is also needed into the importance of context in the evolution of drinking, not only the locations in which drinking takes place, but drinking cohorts and the influence of social factors and peers. While peer influence is considered to be particularly important during adolescence, evidence suggests that peer influences are equally important in later life, reinforcing and encouraging particular drinking patterns. Peers in the workplace, social groups of new mothers, or of single men and women all contribute in important ways to the evolution of the drinking trajectory.

The existing evidence on the relationship between drinking and life transitions is predicated on the assumption that transitions are well-defined, sequentially discrete, and often mutually exclusive. Available research has focused largely on individual life stages and their relationship with drinking. Yet significant macro-level shifts have occurred over recent decades, particularly around gender roles, rendering life transitions more fluid, interchangeable, and no longer clearly delineated. The changing role of women and also of men in many societies has been a major factor in this shift, and has changed how women drink, where, with whom, and how much. What has not changed as quickly are society's assumptions about the relationship between life stages and drinking, and views on drinking behaviors that are appropriate with different gender roles. Much more insight is needed into the relationship between drinking by men and women and the reality of their social roles in the twenty-first century.

The need for further research into these relationships is not purely academic. A globalized world means that social constructs about role definitions and drinking are evolving quickly and no longer entirely culture-bound. Competing life roles and pressures, evolving transitions, and changes in their timing relative to each other are also a potential source of problems that can include a rise in harmful drinking among some groups traditionally considered to be protected as a function of their social roles. Better understanding of these linkages creates opportunities for developing targeted interventions to address harmful drinking and can help to identify particular risk and protective factors. Substance use, including harmful drinking, is among the risk factors for a number of health outcomes that have implications for individuals, but also for population health, social cost, and a thriving world for generations to come.

References

Ahlström, S., Bloomfield, K., & Knibbe, R. (2001). Gender differences in drinking patterns in nine European countries: Descriptive findings. *Substance Abuse, 22*(1), 69–85.

Alstveit, M., Severinsson, E., & Karlsen, B. (2011). Readjusting one's life in the tension inherent in work and motherhood. *Journal of Advanced Nursing, 67*(10), 2151–2160.

Amato, P. R., & Kane, J. B. (2011). Life-course pathways and the psychosocial adjustment of young adult women. *Journal of Marriage and the Family, 73*(1), 279–295.

Aseltine, R. H., & Gore, S. (2005). Work, postsecondary education, and psychosocial functioning following the transition from high school. *Journal of Adolescent Research, 20*(6), 615–639.

Balan, S., Widner, G., Chen, H. J., Hudson, D., Gehlert, S., & Price, R. K. (2014). Motherhood, psychological risks, and resources in relation to alcohol use disorder: Are there differences between black and white women? *ISRN Addiction.*

Birditt, K. S., Cranford, J. A., Manalel, J. A., & Antonucci, T. C. (2018). Drinking patterns among older couples: Longitudinal associations with negative marital quality. *The Journals of Gerontology. Series B, Psychological Sciences and Social Sciences, 73*(4), 655–665.

Bowden, J. A., Delfabbro, P., Room, R., Miller, C., & Wilson, C. (2018). Parental drinking in Australia: Does the age of children in the home matter? *Drug and Alcohol Review, 38*(3), 306–315.

Breslow, R. A., Castle, I. P., Chen, C. M., & Graubard, B. I. (2017). Trends in alcohol consumption among older Americans: National health interview surveys, 1997 to 2014. *Alcoholism, Clinical and Experimental Research, 41*(5), 976–986.

Brunborg, G. S., Norstrom, T., & Storvoll, E. E. (2018). Latent developmental trajectories of episodic heavy drinking from adolescence to early adulthood: Predictors of trajectory groups and alcohol problems in early adulthood as outcome. *Drug and Alcohol Review, 37*(3), 389–395.

Chapman, S. L., & Wu, L. T. (2013). Substance use among adolescent mothers: A review. *Children and Youth Services Review, 35*(5), 806–815.

Currie, C., Zanotti, C., Morgan, A., Currie, D., de Looze, M., Roberts, C., … Barnekow, V. (2012). Social determinants of health and well-being among young people: Health behaviour in school-aged children (HBSC) study— International report from the 2009/2010 survey. *Health Policy for Children and Adolescents* (No. 6, p. 272). Copenhagen: WHO Regional Office for Europe.

De Genna, N. M., Goldschmidt, L., Marshal, M., Day, N. L., & Cornelius, M. D. (2017). Maternal age and trajectories of risky alcohol use: A prospective study. *Alcoholism, Clinical and Experimental Research, 41*(10), 1725–1730.

de Looze, M., Harakeh, Z., van Dorsselaer, S. A., Raaijmakers, Q. A., Vollebergh, W. A., & ter Bogt, T. F. (2012). Explaining educational differences in adolescent substance use and early sexual debut: The role of parents and peers. *Journal of Adolescence, 35*(4), 1035–1044.

Dinescu, D., Turkheimer, E., Beam, C. R., Horn, E. E., Duncan, G., & Emery, R. E. (2016). Is marriage a buzzkill? A twin study of marital status and alcohol consumption. *Journal of Family Psychology, 30*(6), 698–707.

Duncan, G. J., Wilkerson, B., & England, P. (2006). Cleaning up their act: The effects of marriage and cohabitation on licit and illicit drug use. *Demography, 43*(4), 691–710.

Eng, P. M., Kawachi, I., Fitzmaurice, G., & Rimm, E. B. (2005). Effects of marital transitions on changes in dietary and other health behaviours in US male health professionals. *Journal of Epidemiology and Community Health, 59*(1), 56–62.

Frone, M. R. (2016). Work stress and alcohol use: Developing and testing a biphasic self-medication model. *Work Stress, 30*(4), 374–394.

Geisner, I. M., Koopmann, J., Bamberger, P., Wang, M., Larimer, M. E., Nahum-Shani, I., & Bacharach, S. (2018). When the party continues: Impulsivity and the effect of employment on young adults' post-college alcohol use. *Addictive Behaviors, 77*, 114–120.

Grant, B. F., Chou, S. P., Saha, T. D., Pickering, R. P., Kerridge, B. T., Ruan, W. J., ... Hasin, D. S. (2017). Prevalence of 12-month alcohol use, high-risk drinking, and DSM-IV alcohol use disorder in the United States, 2001–2002 to 2012–2013: Results from the National Epidemiologic Survey on Alcohol and Related Conditions. *JAMA Psychiatry, 74*(9), 911–923.

Greene, K. M., Eitle, T. M., & Eitle, D. (2014). Adult social roles and alcohol use among American Indians. *Addictive Behaviors, 39*(9), 1357–1360.

Grittner, U., Nemeth, Z., Kuntsche, S., Gaertner, B., & Bloomfield, K. (2015). What is the role of roles? Exploring the link between social roles and women's alcohol use in low- and middle-income countries. *International Journal of Alcohol and Drug Research, 4*(2), 139–149.

Guo, G., Li, Y., Owen, C., Wang, H., & Duncan, G. J. (2015). A natural experiment of peer influences on youth alcohol use. *Social Science Research, 52*, 193–207.

Hurst, G. (2017). Young women become biggest binge drinkers as boys call time. *The Times.* London.

Keenan, K., Ploubidis, G. B., Silverwood, R. J., & Grundy, E. (2017). Life-course partnership history and midlife health behaviours in a population-based birth cohort. *Journal of Epidemiology and Community Health, 71*(3), 232–238.

Kendler, K. S., Lonn, S. L., Salvatore, J. E., Sundquist, J., & Sundquist, K. (2016). Effect of marriage on risk for onset of alcohol use disorder: A longitudinal and co-relative analysis in a Swedish national sample. *American Journal of Psychiatry, 173*(9), 911–918.

Kendler, K. S., Lonn, S. L., Salvatore, J. E., Sundquist, J., & Sundquist, K. (2018). The impact of parenthood on risk of registration for alcohol use disorder in married individuals: A Swedish population-based analysis. *Psychological Medicine, 49*(13), 1–8.

Kindy, K., & Keating, D. (2016). For women, heavy drinking has been normalized. That's dangerous. *The Washington Post.* Washington, DC.

Kinjo, A., Kuwabara, Y., Minobe, R., Maezato, H., Kimura, M., Higuchi, S., ... Osaki, Y. (2018). Different socioeconomic backgrounds between hazardous drinking and heavy episodic drinking: Prevalence by sociodemographic factors in a Japanese general sample. *Drug and Alcohol Dependence, 193*, 55–62.

4 Life Transitions into Adulthood and the Drinking Trajectory 81

Kitsantas, P., Gaffney, K. F., Wu, H., & Kastello, J. C. (2014). Determinants of alcohol cessation, reduction and no reduction during pregnancy. *Archives of Gynecology and Obstetrics, 289*(4), 771–779.

Kretsch, N., & Harden, K. P. (2014). Marriage, divorce, and alcohol use in young adulthood: A longitudinal sibling-comparison study. *Emerging Adulthood, 2*(2), 138–149.

Kuntsche, S., Astudillo, M., & Gmel, G. (2016). Social roles among recruits in Switzerland: Do social roles relate to alcohol use and does role change have an impact? *Addictive Behaviors, 54,* 59–63.

Kuntsche, S., Knibbe, R. A., & Gmel, G. (2009). Social roles and alcohol consumption: A study of 10 industrialised countries. *Social Science and Medicine, 68*(7), 1263–1270.

Kuntsche, S., Knibbe, R. A., & Gmel, G. (2010). A step beyond—The relevance of depressed mood and mastery in the interplay between the number of social roles and alcohol use. *Addictive Behaviors, 35*(11), 1013–1020.

Kuntsche, S., Knibbe, R. A., & Gmel, G. (2012). Parents' alcohol use: Gender differences in the impact of household and family chores. *European Journal of Public Health, 22*(6), 894–899.

Kypri, K., Paschall, M. J., Maclennan, B., & Langley, J. D. (2007). Intoxication by drinking location: A web-based diary study in a New Zealand university community. *Addictive Behaviors, 32*(11), 2586–2596.

Lee, M. R., & Sher, K. J. (2018). "Maturing out" of binge and problem drinking. *Alcohol Research Current Reviews, 39*(1), e1–e12.

Leigh, B., & Lee, C. (2008). What motivates extreme drinking? In M. Martinic & F. Measham (Eds.), *Swimming with crocodiles: The culture of extreme drinking.* New York: Routledge.

Levy, F., Le Strat, Y., Hoertel, N., Ancelet, C., & Dubertret, C. (2018). Childbirth and alcohol consumption: Impact of recent childbirth on alcohol consumption. *Journal of Child and Family Studies, 27*(7), 2245–2253.

Liang, W. B., & Chikritzhs, T. (2012). Brief report: Marital status and alcohol consumption behaviours. *Journal of Substance Use, 17*(1), 84–90.

Liew, H. (2012). The effects of marital status transitions on alcohol use trajectories. *Longitudinal and Life Course Studies, 3*(3), 332–345.

Little, M., Handley, E., Leuthe, E., & Chassin, L. (2009). The impact of parenthood on alcohol consumption trajectories: Variations as a function of timing of parenthood, familial alcoholism, and gender. *Development and Psychopathology, 21*(2), 661–682.

Liu, W., & Mumford, E. A. (2017). Concurrent trajectories of female drinking and smoking behaviors throughout transitions to pregnancy and early parenthood. *Prevention Science, 18*(4), 416–427.

Martinic, M., & Measham, F. (Eds.). (2008). *Swimming with crocodiles: The culture of extreme drinking.* Routledge: New York.

Matusiewicz, A. K., Ilgen, M. A., & Bohnert, K. M. (2016). Changes in alcohol use following the transition to motherhood: Findings from the National Epidemiologic Survey on Alcohol and Related Conditions. *Drug and Alcohol Dependence, 168,* 204–210.

McCabe, S. E., Veliz, P., & Schulenberg, J. E. (2018). How collegiate fraternity and sorority involvement relates to substance use during young adulthood and substance use disorders in early midlife: A national longitudinal study. *Journal of Adolescent Health, 62*(3s), S35–s43.

Meschke, L. L., Holl, J., & Messelt, S. (2013). Older not wiser: Risk of prenatal alcohol use by maternal age. *Maternal and Child Health Journal, 17*(1), 147–155.

Nelson, P., & Taberrer, S. (2017). Hard to reach and easy to ignore: The drinking careers of young people not in education, employment or training. *Child & Family Social Work, 22*(1), 428–439.

Olson, J. S., Hummer, R. A., & Harris, K. M. (2017). Gender and health behavior clustering among U.S. young adults. *Biodemography and Social Biology, 63*(1), 3–20.

Ostergaard, J., Jarvinen, M., & Andreasen, A. G. (2018). A matter of rules? A longitudinal study of parents' influence on young people's drinking trajectories. *European Addiction Research, 24*(4), 206–215.

Paradis, C. (2011). Parenthood, drinking locations and heavy drinking. *Social Science and Medicine, 72*(8), 1258–1265.

Paradis, C., Demers, A., Nadeau, L., & Picard, E. (2015). Parenthood, alcohol intake, and drinking contexts: *occasio furem facit. Journal of Studies on Alcohol and Drugs, 72*(2), 259–269.

Paschall, M. J., & Saltz, R. F. (2007). Relationships between college settings and student alcohol use before, during and after events: A multi-level study. *Drug and Alcohol Review, 26*(6), 635–644.

Patterson, C., Emslie, C., Mason, O., Fergie, G., & Hilton, S. (2016). Content analysis of UK newspaper and online news representations of women's and men's 'binge' drinking: A challenge for communicating evidence-based messages about single-episodic drinking? *British Medical Journal Open, 6*(12), e013124.

Pocuca, N., Hides, L., Quinn, C. A., White, M. J., Mewton, L., Newton, N. C., ... McBride, N. (2018). The interactive effects of perceived peer drinking and personality profiles on adolescent drinking: A prospective cohort study. *Addiction, 114*(3), 450–461.

Polenick, C. A., Birditt, K. S., & Blow, F. C. (2018). Couples' alcohol use in middle and later life: Stability and mutual influence. *Journal of Studies on Alcohol and Drugs, 79*(1), 111–118.

Qian, L., Newman, I., Yuen, L.-W., Shell, D., & Xu, J. (2018). Variables associated with alcohol consumption and abstinence among young adults in Central China. *International Journal of Environmental Research and Public Health, 15*(8), 1675.

Rolando, S., Taddeo, G., & Beccaria, F. (2016). New media and the old stereotypes: Images and discourses about drunk women and men on YouTube. *Journal of Gender Studies, 25*(5), 492–506.

Rossen, F., Newcombe, D., Parag, V., Underwood, L., Marsh, S., Berry, S., ... Bullen, C. (2018). Alcohol consumption in New Zealand women before and during pregnancy: Findings from the growing up in New Zealand study. *New Zealand Medical Journal,131*(1479), 24–34.

Salvatore, J. E., Lonn, S. L., Sundquist, J., Lichtenstein, P., Sundquist, K., & Kendler, K. S. (2017). Alcohol use disorder and divorce: Evidence for a genetic correlation in a population-based Swedish sample. *Addiction, 112*(4), 586–593.

Scott-Sheldon, L. A., Carey, K. B., Elliott, J. C., Garey, L., & Carey, M. P. (2014). Efficacy of alcohol interventions for first-year college students: A meta-analytic review of randomized controlled trials. *Journal of Consulting and Clinical Psychology, 82*(2), 177–188.

Staff, J., Greene, K. M., Maggs, J. L., & Schoon, I. (2014). Family transitions and changes in drinking from adolescence through mid-life. *Addiction, 109*(2), 227–236.

Staff, J., Schulenberg, J. E., Maslowsky, J., Bachman, J. G., O'Malley, P. M., Maggs, J. L., & Johnston, L. D. (2010). Substance use changes and social role transitions: Proximal developmental effects on ongoing trajectories from late adolescence through early adulthood. *Development and Psychopathology, 22*(4), 917–932.

Taylor, A. W., Bewick, B. M., Makanjuola, A. B., Qian, L., Kirzhanova, V. V., & Alterwain, P. (2017). Context and culture associated with alcohol use amongst youth in major urban cities: A cross-country population based survey. *PLoS ONE, 12*(11), e0187812.

The ESPAD Group (2016). *ESPAD report 2015. Results from the European school survey project on alcohol and other drugs.* Luxembourg. Retrieved 1 November 2019 from http://www.espad.org/sites/espad.org/files/ESPAD_report_2015.pdf.

Virtanen, M., Jokela, M., Nyberg, S. T., Madsen, I. E., Lallukka, T., Ahola, K., … Burr, H. (2015). Long working hours and alcohol use: Systematic review and meta-analysis of published studies and unpublished individual participant data. *British Medical Journal, 350*, g7772.

Wainberg, M., Oquendo, M. A., Peratikos, M. B., Gonzalez-Calvo, L., Pinsky, I., Duarte, C. S., … Audet, C. M. (2018). Hazardous alcohol use among female heads-of-household in rural Mozambique. *Alcohol, 73*, 37–44.

Watt, M. H., Eaton, L. A., Choi, K. W., Velloza, J., Kalichman, S. C., Skinner, D., & Sikkema, K. J. (2014). "It's better for me to drink, at least the stress is going away": Perspectives on alcohol use during pregnancy among South African women attending drinking establishments. *Social Science and Medicine, 116*, 119–125.

Willoughby, B. J., Hall, S. S., & Goff, S. (2015). Marriage matters but how much? Marital centrality among young adults. *The Journal of Psychology, 149*(8), 796–817.

Windle, R. C., & Windle, M. (2018). Adolescent precursors of young adult drinking motives. *Addictive Behaviors, 82*, 151–157.

Wolff, J. M., Rospenda, K. M., Richman, J. A., Liu, L., & Milner, L. A. (2013). Work-family conflict and alcohol use: Examination of a moderated mediation model. *Journal of Addictive Diseases, 32*(1), 85–98.

Part II
Young Adult Drinking in Context

5

Into the Woods: Contextualising Atypical Intoxication by Young Adults in Music Festivals and Nightlife Tourist Resorts

Tim Turner and Fiona Measham

Once upon a time in a faraway land …

The telling of stories and fairy tales is a universal feature of human society, their structure often shaped by the three-phase monomyth of *separation, immersion* and *return*. Leaving the safety of home in order to undertake a journey into the woods is the starting point for innumerable fables; the dark forest is a symbolic place of pleasure, risk, danger and subverted social rules. The magical realms of Lewis Carroll's *Wonderland*, C. S. Lewis's *Narnia* and Tolkien's *Middle Earth*, for example, represent "secondary worlds"

T. Turner (✉)
School of Psychological, Social and Behavioural Sciences, Coventry University, Coventry, UK
e-mail: t.turner@coventry.ac.uk

F. Measham
Department of Sociology, Social Policy and Criminology, University of Liverpool, Liverpool, UK
e-mail: f.measham@liverpool.ac.uk

© The Author(s) 2019
D. Conroy and F. Measham (eds.), *Young Adult Drinking Styles*,
https://doi.org/10.1007/978-3-030-28607-1_5

of mischief and merriment, standing as "allegories of alternatives to the world we know" (Warner, 2014: xx). This chapter draws on this simple allegorical monomyth to explore young adult intoxication within the context of the magical, secondary worlds of UK outdoor music festivals and Ibizan nightlife tourist resorts. Like the dark forest, these leisure spaces represent carnivalesque realms that merge opportunities for transgressive pleasure with elements of risk, danger and subversion. Drawing on a number of empirical studies by the authors, together and individually, of British young adults on holiday in the "freak zone safety net" (Power, 2013) of festivals and nightlife resorts, we consider how, for many of those entering these multi-day play spaces, their usual patterns of alcohol and illegal drug use become distorted, with atypical and "extreme" intoxication integral to the immersive and transformational experiences on offer. Therefore, despite evidence of a broader decline in young adult consumption (discussed in more detail in the chapters in this edited collection), there are still pockets of excess which become even more risky in their atypicalness.

In alignment with the monomyth, the chapter is structured around three key sections. Firstly, the issue of *Separation* is explored, as we consider the motivations, expectations and starting points for journeys into the hedonistic realms of festivals and nightlife tourist resorts. Secondly, under the title of *Immersion*, we consider the sensorial pleasures of intoxication within these secondary worlds, as well as the associated risks. What role does intoxication play in these hedonistic woodland wonderlands and how might young adult drinking and drug use differ from everyday consumption patterns? Thirdly, we examine our protagonists' *Return*, with a focus on the narratives and stories that young people bring back from their journeys into the "wild zones" of dark forest and white isle. We conclude that if young people are to emerge from their journeys into the "woods" unscathed, there is an urgent need to embed innovative and effective harm reduction strategies within the secondary worlds of music festivals, nightlife tourist resorts and other bounded play spaces where regular patterns of drinking and drug use and attitudes to risk can be rapidly, if temporarily, distorted. Thus, these secondary worlds embody an opportunity for engagement as well as for excess.

Separation

> You have a sketch map and a rough guide; the lights are lit in the windows of that house in the deep dark forest ahead of us. We can begin to move in, listening out, eyes open, trying to find our bearings. (Warner, 2014: xxvi)

In Joseph Campbell's seminal deconstruction of myth, *The Hero with a Thousand Faces*, the protagonist's epic journey begins with a "call to adventure" to faraway lands—a dark forest or jungle, a mysterious island or mountain, an underground kingdom—"places of strangely fluid and polymorphous beings, unimaginable torments, superhuman deeds, and impossible delight" (Campbell, 2008: 48). It is easy to see how the carnivalesque secondary worlds of music festivals and nightlife tourist resorts—where conventions are suspended in a social and spatial separation from home (Urry & Larsen, 2011: 12)—can symbolically represent such magical realms of faraway adventure.

Similarly, in the classic novel *Heart of Darkness*, Joseph Conrad's hero's voyage into the African interior is a physical, psychological and metaphorical journey into an alien, primeval landscape focusing on central protagonist Marlow, following in ivory trader Kurtz' footsteps, immersing himself in Kurtz' slow reversion to brutality and degradation. During the geographical journey up the Congo River and into dense jungle, the layers of presumed civilisation are slowly peeled back and the local native culture increasingly embraced and, as Kurtz embarks on a brutal slaughtering of "savages", the reader is led to question the supposed gulf between colonial civilisation and native "savagery". In Ward's consideration of the relative importance of rational and emotive drivers for cruelty in colonial state crime, he draws together Conrad's novel and Katz' (1988) criminology of seduction, noting that "what Marlow cannot articulate but Conrad's narrative implies about Kurtz's relationship with the wilderness is better captured in a phrase by Jack Katz: it is a 'dialectic process through which a person empowers the world to seduce him to criminality' (Katz, 1988: 7)" (2005: 438). Thus, embarking on a journey into the woods or wilderness means offering oneself up to this seduction into transgression.

In Hayward's (2002) discussion of transgressive leisure, he notes that the thrill of transgression comes in part from this individual excitement to commit crime, Katz' (1988) seduction of the offender. However, for both Hayward and Ferrell, there is more to transgressive leisure than simply the individual thrill created by a break from monotony. For Ferrell, in the collective reaction to boredom, there are not only "ephemeral crimes committed against boredom itself—but larger efflorescences of political and cultural rebellion" (2004: 287) suggesting that music holidays—to forest festivals or Balearic superclubs—could be in themselves a form of cultural resistance to the monotony of the everyday. Additionally, Hayward (2002: xx) notes how transgressive leisure and carnivalesque pleasure offer an opportunity for escapism not just from boredom but also the from the insecurity and "hyper-banalization" of everyday life in which people feel increasingly over-controlled not just by agents of the state but also in a cultural and economic sense.

Prior to the turn of the millennium, UK music festivals were relatively small in scale and few in number. Such festivals may have been counter-cultural in nature, if only for the brief period of their existence, inverting the usual social order to suffuse the tensions of everyday life (Presdee, 2000) and providing a "temporary autonomous zone" (Bey, 1985) from the outside world for a form of carnivalesque social anarchism. The threads of cultural resistance and commercial exploitation are increasingly intertwined, however, with carnivalesque "urban spectacles" (Gotham, 2005) proliferating as key sites of experiential consumption for the millennial generation now reaching young adulthood. For example, Mintel (2018) estimates that there were 918 UK festivals in 2018, more than double that of a decade earlier, and CGA (2019) estimates that there were 700 UK music festivals attended by 7.1 million customers in 2018. Almost a quarter of UK adults report going to a music festival in the previous year, whilst for young men aged 16–24, the figure rises to half (Mintel, 2018). Such exceptional demand for festival tickets is exemplified by *Glastonbury*, with 135,000 tickets for the 2019 festival selling within the first 30 minutes (Heal, 2018). Given the growing financial significance of UK festivals for the events industry—with the festival industry estimated by Mintel to be worth £2459 million in 2018—festivals are replacing traditional package holidays abroad for young people with limited expenditure. The value of festival-goers as consumers is not lost on the hospitality, food and beverage industries: CGA (2019) estimates that £114m is spent on alcohol sales alone at UK music festivals each year and festivals are considered to be the number one marketing target for drinks suppliers, with alcohol industry-sponsored bars and stages, free samples and other promotional activities.

Festivals and superclubs are now global destinations, drawing party-goers from across the world. In the UK, the average travel time to festivals is around four hours, whilst a third of adults are willing to travel abroad (Mintel, 2018). Nearly two-thirds (62%) of UK festival-goers travelled over 100 km to reach their festival of choice, 12% attended a festival abroad, and only 10% considered proximity to their home a major factor when deciding on which festivals to attend (CGA, 2019). This growing internationalisation of festivals and carnivals sees their transition from indigenous cultural celebrations into "experience production systems" developed by international entrepreneurs (Ferdinand & Williams, 2013).

Within consumer culture, transgression leisure is facilitated, commodified and rebranded for youth and young adult audiences as part of a growing "experience economy" (Pine & Gilmore, 1999) where people increasingly seek to purchase a meaningful, memorable and "Instagrammable" "experience". Thus, the experience economy exploits the tensions between capitalist consumerism and people's desire for authenticity, freedom and self-fulfilment. Haydock (2015), echoing Stallybrass and White (1986), notes an ambivalence at the heart of carnival precisely because of this combination of radicalism and conservatism, suggesting that it "makes little sense to fight out the issue of whether or not carnivals are intrinsically radical or conservative, for to do so automatically involves the false essentializing of carnivalesque transgression" (Stallybrass & White, 1986: 14). "Instagrammable" festivals and nightlife resorts are now spectacular themed and branded environments curated and marketed for social media feeds and glossy magazine festival guides (Baxter-Wright, 2019), furnished with everything from forest art installations to brightly coloured dip-dyed sheep and ubiquitous giant-sized letters demanding social media attention. For the events industry, this means designing festivals and superclubs with increasing innovation and differentiation (Sipe, 2018), to elicit "socially approved arousal of moderate excitement" with the end goal of "maximising profit through consumer enjoyment" (O'Sullivan, 2016: 3). For festival and club-goers, in their quest for experiential consumption within and yet potentially at odds with the highly structured nature of such leisure, this can lead to the hijacking of "brandfests" in the pursuit of more spontaneous, subversive and less sanitised excitement (O'Sullivan, 2016). "Excitement, even ecstasy (the abandonment of reason and rationale), is the goal" (Presdee, 2000: 7) and intoxication is a key vehicle for young adults to achieve this "controlled loss of control" within these performance zones (Hayward, 2002; Measham, 2002).

In general, prevalence of use of illegal drugs is higher amongst festival and club-goers than the general population. In the UK, 20.9% of festival-goers in a self-selecting online survey reported having taken any drugs at festivals that year (UKFA, 2017), compared with 9% of 16- to 59-year-olds and 19.8% of 16- to 24-year-olds in the general population, in the previous 12 months (Home Office, 2018). International surveys (Hesse & Tutenges, 2008; Lim, Hellard, & Hocking, 2008; Martinus, McAlaney, McLaughlin, & Smith, 2010) also indicate that festival-goers have a higher prevalence of drug use than the general population. Similarly, attendance at dance clubs is consistently correlated with higher levels of drug use than in the general population: in self-report studies of club-goers in the 1990s and 2000s (Measham, Aldridge, & Parker, 2001; Measham & Moore, 2009), and in annual household surveys, with adults who attended nightclubs four times or more in the previous month nearly six times more likely to report having taken drugs in the past year than those not attending nightclubs in the past month (Home Office, 2018). In relation to British holidaymakers, Bellis, Hughes, Bennett, and Thomson (2003) Bellis, Hughes, Calafat, Montse, and Schnitzer (2009) found that young adults going to Ibiza, a nightlife tourist destination with a much higher density of electronic dance music (EDM) superclubs than other Balearic islands, had significantly higher levels of drug use and lower levels of alcohol consumption and alcohol-related violence. The contrasting backdrop to festival and nightlife consumption is that young adult drug use (Home Office, 2018), drinking and drunkenness more generally have been stable or falling in the UK in recent years (Measham, 2008), as discussed elsewhere in this collection.

5 Into the Woods: Contextualising Atypical Intoxication … 93

This desire to seek the excitement of carnivalesque experiences is reflected in a continued demand for young adult-orientated holidays, although it has shifted away from cheap package holidays—symbolised by the death of the iconic "Club 18-30" (Mackay, 2018)—towards millennial preferences for festivals, adventure holidays and independent travel, creating photogenic experiences, health-conscious images and social kudos in their place. Similarly, the value of the UK nightclub industry has fallen by £200 million in five years due to a shift in leisure preferences away from late-night dancing to gyms, restaurants and coffee shops (Booth & Halliday, 2018). Festivals and clubbing holidays, however, retain opportunities for young adult experimentation and excess as they escape the panoptic gaze of parents in the neon party enclaves of Spain, Greece, Croatia and Bulgaria, with the exotic, other-worldly EDM superclubs of Ibiza drawing young tourists from across the globe. For some, the *journey* to these secondary worlds is part of the appeal—leaving the humdrum routines of home and life in the "real world" (Dilkes-Frayne, 2016) for faraway adventures with friends and "randoms". In *Altered State*, the seminal account of Acid House by a promoter, Collin (1998: 51) identifies how for many young people such escapism represents "an extended vacation in an alternate reality … a peak experience that allows for utopian dreaming", echoed by our research participants:

> We save for this all year, we count down the days. It's a week where we don't have to think about anything apart from getting fucked up and having a laugh. (Harry, tourist, Ibiza)

> All year, you get up, go to work, come home. It's fucking boring, man. This is my ten days to get lost. It's what keeps me going for the rest of the year. (Rob, tourist, Ibiza)

> This is an escape. You can act differently here, no one knows who you are. (Alex, tourist)

For young people travelling to these secondary worlds, entering the "liminal travel space" (Pritchard & Morgan, 2006: 762) of airports, motorway service stations and train stations can be an important first stage of the journey. In the monomyth structure, this represents the "crossing of the first threshold" as the traveller begins to cross from "the veil of the known into the unknown" (Campbell, 2008: 67). These transitional travel hubs represent intriguing spaces defined by the performance of departure, arrival and mobility. The liminal traveller is "neither here nor there; they are betwixt and between", positioned in a liminal zone alikened "to death, to being in the womb, to invisibility, to darkness, to bisexuality, to the wilderness, and to an eclipse of the sun or moon" (Turner, 1997: 95), out of time and out of place. Here, as social conventions begin to fall away, structure and order are replaced with a sense of "playfulness, chance and the possibilities of subversion" (Carlson, 1996: 24). As these interviewees exemplify, for many young people these travel hubs represent the first stage of hedonistic intoxication:

> We were drinking Stella at the airport for 3 hours, then we thought we might as well warm up properly for the holiday, so we ordered three bottles of Champagne. (Mark, tourist, Ibiza)

> I was slaughtered at the airport. (Jed, tourist)

> We had to carry him off the plane cos he was so drunk. We had to put him to bed, and then me and my other mate went out. (George, tourist).

Allusions to the binge consumption of alcohol at airports, on flights and on long car journeys were a common feature of interviews for this fieldwork. This seemed to be symbolic of social and spatial separation from "reality" (Turner, 1997) and a permissible prelude to the (often illegal) excesses of the experience ahead. Travel hubs are ambiguous, however, splicing notions of freedom with hyper-securitisation, control and surveillance. The condition of entry into wonderland entails running a gauntlet of security staff, metal detector gates, searches of one's person and possessions, and possibly even drug detection dogs. However, as Campbell (2008: 65) states, the rewards of crossing such thresholds are entry to the "regions of the unknown" and the untold pleasures of the secondary world. For many of our participants, the immersive nature of this experience was akin to dropping down the rabbit hole into wonderland, as Garratt (1998) noted in relation to dance clubs and as research participant Maria noted in relation to taking ketamine:

> I took this big line of ket. To say it was euphoric isn't enough. It was like falling into another world. Down the rabbit hole, I was lost and falling, falling, falling. It was almost *beyond* happiness. (Maria, tourist)

Immersion

Suspension of Rules in the Secondary World

> Entering the grounds of the music festival was like entering another world for the day. Although the tickets say things about rules of the festival being like rules of the outside world, there is a sense that social rules and ways of relating to each other were quite different from the outside world, allowing people to engage with each other with a sense of freedom, free from the formality of being among strangers in the 'real world'. (Borlagdan, Freeman, Duvnjak, Bywood & Roche, 2010: 97)

For many young people, the magical realms of festivals and nightlife tourist resorts feel like they exist outside the parameters of "real life"; the world no longer operates in the same way (Warner, 2014: 20). As in the mythological secondary worlds of Carroll, Lewis and Tolkien, many of our participants described a distorted sense of reality, as notions of space and time seemed to shrink and stretch:

> I don't know how long I've been here. It feels like years, but it's just a few days. The whole place is just surreal. It's like nowhere else. (Ashley, Ibiza)

> I love it here. I don't want to leave. It's not real though. (Bianca, Ibiza)

The creeping sense of the surreal described within these narratives is enhanced by the deeply immersive spectacles that characterise such space.

The late-night dance tents at festivals and the superclub dance floors of Ibiza are bound by their ability to create profoundly sensual *atmospheres* that can saturate space to completely transform the affective experience of those present (Edensor & Sumartajo, 2015; Shaw, 2013: 88). This is exemplified in the *Secret Garden Party* festival, a "hedonistic woodland wonderland" (Time Out, 2015) with 24-hour forest raves in its "Lost Woods", quirky art installations and immersive entertainment; and the *Shangri-La* sector of Glastonbury festival, described as a dystopian pleasure city that comes alive after midnight in "a great swell of music, art, drugs, joy, fear and wild abandonment" (Barton, 2012). For those present, this "magical alternate reality" (Braverman, 2000: 104) opens up new possibilities of transgression as they step into a "temporary sphere of behaviour" (Shaw & Williams, 2004: 151), to combine alcohol with the illicit pleasures of drugs such as MDMA, cocaine, ketamine and LSD. In these "phantasmagoric realms" (Edensor, 2015: 332), the world of illegal drugs that usually operates on a veiled, subterranean level is inverted and woven into the consumer experience, blurring the boundaries between permissible and impermissible behaviours. As Steeves (2003: 185) suggests, in the hyper-real "fantasyscapes" of Disneyland, "a different kind of conscious engagement with the world is at work [and] one cannot help but be altered by the environment". Consequently, as our fieldwork in festivals and dance clubs consistently revealed, this opened up opportunities to engage in patterns of psychoactive consumption that were significantly different from their everyday lives back home (Measham, 2004a; Measham & Shiner, 2009: 507).

Pushing the Boundaries: Intoxication in the Secondary World

What role does intoxication play in these performance zones and to what extent is this atypical of everyday consumption patterns? Consumption within festivals and nightlife tourist resorts can be both everyday and atypical: a carnival of excess during a temporal and geographical dislocation from the usual constraints of work, home and family that is accepted, expected and even normalised within that space (Measham,

2004a; Measham et al., 2001). In situ surveys of festival and club-goers offer an opportunity to shed light on intoxication at play within these contexts.

The UK's largest ongoing study of festival drinking and drug use, conducted by Measham and colleagues, utilises an in situ research design previously used in dance clubs (Measham et al., 2001; Measham, Wood, Dargan, & Moore, 2011), "High Street" nightclubs (Measham, Moore, & Welch, 2012) and bars (Measham & Brain, 2005). The study includes annual convenience sample surveys, interviews and focus groups with festival-goers and staff each summer from 2010 onwards at outdoor music festivals by teams of mixed gender, ethnicity, age, social class and sexual orientation researchers. In 2018, 2250 respondents completed the annual survey at 11 UK outdoor music festivals chosen as contrasting examples of festivals in operation annually in the UK, ranging from urban parks to remote rural farms, from one to five days in length, from over-18s to family-friendly admission policies, and from specialist EDM to live music, comedy and theatrical entertainment. Short surveys were conducted with individuals across all show days and across the full footprint of each festival, including entertainment and camping areas, with over 9 in 10 surveys conducted between 12 and 6 p.m. Over half (51.1%) of respondents were identified as female and the mean age was 25.3.

Regarding alcohol consumption, nearly two-thirds (63.3%) of respondents in the 2018 festival survey had been drinking alcohol on the day of interview and reported consuming an average of 7.6 units of alcohol (a UK unit of alcohol is equivalent to 10 ml of pure alcohol) by the time of interview. Female respondents had consumed an average of 6.2 units of alcohol and male respondents 8.8 units, meaning that both women and men had already exceeded binge drinking levels (NHS, 2019) by late afternoon and before the evening's entertainment had started. When including both those who had already consumed alcohol by the time of interview and those who intended to drink later, it rises to nearly nine in ten (86.8%) festival-goers either having had a drink or intending to drink that day. Indeed, a notable feature of festival and holiday consumption is the preponderance of people drinking alcohol throughout the day who would not usually drink alcohol in the morning and at lunchtime in their everyday lives. As one respondent stated, "I only usually drink on Friday nights, but here, you just wake up and think, 'right, let's have a Stella'" (Rob, tourist, Ibiza).

If we explore festival drinking in more detail for different categories of respondents according to their self-reported usual drinking patterns, we can see that whilst more frequent drinkers are more likely to drink larger quantities of alcohol at festivals than their less frequently drinking peers, occasional drinkers also drank not insignificant amounts onsite. Looking at daily drinkers, 6.9% of festival-goers said that they usually drank alcohol every day in their everyday lives and over eight in ten (81.1%) of these daily drinkers had already had a drink on the interview day, consuming an average of 10.3 units of alcohol by late afternoon. At the other end of the scale are occasional drinkers (here defined as those who identify as drinkers but report usually drinking alcohol less than once a month): whilst only 2.9% of festival-goers considered themselves to usually drink alcohol less than once in a month, 60% of these had already had a drink that afternoon and had already consumed on average 4.5 units of alcohol. When we look at consumption on both the fieldwork day and the previous day, this rises to over three quarters (76.9%) of occasional drinkers having consumed alcohol at the festival either that day or the previous day. This illustrates the elevated prevalence and quantity of alcohol consumed by young adults, from daily drinkers through to even very occasional drinkers, whilst attending festivals.

UK festivals can be atypical of everyday consumption patterns not only in respect of alcohol, as above, but also illegal drugs, most often with both combined. Drug use was strongly correlated with drinking: over half (52.4%) of festival-goers either had already taken or intended to take a drug at the festival on the day they were interviewed. Looking more closely at those reporting taking drugs "today or tonight", over nine in ten (91.8%) also had already drank or intended to drink alcohol that day, compared with only 8.2% of drug users not planning on drinking. Drug users were also asked how typical their festival drug use was: over half (54.1%) said that they took a larger quantity of drugs than they usually consumed and a quarter (24.3%) said that they took a wider range of different drugs than they usually consumed.

Regarding festivals as sites of atypical drug use, 7.9% of all survey respondents reported that they *only* took drugs at festivals and over eight

5 Into the Woods: Contextualising Atypical Intoxication ...   99

in ten (80.3%) of those either had taken drugs or intended to that day. Nevertheless, whilst nearly half (46.9%) of all festival-goers reported either already having consumed both alcohol and illegal drugs on the fieldwork day or intending to, there is also a small but not insignificant group of festival-goers who do not take any psychoactive substances when they go to festivals: nearly one in ten (9.1%) festival-goers reported having consumed neither alcohol nor other drugs and not intending to that day.

Greater access and availability of illegal drugs at festivals and in nightlife resorts, as well as greater availability of holiday spending money and free time, all help to facilitate these higher levels of drug use:

> I've been offered pills about forty times. Even sitting around here [by the hotel swimming pool] you'll get people coming and asking if you want anything. One of the mates I'm with is clean living at home, goes down the gym and all that. He took three pills yesterday afternoon, just sat by the pool. (Rob, tourist)

> The only thing I took was a pill and a bit of M-Cat [mephedrone], because I'd never tried it before. We were in the hotel room with some guys who'd moved into the room next door half way through the week, and I said I'll try a bit, just to see what it did. (Ashley, tourist)

In this section, we have demonstrated how alcohol and drug use are intricately woven into the immersive secondary worlds of festivals and nightlife tourist resorts, with many participants describing patterns of usage that were very different to their everyday lives, characterised by researchers as "calculated hedonism", "determined drunkenness" (Measham, 2004b), "extreme drinking" (Martinic & Measham, 2008) and a "new culture of intoxication" (Measham & Brain, 2005). To understand the experiential context of these atypical patterns of intoxication, it is important to consider participants' narratives of pleasure, an issue that has been described by Hunt, Moloney, and Evans (2010: 119) as "unseeable" in drugs research.

Pleasure in the Secondary World

The fine point of seldom pleasure has been blunted. (Huxley, 1954: 117)

Researching pleasure, particularly the "impermissible pleasures" of intoxication (Moore & Measham, 2012), remains "the great unmentionable" (Hunt & Evans, 2008) in the drugs field. The pull of professional self-preservation combined with the challenge of capturing psychoactive pleasure in print means that many researchers feel tempted to sidestep such narratives, fearing they may be condemned as unscientific, "pro-drugs", or both (Duff, 2008: 385; Moore, 2008: 355). Given that, for many people, pleasure is the principal motivation behind the atypical intoxication identified above, this obfuscates the entangled sensual pleasures of music, dancing, drugs, alcohol and risk within the secondary worlds of festivals and nightlife resorts, where alcohol and drugs represent an immersive component of the assembled space. This reflects Deleuze and Guattari's (1998: 476) concept of assemblage, defined as an "amorphous collection of juxtaposed pieces that can be joined together in an infinite number of ways". This is demonstrated in the interview narratives below, reflecting recent scholarship on the embodied, affective and sensorial aspects of intoxication (see Bohling, 2015; Demant, 2013; Duff, 2008; Jayne, Valentine, & Holloway, 2008):

> All I know, is I had the best time in there. It was so good. Loved it. Absolutely loved it. I saw Tiesto [superstar DJ]. I was in my element. It was the imagery on stage, his presence in the middle of it all, the visuals behind him and all the people around me. I was just so happy that these people were next to me. We all had our arms around each other, everyone on pills, everyone at the same level. (Jack, bar worker)

> The music, the pills, the DJs, the crowd, the whole aura. Everything was just perfect. Absolutely incredible. (Ella, ticket seller)

In these accounts, we see how intoxication can represent a key component of the immersive atmosphere generated within festivals and nightlife resorts. In deconstructing the sensorial pleasures of psychoactive drugs,

5 Into the Woods: Contextualising Atypical Intoxication ...   101

light and sound represent two crucial features of the assemblage. Light is an aspect of the sensory environment that can "envelop, guide, invite, deter and otherwise subtly influence our patterns of sociability" in urban space (Atkinson, 2007: 1907). The changing nature of cities at night has been explored within criminology, sociology and geography; however, recent scholarship has focused on the affective and atmospheric dimensions of night time space (Shaw, 2013: 87). In our fieldwork, darkness was one of the most powerful precursors of atmosphere. As the sun goes down in the party spaces of music festivals and nightlife tourist resorts, the playful aspects of liminality and hyper-reality are intensified. Here, the temporal boundaries of light pull bodies in to create a "flexible atmosphere [...] intensified within a small time-space" (Shaw, 2013: 92). This alters the social relations between those present, with alcohol and drugs interwoven aspects of the assemblage.

Sound is also a powerful sensorial component of atmosphere and has been defined by Hill and Saroka (2010: 509) as the fourth dimension of the present. The "sonic ecology" (Atkinson, 2007) of atmosphere is important in understanding intoxication, because sound can break open practices of interaction and experimentation (Edensor & Sumartajo, 2015: 253). From Glastonbury to Ibiza, music defines both the meaning and the boundaries of themed space, sonically promoting culture, lifestyle and [drug] consumption (Hayward, 2012). This immersive symbiosis of sound and drugs featured regularly in participant narratives:

I took the best pill I've ever taken in my life in there [super-club]. The music was amazing. I had about two hours just next to the bass bins with my eyes closed. (Jack, bar worker)

We did gold leaf [ecstasy]. It was so intense, so good, like dancing inside some claustrophobic sweatbox. I felt the bass through every part of my body, like it had passed through every one of us in the club. It connected us, like we were inside the music. (Maria, tourist)

The *connection* described here by Maria was a narrative of pleasure that emerged consistently in fieldwork. It seems that when we enter within these secondary worlds, the fear and distrust of strangers that we experience in the late modern landscapes of the *"soft city"* (Raban, 1974) ebb away. As Bauman (2000: 95) states:

> the meeting of strangers is an event without a past. More often than not, it is also an event without a future ... a story most certainly 'not to be continued', a one-off chance, to be consummated in full while it lasts.

The pleasure of connection at festivals and nightlife resorts is of course enmeshed with the socialising effects of alcohol and drug use. This desire for sociability has been described as a core aspect of the tourist experience, with fleeting temporary bonds formed during travel leaving indelible cherished memories (Harrison, 2003), as indicated in these excerpts:

> You get so loved up. It's unbelievable. We were dancing last night, and we all got in a circle and just starting hugging. (Paul, tourist)

> People you meet here are wicked. People you wouldn't meet every day at home. The best thing about being here has been meeting these [points to two friends made whilst on holiday]. (Matt, tourist)

Connection with friends is only one aspect, however. Many respondents gave vivid accounts of moments where they felt deeply connected to themselves and to the crowd, as a consequence of the synergy between dancing, music and intoxication. This "oceanic experience"—the feeling of deep connection to the crowd—is rarely attained with the music alone (Malbon, 1999: 110). For some, it was their consumption of MDMA that intensified this oceanic state and led them to lose themselves in moments of benevolent euphoria:

> I wandered through the different rooms in the club, and it was just like I was floating. I put my hand up for people to touch as they passed me. Everyone's just smiling at each other, everyone. Then I walk into this room and Primal Scream came on. I've never felt so happy. I just started dancing on my own – but not on my own – like the whole crowd is with me. (Carla, tourist)

Risk and Rationalisation in the Secondary World

> Having traversed the threshold, the hero moves in a dream landscape of curiously fluid, ambiguous forms, where he must survive a succession of trials. (Campbell, 2008: 81)

In the monomyth structure, having crossed the threshold and entered the secondary world, the protagonist is open to the ambiguity of untold pleasures merging with trial, risk and danger (Campbell, 2008: 81). As Mark (tourist, Ibiza) stated:

> It's totally different here. It's unlike any other place I've ever been to, but it's hard work. It's an amazing experience, but it is *hard* work.

The sentiment expressed here demonstrates that whilst our participants were immersed in the transgressive sensorial pleasures of the secondary world, they were simultaneously exposed to a multitude of potential harms including exhaustion from lack of sleep; sunburn; dehydration; sexual risk-taking; alcohol intoxication; drug-related harm; violent crime; theft; sexual assault; and intimidation from security, police or other staff.

Whereas mainstream criminology invariably foregrounds the risks of alcohol and drug use for both offender and victim, it is important to maintain perspective and view this as only one aspect of a number of issues that potentially impact on the health, safety and well-being of young people acting within the boundaries of festivals and nightlife resorts. Furthermore, this exposure to harm is compounded by the way in which such contexts can rapidly distort perceptions of risk that characterise life in the "real world". It seems that, for many of our participants, the hyper-reality of the secondary world instils an overwhelming sense of ambivalent well-being:

> Drugs are just accepted here, simple as that. It's not the same as home, people just don't worry about it here. (Nick, bar worker/drug dealer)

> A lot of people will come out here and say, 'this is the first time I've ever taken a pill'. I met this couple here on holiday last week, they were so straight laced at home, and here they'd been doing pills for the first time. It's just seen as acceptable out here. It's just the done thing. (Karen, PR Manager)

These excerpts reveal how interpretations of risk are not shaped in a cultural vacuum, rather they are grounded within the social milieu (Kelly, 2005: 1444). It is therefore important to appreciate how, for some young people, their usual patterns of psychoactive consumption may be rapidly transformed within the boundaries of festivals and nightlife resorts. This distortion is not necessarily founded on a lack of awareness about the risks of increased consumption, but rather the *perception* that they are unlikely to be harmed on holiday in wonderland, an issue that permeates the hyper-real, secondary world of Disney theme parks too, as Koenig (2006: 179) states: "guests get reckless, thinking, 'This is Disneyland. Nothing bad can happen to me'".

Perceptions of the potential consequences of intoxication therefore influence intent, both in terms of deciding to try certain drugs for the first time and in continuing to use them (Martins, Carlson, Alexandre, & Falke, 2011: 551). These perceptions are shaped by the bounded normalisation of illicit drugs within the sociocultural context of festivals and nightlife resorts (Measham & Shiner, 2009). Gamma, Jerome, Liechti, and Sumnall (2005: 390) argue that one of the strongest behavioural determinants of drug use is witnessing immediate adverse effects. However, despite a number of MDMA-related deaths within the festivals and dance clubs that were our fieldwork sites, the reactions of festival and club-goers to such fatalities on site were nonplussed. Despite the cause of death being unconfirmed for many months, and the details of the incidents sketchy and unclear, drug users reassured themselves by utilising distancing strategies such as rationalising that they were not at risk because they had not made the same (presumed) mistake: for example, "I had the red pills, not the green pills, so I'm okay" or "I bought my drugs from my regular dealer not from the onsite dealer, so I'm okay". This sort of post hoc rationalisation on risk-taking is illustrated in the following excerpts:

> I'd been told not to buy pills from people inside the club but I still bought a rockstar [ecstasy pill] from a random lad. You know, it's not a very sensible thing to do, I'd been warned against it, but at the time I was partying and needed to go for another few hours and I needed to get another one, so it's just like [shrugs shoulders to show ambivalence]. (Matt, tourist)

> I mean we read the paper about the lass dying [in X superclub], and not one person flinched. Not one of the group said 'oh I'm not going to have a pill tonight'. Then the group next to us started talking about it and they said the exact same thing, not one of them said they weren't going to have one that night. (Ben, tourist)

This apparent ambivalence did not mean that tourists were unaware of the potential harms associated with their use of drugs, but rather that they balanced perceived potential risks against already experienced benefits (Kelly, 2005: 1454; Parker, Aldridge, & Measham, 1998). Yet the spectre of the unknown content and strength of drugs in circulation in the illegal drug market hovered over them: over two-thirds (68.7%) of all respondents in the 2018 UK festival survey reported that they worried about the contents or strength of illegal drugs and, with public drug safety testing introduced to UK festivals two years earlier (Measham, 2019), 8.2% of respondents had used a festival drug testing service within the previous 12 months.

Despite this ambivalence to safety, it is important to recognise that young adult atypical intoxication within their time-limited immersion in the hedonistic pleasures of festivals and nightlife resorts created multiple levels of additional risk by comparison with their everyday lives. As fieldwork frequently revealed, moments of danger punctured the atmosphere at times, whether it was explosions of violence, robbery, sexual assault, or alcohol or drug-related harm:

> A woman in her 20s collapses on the floor, and in that moment the spell of the club is broken. She looks terrible. Her eyes have rolled back, and her mouth hangs limply open. Those in the vicinity look shocked as two visibly shaken male friends grasp her under the shoulders and drag her limp body off the dance floor. As she disappears into the crowd, the group around me shake off their concern, turn to face the DJ and start dancing again. Out

of sight and out of mind, the bubble is restored. (Tim Turner, field notes, Ibiza)

Return

I stood before a dark cave, wanting to go in [...] and I shuddered at the thought that I might not be able to find my way back. (Campbell, 2008: 85)

As the hero accomplishes their transcendental quest, so they must return back home from the woodland wonderland and readjust to life back in the "real world". As Campbell (2008: 189) states: "the first problem of the returning hero is to accept as real, after an experience of the soul satisfying vision of fulfilment, the passing joys and sorrows, banalities and noisy obscenities of life". The difficulties of returning to the humdrum schedules of home after the hedonistic freedom of festivals and nightlife resorts was a recurring theme within our fieldwork, exemplified in the following excerpts:

It's so different from home. None of us want to leave. (Sarah, tourist)

On the flight out, everyone is happy and wants to party. Coming back, they're all different. Everyone is tired and fed up about going home. (Dominika, cabin crew)

I don't know how much I've spent. I haven't checked my balance once, and I've been waving my credit card around all week. The consequences are gonna kick me in the face when I get home ... financial consequences, health consequences. (Paul, tourist)

For many, the gradual transition back into the rhythms of everyday life seemed to be characterised by a brief but powerful stage of liminality—a temporal period of readjustment where the "stickiness" of their experience in the secondary world seemed to cross over and seep into normal life:

5 Into the Woods: Contextualising Atypical Intoxication … 107

When I got home, things were bad for a few days. I kept waking up in the middle of the night, I was convinced that the demon from 'Insidious' [a horror film] was in the room - *absolutely convinced*. And that was for three or four days. I couldn't shake it. (Alex, tourist)

I swear I could still hear the music when I got home, I'd be in that weird state of half-sleep and I could hear the distant thud of techno. I'd wake up and be really confused, thinking I was still there. (Maria, tourist)

As this sense of being caught in-between reality and non-reality dissipated, our participants talked of the importance of stories that they could draw upon. These represented cherished memories, a key feature of a late modern experience economy that offers sensation gathering opportunities that provide social kudos, identity and social bonds. In this respect, festivals and nightlife resorts represent experiential spaces where actors can generate "Instagrammable" stories of their transgressive interludes. These stories—retold and reshaped over a lifetime—can help to strengthen the social ties between those involved (Tutenges & Rod, 2009; Tutenges & Sandberg, 2013). Intoxication is not simply for the fun of the moment, then, but "to create stories of transgression that they can later use as a form of entertainment and as a token of their capacity to modify and partly suspend their ingrown habits of self-censorship" (Tutenges, 2012: 147):

We've had *the best time* here, so many memories to take home. (George, tourist)

It's about the experience and the journey. It's a story to share with my friends – like, 'listen to what happened to me' – it's about getting away from boring, mundane life. You can be someone else for a while. (Christopher, Ibiza)

It's all we come to do; we hope to come back with stories to tell. Good stories. It's like we come out here to be able to say, 'do you remember that moment we shared?' I think it builds relationships. I've got a huge cork board, like a half wall, dedicated to times on the island. Little mementoes, ticket stubs, stuff like that. I can pick out moments to draw back on to remember that time. (Alex, tourist)

The question here is, does this transgressive interlude, this atypical excess in festival fields and superclubs, result in any lasting change for young adult attitudes, values or behaviours? What do participants take back home with them from wonderland, aside from their stories, photographs and memories? In contrast to the career, skills and self-enhancement prospects of "serious leisure" (Sachsman, 2007), "casual leisure" at festivals and nightlife resorts requires relatively little planning or commitment, and instead, it is its very serendipity that offers sociability, creativity and potential self-discovery, as this Ibizan tourist noted:

> I think the place really opened my eyes. Big time. I'd experienced lots of things at home, but going there for the first time, it changed me. My eyes were well and truly opened. (Ben, tourist)

This chapter has presented previously unpublished data suggesting that festivals and nightlife resorts are an important feature of leisure time for over half of UK young adults, and for the majority of them, intoxication is an integral part of the experience within these deeply immersive secondary worlds. Festivals and nightlife resorts operate as performance zones for transgressive leisure bounded by time and space: within them, our research suggests, regular, everyday patterns of alcohol and drug use are rapidly and drastically transformed. For nearly half of festival-goers, these polydrug repertoires include both the impermissible pleasures of drugs and the permissible pleasures of alcohol, with *atypical* intoxication across the course of the day and across multiple days. Not only do we see "extreme drinking" (Martinic & Measham, 2008) but extreme drug use: with secondary world drug use reportedly different to everyday drug use because firstly, prevalence is higher amongst festival and club-goers than the general population; secondly, occasional users are more likely to make an exception and consume in these spaces; thirdly, larger quantities of drugs are consumed; and fourthly, wider repertoires of different drugs are consumed. These four features of atypical consumption are likely to result in lower individual tolerance for alcohol and illegal drugs; more limited knowledge of current local drug markets and contents; greater likelihood of drug transactions involving unknown street dealers rather than regular neighbourhood ones; and an associated greater likelihood of being missold unwanted substances by onsite festival dealers compared to offsite dealers (Measham, 2019). All of these risk factors combine with binge drinking in an age group for whom the indicators suggest that these behaviours are all increasingly atypical features of their lives, leading us to conclude that festivals and nightlife resorts are sites of particular concern for young adult health, well-being and safety. Despite and indeed because of the broader downturn in drinking, drunkenness and drug use, these pockets of excess become even more risky in their atypicalness.

Furthermore, our research suggests, many young adults' usual attitudes to risk change alongside their consumption patterns in their temporary immersion in festivals and nightlife space. Festival and club-goers protect themselves from acknowledging the risks of what they do with post hoc rationalisation and distancing strategies, despite not knowing the contents of their own illegal drugs or those of fatalities within those same venues. It is important to note that the majority of young adults *do* worry about the consequences of illegal, if not legal, drugs, however, and do engage with onsite harm reduction services indicated by demand for drug safety testing outstripping supply (Measham, 2019). Therefore, if young adults are to emerge from their journeys into the "woods" unscathed, we suggest embedding harm reduction strategies within these immersive secondary worlds where psychoactive consumption, as well as wider attitudes to risk, is rapidly distorted in spaces where they are far away from the potential safety net of home. Our research highlights the value, therefore, to expanding the scale and range of information, support, medical and welfare services located in or near points of consumption. Thus, these sites of atypical intoxication can be sites of opportunity for engagement, as well as cause for concern, regarding young adult consumption practices.

References

Atkinson, R. (2007). Ecology of sound: The sonic order of urban space. *Urban Studies, 44*(10), 1905–1917.

Barton, L. (2012, June 13). Julien Temple: The dark side of Glastonbury. *The Guardian* [online]. https://www.theguardian.com/music/2012/jun/13/julien-temple-dark-side-of-glastonbury. Accessed 3 July 2016.

Bauman, Z. (2000). *Liquid modernity*. Cambridge: Polity Press.

Baxter-Wright, D. (2019, January 28). 10 of the most Instagrammable UK festivals: Sequins, sunsets and glitter galore. *Cosmopolitan*. https://www.cosmopolitan.com/uk/entertainment/travel/g9930311/festivals-instagram/.

Bellis, M. A., Hughes, K., Bennett, A., & Thomson, R. (2003). The role of an international nightlife resort in the proliferation of recreational drugs. *Addiction, 98*, 1713–1721.

Bellis, M. A., Hughes, K., Calafat, A., Montse, J., & Schnitzer, S. (2009). Relative contributions of holiday location and nationality to changes in recreational drug taking behaviour: A natural experiment in the Balearic Islands. *European Addiction Research, 15*, 78–86.

Bey, H. (1985). *TAZ: The temporary autonomous zone, ontological anarchy, poetic terrorism*. New York: Autonomedia.

Bohling, F. (2015). Alcoholic assemblages: Exploring fluid subjects in the night-time economy. *Geoforum, 58*, 132–142.

Booth, R., & Halliday, J. (2018, December 31). UK's nightclubs suffer as young people seek less hedonistic pursuits: Games, food and even gyms are becoming more popular than hitting the dance floor. *The Guardian*. https://www.theguardian.com/music/2018/dec/31/uk-nightclubs-suffer-young-people-seek-less-hedonistic-pursuits.

Borlagdan, J., Freeman, T., Duvnjak, A., Bywood, P. T., & Roche, A. M. (2010). *From ideal to reality: Cultural contradictions and young people's drinking*. Adelaide: National Centre for Education and Training on Addiction, Flinders University.

Braverman, B. (2000). Libraries and theme parks: Strange bedfellows. *Research Strategies, 17*, 99–105.

Campbell, J. (2008). *The hero with a thousand faces* (3rd ed.). Novato, CA: New World Library.

Carlson, M. (1996). *Performance: A critical introduction*. London: Routledge.

CGA (2019), *Your future in festivals: How to stand out from the crowd* [online]. https://www.cga.co.uk/wp-content/uploads/2019/05/YourFutureinFestivals-CGA-Insights.pdf.

Collin, M. (1998). *Altered state: The story of ecstasy and acid house*. London: Serpent's Tail.

Deleuze, G., & Guattari, F. (1998). *A thousand plateaus: Capitalism and schizophrenia*. Minneapolis: University of Minnesota Press.

Demant, J. (2013). Affected in the nightclub. A case study of regular clubbers' conflictual practices in nightclubs. *International Journal of Drug Policy, 24*, 196–202.

Dilkes-Frayne, E. (2016). Drugs at the campsite: Socio-spatial relations and drug use at music festivals. *International Journal of Drug Policy, 33,* 27–35.

Duff, C. (2008). The pleasure in context. *International Journal of Drug Policy, 19,* 384–392.

Edensor, T. (2015). Light, design and atmosphere. *Visual Communication, 14*(3), 331–350.

Edensor, T., & Sumartojo, S. (2015). Designing atmospheres: Introduction to special issue. *Visual Communication, 14*(3), 251–265.

Ferdinand, N., & Williams, N. (2013). International festivals as experience production systems. *Tourism Management, 34,* 202–210.

Ferrell, J. (2004). Boredom, crime and criminology. *Theoretical Criminology, 8*(3), 287–302.

Gamma, A., Jerome, L., Liechti, M. E., & Sumnall, H. R. (2005). Is ecstasy perceived to be safe? A critical survey. *Drug and Alcohol Dependence, 77,* 185–193.

Garratt, S. (1998). *Adventures in wonderland: A decade of club culture.* London: Headline.

Gotham, K. (2005). Theorizing urban spectacles. *City, 9*(2), 225–246.

Harrison, J. (2003). *Being a tourist: Finding meaning in pleasure travel.* Vancouver: University of British Columbia Press.

Haydock, W. (2015). Understanding English alcohol policy as a neoliberal condemnation of the carnivalesque. *Drugs: Education, Prevention and Policy, 22*(2), 143–149.

Hayward, K. (2002). The vilification and pleasures of youthful transgression. In J. Muncie, G. Hughes, & E. McLaughlin (Eds.), *Youth justice: Critical readings.* London: Sage.

Hayward, K. (2012). Five spaces of cultural criminology. *British Journal of Criminology, 52,* 441–462.

Heal, A. (7 October 2018). Glastonbury tickets for 2019 sell out in half an hour. *The Guardian.* https://www.theguardian.com/music/2018/oct/07/glastonbury-tickets-2019-sell-out-in-half-an-hour.

Hesse, M., & Tutenges, S. (2008). Music and substance preferences among festival attendants. *Drugs and Alcohol Today, 12*(2), 82–88.

Hill, D., & Saroka, K. (2010). Sonic patterns, spirituality and brain function: The sound component of neurotheology. *NeuroQuantology, 8*(4), 509–516.

Home Office. (2018, July) *Drug misuse: Findings from the 2017/18 crime survey for England and Wales,* Statistical Bulletin 14/18, London: Home Office.

Hunt, G., & Evans, K. (2008). 'The great unmentionable': Exploring the pleasures and benefits of ecstasy from the perspectives of drug users. *Drugs: Education, Prevention and Policy, 15*(4), 329–349.

Hunt, G., Moloney, M., & Evans, K. (2010). *Youth, drugs, and nightlife.* London: Routledge.

Huxley, A. (1954). *The doors of perception and heaven and hell.* New York: Harper.

Jayne, M., Valentine, G., & Holloway, S. (2008). Emotional, embodied and affective geographies of alcohol, drinking and drunkenness. *Transactions of the Institute of British Geographers, 35,* 540–555.

Katz, J. (1988). *Seductions of crime.* New York: Basic Books.

Kelly, B. C. (2005). Conceptions of risk in the lives of club drug-using youth. *Substance Use and Misuse, 40,* 1443–1459.

Koenig, D. (2006). *Mouse tales: A behind-the-ears look at Disneyland.* Irvine, CA: Bonaventure Press.

Lim, M., Hellard, M., & Hocking, J. (2008). A cross-sectional survey of young people attending a music festival: Associations between drug use and musical preference. *Drug Alcohol Review, 27,* 439–441.

Mackay, H. (14 May 2018). *Club 18-30: Are millennials responsible for its downfall?* BBC News [Online]. https://www.bbc.co.uk/news/uk-44109100.

Malbon, B. (1999). *Clubbing: Dancing, ecstasy, vitality.* London: Routledge.

Martinic, M., & Measham, F. (Eds.). (2008). *Swimming with crocodiles: The culture of extreme drinking, ICAP series on alcohol in society* (Vol. 9). New York and Abingdon: Routledge.

Martins, S., Carlson, R., Alexandre, P., & Falke, R. (2011). Perceived risk associated with ecstasy use: A latent class analysis approach. *Addictive Behaviours, 36,* 551–554.

Martinus, T., McAlaney, J., McLaughlin, L., & Smith, H. (2010). Outdoor music festivals: Cacophonous consumption or melodious moderation? *Drugs: Education Prevention and Policy, 17*(6), 795–807.

Measham, F. (2002). 'Doing gender'-'doing drugs': Conceptualising the gendering of drugs cultures. *Contemporary Drug Problems, 29*(2), 335–373.

Measham, F. (2004a). Play space: Historical and socio-cultural reflections on drugs, licensed leisure locations, commercialisation and control. *International Journal of Drug Policy, 15*(5–6), 337–345.

Measham, F. (2004b). The decline of ecstasy, the rise of 'binge' drinking and the persistence of pleasure. *Probation Journal, 51*(4), 309–326.

Measham, F. (2008). The turning tides of intoxication: Young people's drinking in Britain in the 2000s. *Health Education, 108*(3), 207–222.

Measham, F. (2019). Drug safety testing, disposals and dealing in an English field: Exploring the operational and behavioural outcomes of the UK's first onsite 'drug checking' service. *International Journal of Drug Policy, 67,* 102–107.

Measham, F., Aldridge, J., & Parker, H. (2001). *Dancing on drugs: Risk, health and hedonism in the British club scene.* London: Free Association Books.

Measham, F., & Brain, K. (2005). 'Binge' drinking, British alcohol policy and the new culture of intoxication. *Crime, Media, Culture: An International Journal, 1*(3), 263–284.

Measham, F., & Moore, K. (2009). Repertoires of distinction: Exploring patterns of weekend polydrug use within local leisure scenes across the English night time economy. *Criminology and Criminal Justice, 9*(4), 437–464.

Measham, F., Moore, K., & Welch, Z. (2012). *Emerging drug trends in Lancashire: Nightclub surveys—Phase three report* (pp. 1–92). Lancaster: Lancaster University and Lancashire Drug and Alcohol Action Team.

Measham, F., & Shiner, M. (2009). The legacy of normalisation: The role of classical and contemporary criminological theory in understanding young people's drug use. *International Journal of Drug Policy, 20*(6), 502–508.

Measham, F., Wood, D., Dargan, P., & Moore, K. (2011). The rise in legal highs: Prevalence and patterns in the use of illegal drugs and first and second generation 'legal highs' in South London gay dance clubs. *Journal of Substance Use, 16*(4), 263–272.

Mintel. (2018). *Music concerts and festivals—UK—August 2018.* Mintel Group Ltd.

Moore, D. (2008). Erasing pleasure from public discourse on illicit drugs: On the creation and reproduction of an absence. *International Journal of Drug Policy, 19,* 353–358.

Moore, K., & Measham, F. (2012). Impermissible pleasures in UK leisure: Exploring policy developments in alcohol and illicit drugs. In C. Jones, E. Barclay, & R. Mawby (Eds.), *The problem of pleasure: Leisure, tourism and crime* (pp. 62–76). London: Routledge.

NHS. (2019). *Binge drinking.* https://www.nhs.uk/live-well/alcohol-support/binge-drinking-effects/.

O'Sullivan, S. (2016). The branded carnival: The dark magic of consumer excitement, *Journal of Marketing Management, 32.*

Parker, H., Aldridge, J., & Measham, F. (1998). *Illegal leisure: The normalization of adolescent recreational drug use.* London: Routledge.

Pine, J., & Gilmore, J. (1999). *The experience economy: Work is theatre & every business a stage.* Boston: Harvard Business Press.

Power, M. (2013). *Drugs 2.0: The web revolution that's changing how the world gets high*. London: Portobello Books.

Presdee, M. (2000). *Cultural criminology and the carnival of crime*. London: Routledge.

Pritchard, A., & Morgan, N. (2006). Hotel Babylon? Exploring hotels as liminal sites of transition and transgression. *Tourism Management, 27*, 762–772.

Raban, J. (1974). *Soft city*. Oxford: Picador.

Sachsman, D. (2007). *Serious leisure: A perspective for our time*. New York: Routledge.

Shaw, G., & Williams, A. (2004). *Tourism and tourism spaces*. London: Sage.

Shaw, R. (2013). Beyond night-time economy: Affective atmosphere of the urban night. *Geoforum, 51*, 87–95.

Sipe, L. (2018). Leveraging neo-localism for experience innovation: A case study of an urban park and entertainment venue. *Journal of Themed Experience and Attractions Studies, 1*(1), 29–37.

Stallybrass, P., & White, A. (1986). *The politics and poetics of transgression*. Ithaca, NY: Cornell University Press.

Steeves, H. (2003). Becoming disney: Perception and being at the happiest place on earth. *Midwest Quarterly, 44*(2), 176–194.

Time Out. (26 February 2015). *A hedonistic woodland wonderland in Cambridgeshire full of bands, DJs and cool installations*. https://www.timeout.com/london/music-festivals/secret-garden-party.

Turner, V. (1997). *The ritual process: Structure and anti-structure*. Livingston, NJ: Transaction.

Tutenges, S. (2012). Nightlife tourism: A mixed methods study of young tourists at an international nightlife resort. *Tourist Studies, 12*(2), 131–150.

Tutenges, S., & Rod, M. H. (2009). 'We got incredibly drunk … it was damned fun': Drinking stories among Danish youth. *Journal of Youth Studies, 12*(4), 355–370.

Tutenges, S., & Sandberg, S. (2013). Intoxicating stories: The characteristics, contexts and implications of drinking stories among Danish youth. *International Journal of Drug Policy, 24*, 538–544.

UK Festival Awards. (2017). *Market Report 2017*. UKFA. https://www.festivalawards.com/wp-content/uploads/2018/08/UK-Festival-Market-Report-2017.pdf.

Urry, J., & Larsen, J. (2011). *The Tourist Gaze 3.0*. London: Sage.

Ward, T. (2005). State crime in the heart of darkness. *British Journal of Criminology, 45*(4), 434–445.

Warner, M. (2014). *Once upon a time: A short history of fairy tale*. Oxford: Oxford University Press.

6

Drinking Norms and Alcohol Identities in the Context of Social Media Interactions Among University Students: An Overview of Relevant Literature

Brad Ridout

Introduction

Addressing problematic drinking among university students presents well-documented challenges given alcohol is a normative element of the university experience (Presley, Meilman, & Leichliter, 2002) and can be an important feature of young adult identity development (Donovan, Jessor, & Jessor, 1983; Wechsler et al., 1998). In this chapter, I intend to describe research concerning alcohol use in the context of social media interaction among young adults. This discussion will involve considering particular characteristics of young adulthood and young adult identity that might help explain aspects of drinking behaviour, leading into a broader discussion of the relationship between alcohol content on social networking sites (SNSs), social norms relevant to young adults and drinking practices themselves.

B. Ridout (✉)
Cyberpsychology Research Group, University of Sydney, Sydney, NSW, Australia
e-mail: brad.ridout@sydney.edu.au

© The Author(s) 2019
D. Conroy and F. Measham (eds.), *Young Adult Drinking Styles*,
https://doi.org/10.1007/978-3-030-28607-1_6

Young Adult Identity Construction in the Context of Drinking Practices

The advent of social media, and SNSs in particular, has fundamentally changed the conditions under which young adult identity development takes place. The ubiquity of SNSs such as Facebook means students now have tangible online identities to communicate information about themselves and depictions of their online and offline behaviours. Research into online alcohol identities suggests that portraying oneself as a drinker is considered by many university students to be a socially desirable component of their online identity, perpetuating and exaggerating perceptions of a binge drinking culture. Not surprisingly, both the posting and viewing of alcohol-related content on SNSs has been associated with adverse alcohol outcomes, including over-consumption, alcohol-related problems, and increased risk for alcoholism (Fournier & Clarke, 2011; Litt & Stock, 2011; Moreno, Christakis, Egan, Brockman, & Becker, 2012; Ridout, Campbell, & Ellis, 2012). However, emerging research is showing that social media can also be used to positively influence young people's drinking behaviour, via prevention and intervention efforts such as social norm interventions, which aim to correct the inflated perceptions that young people have about how much their peers drink (Ridout, 2016; Ridout & Campbell, 2014). Young adulthood is a time of radical change that involves an emerging sense of self in social/societal context; this phenomenon has been covered in detail in classical writings (e.g. Erikson, 1994) and demonstrated in recent empirical work (e.g. Kroger, Martinussen, & Marcia, 2010). However, this period is also seen as a delay of adult commitments, characterised as a period when a person can explore and experiment with emergent identity. University provides a 'safe haven' for identity exploration (Arnett, 2000), where young people have a fresh start to experiment with different behaviour, values and lifestyle in a new environment (Eccles et al., 1993). Experimentation with alcohol has long been recognised as identity-relevant among university students, for whom alcohol consumption is frequently a normative element of the university experience associated with gaining rites of passage to becoming a student (e.g. Crawford & Novak, 2006; Presley et al., 2002). There are a range of key factors identified in the research literature which highlight particular

6 Drinking Norms and Alcohol Identities in the Context ...

characteristics of alcohol consumption during young adulthood. These factors include physiological changes that allow an individual to more quickly overcome alcohol's effects (Spear, 2000), the role of dynamic and reciprocal individual–peer relations including perceived peer norms (Coggans & McKellar, 1994; Varela & Pritchard, 2011), and developmental neurophysiology (e.g. a developing prefrontal cortex) that may explain more impulsive decision-making during young adulthood relative to older adults.

The consumption of alcohol is inextricably linked to social relationships, perhaps no more so than at university (Seaman & Ikegwuonu, 2011). Most social activities between university students occur in the context of drinking (Thombs, 1999). Young people come to university with cultural preconceptions about the 'party' reputation of university campuses and a belief that heavy drinking in undergraduate years is a rite of passage (Prentice & Miller, 1993). This is particularly the case in the United States, where many students leave their family homes to live in on-campus residential halls, which Hollywood films frequently depict as the site of never-ending parties where heavy drinking is the norm and socially expected. Students therefore often start university keen to make new friends and partake in the mythical 'college experience', leading to socially motivated heavy drinking (Maggs, 1999). Increased alcohol consumption during university might be accounted for by increased motivation to conform with (increasingly valued) peer relationships but may also reflect students' response to a novel situation (e.g. starting university) where expected behaviour is unclear or ambiguous (Caspi & Moffitt, 1993). According to social norms theory, students may overestimate the prevalence of heavy drinking on campus (Schultz, Nolan, Cialdini, Goldstein, & Griskevicius, 2007), increasing the likelihood of hazardous drinking to 'fit in' with what is perceived as a dominant social norm. However, it is noted that this traditional theory of peer influence does not reflect more complex, agentic and reciprocal relationships between individuals and their peers discussed elsewhere in this book (see Conroy and Maclean, Chapter 8).

Alcohol Identity Construction on SNSs

Few studies have investigated how young people actively construct their identities during this transition, and what role—if any—alcohol plays in this process. Identity construction refers to intentional aspects of identity formation and is often defined as how people attempt to mould the impression others have of them by choosing to align with particular social norms (Zhao, Grasmuck, & Martin, 2008). In the context of social drinking norms, it is proposed that alcohol consumption motivated by the need to portray oneself as a drinker to one's peers constitutes an 'identity announcement', while positive reinforcements received from peers edifying the 'self as drinker' identity are considered to be 'identity placements'. It could therefore be said that identity is what students are attempting to define when they adhere to social drinking norms, whether they are conscious of this or not.

An investigation by Casey and Dollinger (2007) aimed to operationalise the 'self as drinker' component of identity using an innovative identity assessment method known as the *autophotographic essay*. University students created photo essays in response to the identity question 'who are you?' which were then coded for alcohol content. The resulting 'alcohol identity' score was not only related to self-reported alcohol consumption, but significantly predicted alcohol-related problem behaviours. These findings suggested that the autophotographic essay was a promising methodology for exploring the relationship between identity and alcohol use. Since this study, the rapid rise of online social networking has altered the conditions of identity construction, allowing individuals to interact in fully disembodied text and images, revealing only the physical characteristics they choose. Unlike anonymous settings where individuals are free to present online identities different to their real-life identities (Stone, 1996), 'nonymous' environments such as SNSs place constraints on identity announcements, as the online relationships are 'anchored' in offline relationships (Zhao, 2006). People therefore tend to express what has been dubbed their 'hoped-for possible self' on SNSs; a socially desirable identity one would like to establish and believes is possible under the right conditions (Yurchisin, Watchravesringkan, & McCabe, 2005). Facebook, the world's most popular SNS with almost 2.4 billion monthly users (Statistica, 2019), provides ideal conditions for examining identity construction (Zhao et al., 2008). Unlike other SNSs, information on Facebook regarding identity construction is not exclusively controlled by the profile owner, but can be contributed to by other users, presenting both identity announcements and identity placements. The Facebook timeline therefore serves as an up-to-date chronicle of comments and photos about the profile owner and their social interests and behaviours, presenting the ongoing construction of their online identity to their wider social network.

Alcohol Content on SNSs and Impact on Drinking Behaviours

In one of the first studies to examine online identity construction in relation to problem drinking, Ridout et al. (2012) proposed that the Facebook timeline provides researchers with a ready-made 'real life' photographic essay to operationalise the alcohol identity construct established by Casey and Dollinger (2007). A sample of 158 first-year university students completed a range of self-reported alcohol measures and provided access for researchers to view their Facebook profiles for the purpose of tallying alcohol-related content according to autophotographic methodology. Results revealed that students utilised a variety of photographic and textual material to present alcohol as a component of their identity on Facebook, with over half having selected an alcohol-related profile image. After controlling for gender and number of Facebook friends, alcohol identity significantly predicted alcohol consumption and alcohol-related problems. Support for these findings has since been provided by further studies into the link between alcohol content on SNSs and problematic alcohol use. For example, Facebook posts about intoxication among 224 US university students were analysed by Moreno et al. (2012) revealing a correlation between higher AUDIT scores and increased likelihood of alcohol-related injury. In another example, Fournier and Clarke (2011) also found a significant relationship between alcohol content on Facebook and self-reported alcohol use.

Several other studies have demonstrated the pervasiveness of alcohol-related content on SNSs (Griffiths & Casswell, 2010; Kolek & Saunders,

2008; Morgan, Snelson, & Elison-Bowers, 2010). One study revealed that alcohol references were present on 85.3% of male Facebook profiles (Egan & Moreno, 2011). These studies reinforce that not only is student drinking normalised in university populations, it is also a common feature of SNSs, particularly Facebook. While the sheer amount of alcohol content found on the Facebook profiles of university students in concerning, what is more alarming is how positively alcohol content on SNSs is perceived by peers. A series of open-ended questions posed to a group of 314 university students suggested perceptions of alcohol-related postings were generally positive (Morgan et al., 2010). Almost one-third of the sample said that alcohol-related posts can be funny and are a normal part of indicating social group membership. Some participants even noted that many people post alcohol-related photos in order to feel 'normal' and gain social acceptance. A study by Beullens and Schepers (2013) based on the methodology of Ridout et al. (2012) has lent quantitative support to these findings. Results revealed that alcohol use was depicted in a positive light in the majority of photos (72.2%), and that these positive photos received significantly more 'likes' from friends than those showing alcohol use in a neutral context. Comments on photos from friends were also overwhelmingly positive (87.2%). Interestingly, 86.4% of alcohol photos showed alcohol use implicitly, compared to only 10.2% explicitly, suggesting that drinking is usually presented on SNSs as an accepted and integral component of social gatherings, rather than an act to be explicitly captured as the subject of photos. Taken together, these findings suggest that online drinking identities are not only commonplace among university students, they elicit almost universally positive responses from their peers on SNSs.

The use of SNSs by young people, particularly university students, is now so well integrated into everyday social gatherings that the distinction between the online and offline world is becoming less and less meaningful. Facebook is also an important part of the 'social glue' that helps first-year students settle into university life (Madge, Meek, Wellens, & Hooley, 2009). An understanding of student drinking therefore requires an understanding of how drinking cultures are mediated within SNS environments. Brown and Gregg (2012) suggest that the drinking experience and Facebook are often inherently intertwined. They analysed the posting activity of female Facebook users and found that it was common for a narrative thread of a drinking session to be displayed for onlookers. Status updates are often posted during and in anticipation of a binge drinking session (e.g. 'bout to get ready to have total carnage with the girls, errr i mean social drinks.. hahaha..'), with photos documenting the event's progression posted either immediately via mobile phone, or the following day in a memorialising post-mortem of the night's activity. Sharing the experience of a night out with a wider online audience, who in turn provide encouragement in the form of 'likes' and comments, appears to be part of the pleasure of drinking for many young people, in a mutually reinforcing relationship. The authors argued that the ritual of posting photos on Facebook during and following drinking sessions adds a further visual dimension to the pleasure of storytelling that already surrounds heavy drinking experiences (Sheehan & Ridge, 2001), and extends the excitement and drama of a night out for a longer period. It has been argued that the high prevalence of alcohol content on SNSs like Facebook is an artefact of the situations where cameras are present (i.e. social and celebratory occasions that involve alcohol; Seaman & Ikegwuonu, 2011), exaggerating the prevalence of alcohol consumption among peers. In addition, a study by Brock (2007) revealed that 8% of students exaggerated their alcohol or drug use in Facebook posts. However, the accuracy of drinking norms depicted on Facebook is not the issue, rather it is how viewing such content inflates perceptions of how much peers drink, and the influence this has on drinking attitudes and behaviour.

The positive regard for alcohol-related content on SNSs may also encourage others to begin posting alcohol content themselves. A recent longitudinal study by Moreno et al. (2014) investigated the emergence of alcohol references on the Facebook profiles of 338 first-year students at two US universities. Participants were recruited prior to beginning university to allow for the number of alcohol references on their Facebook profiles to be calculated at baseline and then every four weeks until the end of their first year of university. At baseline, only 20.1% of Facebook profiles included alcohol content. However, the proportion increased dramatically over the course of the year to 60.0%, of which one quarter included specific references to being intoxicated. The students who displayed alcohol content prior to beginning university were highly likely to escalate their Facebook displays of alcohol to included references to intoxication and problem drinking. These findings are consistent with an earlier study that showed a large increase in the number of alcohol references by male students after beginning university (Egan & Moreno, 2011).

Given the extent of alcohol content on SNSs and the broader phenomenon of striving for favourable self-presentations in online environments (Chou & Edge, 2012), self-portrayal as a drinker seems likely to offer an important and socially desirable component of SNS identity for many university students. This is very concerning when understood in the context of social norms theory, as the proliferation of positively regarded alcohol content on SNSs, in particular Facebook, may perpetuate the normalisation of heavy drinking among university students (Ridout et al., 2012) and therefore increase pressure to binge drink.

Do SNSs Influence Social Drinking Norms?

While the impact of SNSs on social drinking norms and consequently drinking behaviour is still in its infancy, there is a large body of research suggesting that exposure to alcohol content in advertising (Anderson, de Bruijn, Angus, Gordon, & Hastings, 2009; Ellickson, Collins, Hambarsoomians, & McCaffrey, 2005) and in films (Dal Cin et al., 2009; Hanewinkel et al., 2012; Sargent, Wills, Stoolmiller, Gibson, & Gibbons, 2006) contributes to perceptions of social drinking norms and the uptake of drinking among young people by portraying alcohol use as common and risk-free. Given the pervasiveness of both advertised and user-driven alcohol content on SNSs, the positive regard with which it is perceived, and the fact that the latter allows for the observation of the behaviour of actual peers (as opposed to media depictions of peers), it is suspected that the potential for SNSs to affect perceived alcohol norms may be even greater than for traditional media (Beullens & Schepers, 2013). Fournier and Clarke (2011) suggest that the vicarious learning about student alcohol use that Facebook facilitates poses a major challenge for health professionals and researchers aiming to correct misperceptions about heavy alcohol use among university students. A handful of studies have investigated the influence of viewing alcohol content on SNSs on young people's attitudes towards alcohol and perceptions of social drinking norms. Moreno,

Briner, Williams, Walker, and Christakis (2009) conducted a series of focus groups to investigate how young people interpret alcohol references displayed on SNSs, including Facebook. Not surprisingly, young people and particularly adolescents in their early teens interpreted online alcohol content as evidence of actual use and as attempts to 'look cool'. Furthermore, participants identified viewing alcohol content on SNSs as a factor that may influence drinking decisions.

Litt and Stock (2011) investigated younger teens' views of old teens' drinking by asking 189 adolescents aged 13–15 to view experimenter-created Facebook profile pages of four fictional high-school students. As predicted, compared to a control group, those exposed to more alcohol content perceived descriptive drinking norms to be higher and reported more favourable attitudes towards drinking and drinker prototypes, lower perceived vulnerability to the consequences of alcohol use and a greater willingness to use alcohol. Another between subjects study by Fournier, Hall, Ricke, and Storey (2013) found that perceptions of descriptive drinking norms were significantly higher after only 10 minutes of viewing a Facebook profile featuring alcohol content, compared to viewing a profile without alcohol content. These results demonstrate that younger adolescents' beliefs around normative drinking behaviour are easily influenced by exposure to alcohol content on Facebook, that could put them at a higher risk of cognitions that predict problematic alcohol use later (Gerrard, Gibbons, Houlihan, Stock, & Pomery, 2008). Stoddard, Bauermeister, Gordon-Messer, Johns, and Zimmerman (2012) asked students to report their perceptions of peer attitudes to the posting of alcohol and drug use online. Results suggested that while perceptions of attitudes towards posting alcohol use on SNSs (i.e. injunctive norms) are associated with higher alcohol use, it is the sheer quantity of SNS alcohol content (i.e. descriptive norms) that has the most significant effect on a student's own alcohol use. A longitudinal study by Huang et al. (2014) supports this view, with the amount of exposure to friends' alcohol-related photos on SNSs found to be significantly associated with alcohol consumption. They also found that drinkers pursued more online friendships with fellow drinkers than non-drinkers, providing empirical support for alcohol and selection effects when constructing online identities and networks.

Alcohol advertising also has a prominent place in the social media environment. Alcohol brands use Facebook in a variety of ways to target young people in particular (Niland, McCreanor, Lyons, & Griffins, 2017). These include alcohol-themed games that automatically share users' scores with their Facebook friends, sponsored events and competitions, along with regular posting of branded images that appear in Facebook news feeds. All of these strategies generate further user-driven viral marketing activity through 'shares', 'likes' and comments. The most concerning aspect of alcohol advertising on Facebook is that at present it is essentially unregulated, allowing alcohol brands to embed themselves in the daily online experience of young Facebook users (Brodmerkel & Carah, 2013). The potential revealed in the above studies for SNSs to negatively affect young people's drinking behaviours is concerning. Furthermore, there is potential for the exposure to heavy drinking on social media to interact with depictions in traditional media, as previous research has indicated that when images in the media are similar to one's own experience in the social environment, the influential effects of the media are more powerful (Greene et al., 2012). These factors, the general ubiquity of SNSs, not to mention associations between Internet addiction and high alcohol consumption (Yen, Ko, Yen, Chen, & Chen, 2009), all suggest that the role of SNSs should not be underestimated in public health research.

Social Networking Sites as a Means of Promoting Safer Drinking Practices

Today's university students are 'digital natives' who spend a considerable proportion of their time using SNSs. SNSs are also used as an advertising tool, allowing for unprecedented targeting of personalised ad content based on users' SNS activity. While used by the alcohol advertising industry to great effect (Carah, 2014; Online Circle, 2013), the public health sector has yet to harness the power of SNS to effectively target university students showing signs of problematic drinking behaviour through their online 'alcohol identity'. The findings of studies discussed in this chapter (e.g. Moreno et al., 2012; Ridout et al., 2012) suggest there is huge potential to harness the identity and behavioural data presented on Facebook profiles to identify students at risk of alcohol-related harm using predictive analytic techniques. However, this has yet to be tested empirically. While using a predictive tool to label students as 'at-risk' could potentially be problematic and stigmatising, this needs to be weighed up against the negative alcohol-related consequences that these students may experience if the opportunity for early intervention is missed (Rosenbloom, 2015).

SNSs have been successfully used to deliver health information in other areas of e-health promotion (Park & Calamaro, 2013; Uhrig, Bann, Williams, & Evans, 2010; Woolley & Peterson, 2012), so it is somewhat surprising that until relatively recently no study had sought to utilise SNSs to deliver an intervention to reduce problematic drinking behaviour. Ridout and Campbell (2014) aimed to address this gap in the literature by testing the feasibility of delivering a personalised feedback intervention (PFI) using Facebook. Based on social norms theory, PFIs are designed to motivate students to reduce their alcohol consumption by highlighting discrepancies between self-reported alcohol consumption and peer drinking norms (Walters & Neighbors, 2005). Online PFIs are particularly well-suited to university students, as they allow for anonymity, and are quick and convenient to administer to large samples (Koski-Jännes & Cunningham, 2001; Kypri & Langley, 2003). Ridout and Campbell collected actual and perceived descriptive and injunctive drinking norms of 244 Australian university students. Ninety-five screened positive for hazardous drinking and were randomly allocated to a control group or intervention group that received personalised feedback via Facebook private messages, comparing their perception of their classmates' drinking norms and their own drinking levels with the actual drinking norms of their classmates. One month post-intervention, the intervention group significantly reduced their monthly alcohol consumption compared to baseline and controls, and reductions were maintained after three months. Furthermore, the intervention group's perceived peer drinking norms were significantly more accurate post-intervention, with analyses confirming improvements in norm accuracy were positively associated with clinically significant reductions in participants' own alcohol consumption. This was the first and to date only published study to use Facebook to successfully deliver a PFI, suggesting that SNSs may be an effective medium for positively influencing drinking norms and online drinking identities.

It should be kept in mind though that the most defining aspect of social media—peer-to-peer sharing—can be much more effective than traditional organisation-driven persuasion (Freeman & Chapman, 2008). The advertising industry has known this for some time, with alcohol brands utilising the peer-to-peer shareability of social media content to embed themselves in the everyday online experience of young people (Brodmerkel & Carah, 2013). Health promotion professionals need to follow this lead and leverage the shareability of social media content to get their messages across. Temporary abstinence initiatives such as 'febfast', 'Dry January', 'Dry July' and 'Hello Sunday Morning' (Febfast, 2019; Alcohol Change UK, 2019; Dry July, 2019; Hello Sunday Morning, 2019) are already utilising peer-to-peer sharing to create culture change regarding alcohol behaviour and online drinking identities, by encouraging participants to share their experiences of reducing their alcohol consumption via social media. The evidence-base for these approaches is not yet developed, but early indications suggest participants often make lasting positive changes and engage in increased conversation with peers about the benefits of periodically reducing alcohol consumption (Hillgrove & Thomson, 2012). These approaches are likely to be especially suitable for university students, who are not only heavy users of social media, but more susceptible to the influence of peers than at any other point in their identity development (Caspi & Moffitt, 1993; Steinberg & Silverberg, 1986).

Conclusion

Alcohol has long been a feature of young adult identity construction, especially for university students, who often find themselves in a new environment where heavy drinking is perceived to be the dominant social norm. The advent of social media has not only changed the traditional conditions in which young people's identity construction takes place, it has provided researchers with a vast amount of tangible data on the phenomenon. Discussion in this chapter draws attention to research that reveals alcohol as a feature of the online identity of many students, and that posting and viewing alcohol-related content is linked to both actual and perceived norms concerning drinking behaviour. Understanding the role SNSs currently play in the identity development of university students and the perpetuation of an exaggerated heavy drinking culture is important for developing applied interventions that can capitalise on the influence social media has in the lives of students.

References

Alcohol Change UK. (2019). *Dry January*. Retrieved from https://alcoholchange. org.uk/get-involved/campaigns/dry-january.

Anderson, P., de Bruijn, A., Angus, K., Gordon, R., & Hastings, G. (2009). Impact of alcohol advertising and media exposure on adolescent alcohol use: A systematic review of longitudinal studies. *Alcohol and Alcoholism, 44*(3), 229–243.

Arnett, J. J. (2000). Emerging adulthood: A theory of development from the late teens through the twenties. *American Psychologist, 55*(5), 469–480.

Beullens, K., & Schepers, A. (2013). Display of alcohol use on Facebook: A content analysis. *Cyberpsychology, Behavior, and Social Networking, 16*(7), 497–503.

Brock, R. (2007, January 12). *Online: Chronicle of Higher Education, 53*(19), A31.

Brodmerkel, S., & Carah, N. (2013). Alcohol brands on Facebook: The challenges of regulating brands on social media. *Journal of Public Affairs, 13*(3), 272–281.

Brown, R., & Gregg, M. (2012). The pedagogy of regret: Facebook, binge drinking and young women. *Continuum: Journal of Media & Cultural Studies, 26*(3), 357–369.

Carah, N. (2014). *Like, comment, share: Alcohol brand activity on Facebook.* Deakin, ACT: Foundation for Alcohol Research & Education.

Casey, P. F., & Dollinger, S. J. (2007). College students' alcohol-related problems: An autophotographic approach. *Journal of Alcohol and Drug Education, 51*(2), 8–25.

Caspi, A., & Moffitt, T. E. (1993). When do individual differences matter? A paradoxical theory of personality coherence. *Psychological Inquiry, 4*(4), 247–271.

Chou, H.-T. G., & Edge, N. (2012). "They are happier and having better lives than I am": The impact of using Facebook on perceptions of others' lives. *Cyberpsychology, Behavior, and Social Networking, 15*(2), 117–121.

Coggans, N., & McKellar, S. (1994). Drug use amongst peers: Peer pressure or peer preference? *Drugs: Education, Prevention and Policy, 1*(1), 15–26.

Crawford, L. A., & Novak, K. B. (2006). Alcohol abuse as a rite of passage: The effect of beliefs about alcohol and the college experience on undergraduates' drinking behaviors. *Journal of Drug Education, 36*(3), 193–212.

Dal Cin, S., Worth, K. A., Gerrard, M., Gibbons, F. X., Stoolmiller, M., Wills, T. A., & Sargent, J. D. (2009). Watching and drinking: Expectancies, prototypes, and friends' alcohol use mediate the effect of exposure to alcohol use in movies on adolescent drinking. *Health Psychology, 28*(4), 473–483.

Donovan, J. E., Jessor, R., & Jessor, L. (1983). Problem drinking in adolescence and young adulthood: A follow-up study. *Journal of Studies on Alcohol, 44*(1), 109–137.

Dry July. (2019). *About Dry July.* Retrieved from https://au.dryjuly.com/about.

Eccles, J. S., Midgley, C., Wigfield, A., Buchanan, C. M., Reuman, D., Flanagan, C., & Mac Iver, D. (1993). Development during adolescence: The impact of stage-environment fit on young adolescents' experiences in schools and in families. *American Psychologist, 48*(2), 90–101.

Egan, K. G., & Moreno, M. A. (2011). Alcohol references on undergraduate males' Facebook profiles. *American Journal of Men's Health, 5*(5), 413–420.

Ellickson, P. L., Collins, R. L., Hambarsoomians, K., & McCaffrey, D. F. (2005). Does alcohol advertising promote adolescent drinking? Results from a longitudinal assessment. *Addiction, 100*(2), 235–246.

Erikson, E. H. (1994). *Identity: Youth and crisis.* New York, NY: W. W Norton.

Febfast. (2019). *About us.* Retrieved from https://febfast.org.au/about/.

Fournier, A. K., & Clarke, S. W. (2011). Do college students use Facebook to communicate about alcohol? An analysis of student profile pages. *Journal of Psychosocial Research on Cyberspace, 5*(2), article 1. Retrieved from http://www.cyberpsychology.eu/view.php?cisloclanku=2011121702.

Fournier, A. K., Hall, E., Ricke, P., & Storey, B. (2013). Alcohol and the social network: Online social networking sites and college students' perceived drinking norms. *Psychology of Popular Media Culture, 2*(2), 86–95.

Freeman, B., & Chapman, S. (2008). Gone viral? Heard the buzz? A guide for public health practitioners and researchers on how Web 2.0 can subvert advertising restrictions and spread health information. *Journal of Epidemiology & Community Health, 62*(9), 778–782.

Gerrard, M., Gibbons, F. X., Houlihan, A. E., Stock, M. L., & Pomery, E. A. (2008). A dual-process approach to health risk decision making: The prototype willingness model. *Developmental Review, 28*(1), 29–61.

6 Drinking Norms and Alcohol Identities in the Context ...   129

Greene, G. W., White, A. A., Hoerr, S. L., Lohse, B., Schembre, S. M., Riebe, D., ... Horacek, T. (2012). Impact of an online healthful eating and physical activity program for college students. *American Journal of Health Promotion, 27*(2), e47–e58.

Griffiths, R., & Casswell, S. (2010). Intoxigenic digital spaces? Youth, social networking sites and alcohol marketing. *Drug and Alcohol Review, 29*(5), 525–530.

Hanewinkel, R., Sargent, J. D., Poelen, E. A., Scholte, R., Florek, E., Sweeting, H., ... Mathis, F. (2012). Alcohol consumption in movies and adolescent binge drinking in 6 European countries. *Pediatrics, 129*(4), 709–720.

Hello Sunday Morning. (2019). *Our Story*. Retrieved from https://www.hellosundaymorning.org/who-we-are/.

Hillgrove, T., & Thomson, L. (2012). *Evaluation of the impact of febfast participation*. Carlton, VIC: VicHealth.

Huang, G. C., Unger, J. B., Soto, D., Fujimoto, K., Pentz, M. A., Jordan-Marsh, M., & Valente, T. W. (2014). Peer influences: The impact of online and offline friendship networks on adolescent smoking and alcohol use. *Journal of Adolescent Health, 54*(5), 508–514.

Kolek, E. A., & Saunders, D. (2008). Online disclosure: An empirical examination of undergraduate Facebook profiles. *Journal of Student Affairs Research and Practice, 45*(1), 1–25.

Koski-Jännes, A., & Cunningham, J. (2001). Interest in different forms of self-help in a general population sample of drinkers. *Addictive Behaviors, 26*(1), 91–99.

Kroger, J., Martinussen, M., & Marcia, J. E. (2010). Identity status change during adolescence and young adulthood: A meta-analysis. *Journal of Adolescence, 33*(5), 683–698.

Kypri, K., & Langley, J. D. (2003). Perceived social norms and their relation to university student drinking. *Journal of Studies on Alcohol, 64*(6), 829–834.

Litt, D. M., & Stock, M. L. (2011). Adolescent alcohol-related risk cognitions: The roles of social norms and social networking sites. *Psychology of Addictive Behaviors, 25*(4), 708–713.

Madge, C., Meek, J., Wellens, J., & Hooley, T. (2009). Facebook, social integration and informal learning at university: 'It is more for socialising and talking to friends about work than for actually doing work'. *Learning, Media and Technology, 34*(2), 141–155.

Maggs, J. L. (1999). Alcohol use and binge drinking as goal-directed action during the transition to postsecondary education. In J. Schulenberg, J. L. Maggs, & K. Hurrelmann (Eds.), *Health risks and developmental transitions during adolescence* (pp. 345–371). Cambridge, UK: Cambridge University Press.

Moreno, M. A., Briner, L. R., Williams, A., Walker, L., & Christakis, D. A. (2009). Real use or "real cool": Adolescents speak out about displayed alcohol references on social networking websites. *Journal of Adolescent Health, 45*(4), 420–422.

Moreno, M. A., Christakis, D. A., Egan, K. G., Brockman, L. N., & Becker, T. (2012). Associations between displayed alcohol references on Facebook and problem drinking among college students. *Archives of Pediatrics and Adolescent Medicine, 166*(2), 157–163.

Moreno, M. A., D'Angelo, J., Kacvinsky, L. E., Kerr, B., Zhang, C., & Eickhoff, J. (2014). Emergence and predictors of alcohol reference displays on Facebook during the first year of college. *Computers in Human Behavior, 30*, 87–94.

Morgan, E. M., Snelson, C., & Elison-Bowers, P. (2010). Image and video disclosure of substance use on social media websites. *Computers in Human Behavior, 26*(6), 1405–1411.

Niland, P., McCreanor, T., Lyons, A. C., & Griffin, C. (2017). Alcohol marketing on social media: Young adults engage with alcohol marketing on facebook. *Addiction Research & Theory, 25*(4), 273–284.

Online Circle. (2013). *Australian Facebook performance report June 2013.* Retrieved from http://theonlinecircle.com/australian-facebook-performance-report-june-2013/.

Park, B. K., & Calamaro, C. (2013). A systematic review of social networking sites: Innovative platforms for health research targeting adolescents and young adults. *Journal of Nursing Scholarship, 45*(3), 256–264.

Prentice, D. A., & Miller, D. T. (1993). Pluralistic ignorance and alcohol use on campus: Some consequences of misperceiving the social norm. *Journal of Personality and Social Psychology, 64*(2), 243–256.

Presley, C. A., Meilman, P. W., & Leichliter, J. S. (2002). College factors that influence drinking. *Journal of Studies on Alcohol, 63*(14), 82–90.

Ridout, B. (2016). Facebook, social media and its application to problem drinking among college students. *Current Opinion in Psychology, 9*, 83–87.

Ridout, B., & Campbell, A. (2014). Using Facebook to deliver a social norm intervention to reduce problem drinking at university. *Drug and Alcohol Review, 33*(6), 667–673.

Ridout, B., Campbell, A., & Ellis, L. (2012). 'Off your Face(book)': Alcohol in online social identity construction and its relation to problem drinking in university students. *Drug and Alcohol Review, 31*(1), 20–26.

Rosenbloom, D. (2015). *Workshop on social media, web & mobile interventions for college drinking*. Boston, MA: Boston University School of Public Health.

Sargent, J. D., Wills, T. A., Stoolmiller, M., Gibson, J., & Gibbons, F. X. (2006). Alcohol use in motion pictures and its relation with early-onset teen drinking. *Journal of Studies on Alcohol, 67*(1), 54–65.

Schultz, P. W., Nolan, J. M., Cialdini, R. B., Goldstein, N. J., & Griskevicius, V. (2007). The constructive, destructive, and reconstructive power of social norms. *Psychological Science, 18*(5), 429–434.

Seaman, P., & Ikegwuonu, T. (2011). 'I don't think old people should go to clubs': How universal is the alcohol transition amongst young adults in the United Kingdom? *Journal of Youth Studies, 14*(7), 745–759.

Sheehan, M., & Ridge, D. (2001). 'You become really close… you talk about the silly things you did, and we laugh': The role of binge drinking in female secondary students' lives. *Substance Use and Misuse, 36*(3), 347–372.

Spear, L. P. (2000). *Adolescent period: Biological basis of vulnerability to develop alcoholism and other ethanol-mediated behaviors*. Bethesda, MD: National Institute on Alcohol Abuse and Alcoholism.

Statistica. (2019). *Number of monthly active Facebook users worldwide as of 1st quarter 2019 (in millions)*. Retrieved at https://www.statista.com/statistics/264810/number-of-monthly-active-facebook-users-worldwide/.

Steinberg, L., & Silverberg, S. B. (1986). The vicissitudes of autonomy in early adolescence. *Child Development, 57*(4), 841–851.

Stoddard, S. A., Bauermeister, J. A., Gordon-Messer, D., Johns, M., & Zimmerman, M. A. (2012). Permissive norms and young adults' alcohol and marijuana use: The role of online communities. *Journal of Studies on Alcohol and Drugs, 73*(6), 968–975.

Stone, A. A. (1996). *The war of desire and technology at the close of the mechanical age*. Cambridge, MA: MIT Press.

Thombs, D. (1999). *An introduction to addictive behaviors* (2nd ed.). New York, NY: Guilford Press.

Uhrig, J., Bann, C., Williams, P., & Evans, W. D. (2010). Social networking websites as a platform for disseminating social marketing interventions: An exploratory pilot study. *Social Marketing Quarterly, 16*(1), 2–20.

Varela, A., & Pritchard, M. E. (2011). Peer influence: Use of alcohol, tobacco, and prescription medications. *Journal of American College Health, 59*(8), 751–756.

Walters, S. T., & Neighbors, C. (2005). Feedback interventions for college alcohol misuse: What, why and for whom? *Addictive Behaviors, 30*(6), 1168–1182.

Wechsler, H., Dowdall, G. W., Maenner, G., Gledhill-Hoyt, J., & Lee, H. (1998). Changes in binge drinking and related problems among American college students between 1993 and 1997 results of the Harvard school of public health college alcohol study. *Journal of American College Health, 47*(2), 57–68.

Woolley, P., & Peterson, M. (2012). Efficacy of a health-related Facebook social network site on health-seeking behaviors. *Social Marketing Quarterly, 18*(1), 29–39.

Yen, J. Y., Ko, C. H., Yen, C. F., Chen, C. S., & Chen, C. C. (2009). The association between harmful alcohol use and Internet addiction among college students: Comparison of personality. *Psychiatry and Clinical Neurosciences, 63*(2), 218–224.

Yurchisin, J., Watchravesringkan, K., & McCabe, D. B. (2005). An exploration of identity re-creation in the context of internet dating. *Social Behavior and Personality: An International Journal, 33*(8), 735–750.

Zhao, S. (2006). *Cyber-gathering places and online-embedded relationships*. Paper presented at the annual meeting of the Eastern Sociological Society, Boston, MA.

Zhao, S., Grasmuck, S., & Martin, J. (2008). Identity construction on Facebook: Digital empowerment in anchored relationships. *Computers in Human Behavior, 24*(5), 1816–1836.

7

Social Media and Young Adults' Drinking Cultures: Research Themes, Technological Developments and Key Emerging Concepts

Ian Goodwin and Antonia Lyons

Over the past 5–10 years, the literature on social media and young adult drinking has developed and diversified remarkably quickly. It shows that social media is now pivotal to the concerns of alcohol researchers, as well as to those interested in youth culture, leisure practices and the life experiences of young adults more generally. While cognisant of the risk of producing premature conclusions, in this chapter we outline four key thematic concerns apparent within this body of literature. We then highlight recent developments in social media technologies and environments that are relevant for researchers seeking to gain insight into young adults' drinking cultures and practices, and outline some of the major conceptual issues that these raise, including a holistic, social media ecology perspective. We

---

I. Goodwin (✉)
Massey University, Wellington, New Zealand
e-mail: I.Goodwin@massey.ac.nz

A. Lyons
Victoria University of Wellington, Wellington, New Zealand

© The Author(s) 2019
D. Conroy and F. Measham (eds.), *Young Adult Drinking Styles*,
https://doi.org/10.1007/978-3-030-28607-1_7

133

suggest how to incorporate these important shifting developments into alcohol-related research with young people.

One important thematic concern in the research links content on social network sites (SNS) to the health and well-being of young people. Numerous researchers have documented the sheer prevalence of positive references to alcohol on young people's SNS profiles (e.g. Beullens & Schepers, 2013; Egan & Moreno, 2011), while others have provided quantitative, correlational analysis of how such user-generated, alcohol-related profile content relates to heavier drinking patterns that pose a health risk (e.g. Stoddard, Bauermeister, Gordon-Messer, Johns, & Zimmerman, 2012). This has resulted in a general concern that SNSs create 'intoxigenic digital spaces' (Griffiths & Casswell, 2010: 525)—online alcohol-promoting environments—that are potentially damaging to public health (McCreanor et al., 2013). Documenting the alcohol-related content of young adult's SNS profiles, and seeking to understand its 'effects' on alcohol consumption, makes sense given the well-documented negative health outcomes associated with alcohol consumption.

In contrast, the second major thematic concern in the literature focuses on gaining understanding of young adults' drinking-related SNS activities as a form of online drinking *culture*. Here, the emphasis has been on investigating how drinking displays on SNS relate to the forging of young adults' identities (e.g. Goodwin & Griffin, 2017; Lindsay & Supski, 2017) and examining the close ties between alcohol consumption, SNS use and the maintenance of young adults' intimate social ties and broader social worlds (e.g. Niland, Lyons, Goodwin, & Hutton, 2015). Focusing on drinking as a leisure practice imbued with power relations, much of this work has usefully documented how class, gender, and ethnicity structures young adults' engagement with online drinking displays (e.g. Atkinson & Sumnall, 2016; Hutton, Griffin, Lyons, Niland, & McCreanot, 2016; Moewaka Barnes, Niland, Samu, Sciasia, & McCreanor, 2017). These studies highlight the deep ambivalence emerging at the heart of research into online young adult drinking cultures. Drinking and its online display are recognised as a means for young adults to exercise considerable autonomy and agency as they engage in leisure practices, narrate their own sense of identity, forge and maintain friendships, and develop sociality. Simultaneously such practices are subject to, and potentially reproductive of, broader power relations that can limit, constrain or shape young adults' lives in problematic or even disempowering ways.

This sense of ambivalence is heightened within the third major thematic concern we see emerging in the contemporary literature: an examination of how commercial alcohol interests have quickly moved to take advantage of young adults' enthusiasm for alcohol-related content on SNSs (Nicholls, 2012; Niland, McCreanor, Lyons, & Griffin, 2017). Contemporary SNS are replete with commercialised messages (McCreanor et al., 2013). Various studies of the wide range of marketing activities by alcohol corporations on SNS have become a focus of analysis. In a systematic review of 47 studies in this growing field, Lobstein, Landon, Thornton, and Jernigan (2017) conclude that branded marketing messages are highly appealing to young adults, and that exposure to marketing via digital channels is associated with higher levels of drinking. This in turn has raised a series of public policy concerns about the difficulties of regulating such activities (Mart, 2017), which may subvert current alcohol marketing codes (Lobstein et al., 2017). In contrast to a lack of effective state-led regulatory developments, various non-governmental experiments in health promotion on SNS aimed at curbing alcohol consumption have developed (e.g. Cherrier, Carah, & Meurk, 2017).

Overarching each of these themes lies the fourth and final issue we wish to highlight: a growing critical awareness of the ways in which the informational architectures and affordances of SNS influence the social interactions and user activities that occur on them, including drinking-related displays and behaviours. While SNS do not simplistically determine what users do, they are far from neutral facilitators of user activities (Bucher, 2018). The particular form and functionality of the 'virtual environments' made available through specific SNS have 'wide-ranging consequences (whether intentional or not) for the types of public interaction and participation made possible' (Wahl-Jorgensen, 2018: 78). For example, Facebook provides new technological affordances for users to edit their displays of alcohol-related sociality before posting them online, allowing them to emphasise only the positive aspects of their nights out that they wish to share, thereby producing 'airbrushed' online drinking cultures that minimise the negative effects of alcohol consumption (Niland, Lyons, Goodwin, & Hutton, 2014). More broadly, SNS are routinely designed to create powerful imperatives to share personal and social information with others in the network (van Dijck, 2013; Wahl-Jorgensen, 2018). Goodwin, Griffin, Lyons, McCreanor, and Moewaka Barnes (2016) have argued that the posting of images of alcohol consumption on Facebook is related to the way that the system's Edge Rank algorithm prioritises content in users' News Feeds. Despite being 'risky' forms of content that can attract social censure from employers and others, drinking photos often generate many more likes and comments from peers than other forms of content. This in turn means that Edge Rank prioritises drinking photos in the News Feed, helping young people attain a greater level of visibility in their online peer networks than they may otherwise be able to achieve. This level of visibility is not guaranteed on Facebook more generally and yet is necessary if young people wish to sustain high levels of sociality online. Thus, drinking photos facilitate a valued 'precarious popularity' for many young people in their social worlds, in a manner inherently encouraged by Facebook's informational architecture (Goodwin et al., 2016).

One of the key aspects of such 'architectural' influences on SNS is therefore the data-driven and algorithmic nature of their interfaces, which are designed to hone in on the data the user provides to shape the user experience (Bucher, 2018). This includes popular user-generated content such as drinking photos (Goodwin et al., 2016). It also encompasses any demographic information supplied, users' professed interests, their specific social network and their geographic location. By using algorithmic code to examine such data, the system comprehensively learns a wide range of 'individual preferences that determine the unique feed of content that the user will see' (Carah & Meurk, 2017: 370). Alcohol corporations now use such algorithmic sorting of content to maximise marketing opportunities. For example, they are producing algorithmically driven promotions that—rather than seeking to control the 'message'—work by stimulating and managing user engagement with branded content (liking, commenting, sharing, tagging), seeking to deeply embed brands in the everyday identity work and sociality of SNS users (Carah, Brodmerkel, & Hernandez, 2014). Users *themselves* therefore come to circulate and help construct alcohol marketing as an inherent part of developing their online drinking cultures, and often enjoy engaging with branded content and sharing this across their peer networks. As users engage with the interface in this manner, the line between user-generated and commercial content becomes fundamentally blurred.

Together these four thematic concerns constitute considerable advancements in our understandings of young adults, alcohol consumption and SNS use. We need to retain the focus they provide and to continue their trajectories of investigation. However, if research in these areas is to remain relevant, it needs to become more fully orientated towards contemporary technological developments, including the rapid growth of diverse and differentiated SNS platforms, the role of the smartphone and the shift to mobile SNS, and the associated rise of real-time social interaction. Much work to date has tended to focus on one or two SNS platforms at a time, investigating the impacts and influences of young people documenting drinking on social media profiles via user-generated content. However, this now paints too static and narrow a picture. The shifts we identify create a more dynamic form of 'cybernetic' sociality, one characterised by real-time feedback loops *across* multiple uses of differentiated and 'always-on' social media. In other words, today's technological context is increasingly characterised by a series of profound, differentiated and dynamic influences over the lived experiences of young people *as* they drink and navigate the night time economy (NTE).

Multiplicity, Mobility and Temporality in a Social Media Ecology

Research into young adults, drinking and SNS has historically focused on Facebook (Boyle, Earle, LaBrie, & Ballou, 2017), which made sense when Facebook dominated online sociality. With over 2.2 billion monthly active users as of March 2018, Facebook remains the largest SNS in the world and retains a central role in many internet users' lives, one that we still need to understand (Sujon, Viney, & Toker-Turnlar, 2018). However, the current conjuncture is marked by an intense proliferation of multiple social media platforms, including popular sites like Instagram and Snapchat which have been enthusiastically embraced by young adults. This has changed user experiences in significant respects. Zhao, Lampe, and Ellison (2016) contend that a broader *social media ecology* perspective is needed to capture the complex ways that users now negotiate multiple platforms to meet their communicative needs. When choosing which SNS to use, users will simultaneously consider the audience they associate with particular platforms and the nature of the content they wish to share. In striving to stabilise their own specific communication ecosystem they will, at times, seek to preserve strict boundaries between platforms (Zhao et al., 2016). For example, users may choose one specific site to share content with intimate friends, and other sites for keeping in touch with family, for maintaining contact with broader social networks or for facilitating professional and working life. At other times, such boundaries may be deliberately breached through sharing content across platforms, for example, when seeking larger audiences for personal achievements or high-profile social events (e.g. birthday celebrations). Researchers need to maintain an investigative focus on the complex whole to avoid analytical blind spots. Focusing on only one platform may conceal important insights into user behaviour (Zhao et al., 2016).

Obtaining a holistic understanding of multiple social media has significant implications for both health orientated and cultural research into young adults', SNS and drinking. Some researchers have attempted to capture the complexity involved, for example, by examining the unique technological affordances of micro-blogging on Twitter as a means for sharing drinking content that may promote alcohol consumption (Alhabash et al., 2018; Cavazos-Rehg, Krauss, Sowles, & Bierut, 2015). This usefully expands our perspectives beyond Facebook, but still only focuses on one SNS. In contrast, a few studies have begun to investigate drinking-related content and activities across SNS. For example, Hendriks, den Putte, Winifed, and Moreno (2018) found that the positive social framing of alcohol use was present on both Facebook and Instagram and suggest this further entrenches the role of alcohol posts in promoting drinking in young adults' everyday lives. In an attempt to tease out differences that may exist across social media platforms, Boyle et al. (2017) created a series of hypothetical, photographic vignettes of alcohol consumption that either glamorised alcohol use or depicted its negative consequences, and asked young adults to rate where they would likely come across this content on social media. They found that 'Instagram was seen as the most probable destination' (p. 63) for photos depicting alcohol use as attractive and glamorous, while Snapchat was the most likely destination for depictions of negative consequences.

These preliminary differences point to the impact of user engagement with a multifaceted social media ecology. They signal differences beyond technological design, hinting at evolving social norms and practices that shape how users perceive and engage with social media multiplicity. Boczkowski, Matassi, and Mitchelstein (2018) refer to these differences as social media repertoires. Tasked with managing increasingly routine engagement with a range of different social media, repertoires refer to shared constellations of meanings that help young adult users stabilise, understand and navigate what is acceptable and desirable on each platform. Repertoires are always dynamic, and particularly subject to change as new platforms are introduced. However, there are key, recognisable differences across social media: WhatsApp is a multifaceted communication space; Facebook is a space for the display of a carefully crafted and socially acceptable self; Instagram is an environment for more stylised forms of self-presentation; Twitter is valued for information and informality; and Snapchat is a platform for more spontaneous and ludic forms of connection (Boczkowski et al., 2018).

There is a certain relational *calculus* involving the entire social media ecology here, one that shapes an understanding of matters such as what to post where, what comments are appropriate, what one should share and what one should not (Boczkowski et al., 2018). This calculus involves both relational and emotional dynamics across a variety of social domains. It appears that young adults' increasingly undertake their sociality, work, cultural lives and leisure practices within this growing sphere of social media, but in a variegated, dynamic and complex fashion that alcohol researchers need to understand. The initial research suggests that glamorous depictions of alcohol use seem to 'fit' with an environment tailored to stylised self-presentation on Instagram, while the spontaneous and ludic nature of Snapchat may logically lend itself to more negative depictions (Boczkowski et al., 2018; Boyle et al., 2017).

Such emergent platform norms produce different online cultures and divergent opportunities that in one sense provide increasing agency for young adults. Yet Buehler (2017) argues that platform norms also produce powerful constraints on users. While Facebook potentially provides a premium resource for emotional support as it facilities access to a diverse range of social contacts, users requesting such support from friends must navigate norms that 'prevent users from explicitly and directly venting their affect and requesting emotional support' (p. 1). Such 'venting' of affect would potentially disrupt the calculated and considered performance of the socially acceptable self that Boczkowski et al. (2018) describe as normative for Facebook. The affective dimensions of drinking cultures, their links to social support and the role of online displays of drinking in self-presentation are key aspects that alcohol researchers need to understand. New 'norms' and repertoires playing out across an expanding social media ecology will affect these processes. Understanding the associated user agencies and constraints that result is important for future research.

Boczkowski et al. (2018) note that social media repertoires are primarily socially shaped and have relative autonomy from technological affordances. Yet the range of growing, novel technological affordances offered by an expanded, divergent social media ecology clearly matters to the cultures emerging within these contexts. This is also important for alcohol researchers. For example, Snapchat's key technological innovation may well be the ephemeral nature of the content posted to the platform: rather than archiving content for ongoing sharing and viewing, it is displayed for a limited time before disappearing. It is the ephemerality of Snapchat that relates to user perceptions of the platform as ludic: that is as more 'lightweight', enjoyable and fun than other platforms (Bayer et al., 2016). Thus, Snapchat ultimately offers less social support than other technologies, but facilitates positive affect, enables the easy sharing of content with close ties, and produces 'reduced self-presentational concerns' (p. 956). It is easy to see why Snapchat may therefore be appropriated by young adults as a key part of their drinking cultures given they view drinking with close friends as pleasurable, involving having fun and being sociable (Lyons & Willot, 2008). The affordances of Snapchat enable this fun to be enhanced, while avoiding the 'context collapse' (boyd, 2007) associated with sites like Facebook. Such 'collapse' occurs because the persistence of content on Facebook and the ease with which it can be replicated and shared means that communication intended solely for friends may end up being viewed by unintended others, such as parents or employers. The perceived appropriateness of Snapchat vis-à-vis sites like Facebook as a destination for 'negative' drinking events (Boyle et al., 2017) therefore makes sense in light of its specific affordances. This is especially so given that such 'negative' events are often reworked by young people into 'good drinking stories' that facilitate fun and social bonding (Griffin, Bengry-Howell, Hackley, Mistral, & Szmigin, 2009).

Better understanding of young people's drinking practices requires more insight into such interconnections between the social and the technological. Detailed analyses of the specific technological affordances offered by divergent social media are required: both singularly in terms of the unique cultures they facilitate *and* in terms of their *relative* place within the whole. Affordances affect the particular repertoires young adults associate with specific platforms and their subsequent comparative position within the social media ecology. While the specific details of how platforms differ from one another are important, the more general shift to an increasingly visual social media ecology is worth highlighting. Many of the most popular new sites, such as Instagram or Snapchat, are 'explicitly framed around the visual' (Highfield & Leaver, 2016: 47). The visual has a long history in Internet culture, and photos are a voluminous and key element of user-generated content on Facebook and a key part of drinking cultures on that platform (Goodwin et al., 2016). Yet the visual is becoming even more critical to 'story-telling and meaning-making' (Highfield & Leaver, 2016: 47) on social media sites that foreground and prioritise photographic over textual content.

As Rose (2014) argues, in such contemporary forms of visual culture photographs do much more than make aspects of the social visible. They are involved in a form of 'visuality' whereby people make *use* of images 'much more as communicational tools than as representational texts' (p. 24). This is a widespread aspect of current shifts, and yet our "research into the visual as a central component of online communication has lagged behind the analysis of popular, primarily text-driven social media" (Highfield & Leaver, 2016: 47). How communicative visuality affects drinking cultures needs to inform our research efforts. The development of social relationships, both in terms of intimate friendships and broader peer networks, is essential to young adult drinking as a leisure practice and certainly involves communicative dimensions (Niland, Lyons, Goodwin, & Hutton, 2013). It is likely increasingly facilitated by communicative visuality, and this points us *away* from maintaining a dominant focus on analysing user-generated content on individual SNS profiles as a means for representation. We need to think more carefully about the social *dynamics* of communication and friendship facilitated through content like drinking photos, and their relationship to lived leisure practices.

Mobility is another key issue in this context. Smartphones now host social media, and they have become more powerful, cheaper, smaller and increasingly part of everyday life (Mackey, 2016). Contemporary SNS are 'mobile first'. Even Facebook, originally accessed through the desktop PC, has evolved into a mobile platform that has enabled it to play a more central role in young people's sociality and the last minute micro-coordination of social events (Bertel & Ling, 2016). This has important implications for young adults' leisure practices, including drinking. Historically, before the release of the first iPhone in 2007 as the initial 'smart' device that made mobile Internet access mundane (Goggin, 2012), the near synchronous use of SMS (text messaging) was central to the sense of 'perpetual contact' (Katz & Aakus, 2002) that mobiles provide to young adults. When young adults send messages through SMS, they expect a quick response, producing anticipation of attention from peers within a shared time frame (Rettie, 2009). This also results in a continual background awareness of others—whether or not you are currently in contact—that Ito and Okabe (2005) name ambient virtual co-presence. These spatial and temporal processes will continue to be important to understanding mobile sociality, and SMS will remain a significant part of them. However, Bertel and Ling's (2016) research suggests that the 'app centric' (Goggin, 2012) smartphone has elevated mobile SNS apps, as opposed to SMS, into the central role in perpetually connected and 'always-on' young adult culture.

The broader social media ecology, with a variety of mobile SNS apps, also enhances the centrality of the visual image through the increased accessibility of the smartphone's camera. For example, Thulin (2017) argues that the rise of Snapchat has meant that images have replaced SMS as the *mainstay* of young adults' peer-to-peer mobile contacts. Images are central to drinking cultures on social media (e.g. Atkinson & Sumnall,

2016). On Snapchat, 'snapping' is not experienced as a means for exchanging images, but rather becomes 'a way of "speaking with" friends as a conversation in images and a few words only' (Thulin, 2017: 7). Social media mobility also adds to the sheer volume and presence of images in everyday life. Participants in Thulin's (2017) study report snapping via smartphone as something they do all the time, with some respondents reporting '50, 70, 100 or even more snaps per day' (p. 7). An everyday, routine visualisation of social contact—sharing the 'small moments' (Bayer et al., 2016: 956)—has therefore accompanied the rise of mobile social media. As smartphones increase the options and opportunities available to users for 'mediated social contact' (p. 12) over and above the original mobile phone/SMS, this further increases young adults' expectations for always-on engagement with their friends. Thus, Thulin (2017) observes, the recourse to images for communication may partly derive from them being 'expressive, in the moment, and faster than words' (p. 8). Images are not only communicatively and representationally rich, but *efficient* ways of maintaining contacts with peers.

New forms of mobility and intensified always-on sociality, driven by the smartphone, combine with social media multiplicity and the shift to visuality to produce significant change in young adult's practices. This will affect drinking cultures and their implications for health, and the rapid developments involved will require more than simply rethinking the role of drinking-related images. The few studies published on smartphones, SNS and drinking suggest that a series of broader, novel, 'real-time' influences on young adults' drinking experiences in the NTE need to become a closer focus of analysis. Truong's (2018) recent study investigating uses of WhatsApp during nights out drinking in Zurich is illustrative in this regard. She argues that, through WhatsApp, 'young people direct their energy and attention towards [physically] absent others' (p. 199) and become more cognisant of possible alternative venues as they navigate their way through a night out. She suggests young adults become aware of 'a broader horizon of friendship practices and wider windows of nightlife experiences' (p. 199). This strengthens 'orientations' towards 'comparison, competition, and optimisation of nightlife' (p. 199) *during* nightlife experiences, or in other words, reinforces a form of entrepreneurial ethics preoccupied with maximising leisure. In the process, the real-time sharing of images, videos and sounds intensifies the synchronisation of young adults' time frames and links disparate drinking spaces.

Researchers have already provided valuable understandings of urban mobility and the influence of space and place on young adults' drinking practices in the NTE (e.g. Demant & Landholt, 2014; Wilkinson, 2017). However, we need to build on work like Truong's (2018) to explore how mobile SNS alter young adults' lived nightlife experiences rather than solely focusing on SNS as a means for *representing* drinking. New forms of 'perpetual contact', 'ambient virtual co-presence' and 'shared time frames' forged through uses of mobile SNS are likely creating new networked, drinking-related leisure *practices* that cut across the physical spaces of the city (streets, parks, malls), leisure venues (pubs and clubs), suburban and rural locations and private homes (especially as they relate to issues like preloading and parties). A rapidly developing mobile, diverse social media ecology is increasingly offering a set of affordances that allow for the dynamic, real-time micro-coordination of drinking practices throughout nights out drinking. The novel geolocative affordances of mobile social media are a key part of these changes, which directly 'impact people's mobility decisions' (Frith, 2013: 248). Varied, rich forms of online content can be posted and feedback received from peers almost instantaneously as young adults navigate urban nightlife spaces and precincts. In sum, social media are becoming a more integral part of the drinking experience, continuously involved in drinking practices, event planning, deciding where and what to drink, and with whom.

The Commercial Dimensions of Mobile Social Media Multiplicity

While the social media ecology is lively and diverse, it remains privatised and commercially driven, and the multiplicity of platforms does not necessarily reflect a multiplicity of ownership. Facebook, for example, owns both Instagram and WhatsApp. This heightens the company's ability to capture user data and offers opportunities for alcohol corporations to increase the power and reach of their promotional campaigns on social media. When we consider the new capacities that novel technological affordances offer 'users' of social media, it is important that we do not confine ourselves to end-users alone but equally explore developers and advertisers as important user groups (Bucher & Helmond, 2017). Social media platforms continue to be programmable informational architectures built on an economic model that relies on connecting end-users to advertisers-as-users in increasingly efficient and effective ways (Helmond, 2015).

Global alcohol corporations such as Diageo have been innovative and proactive in their use of social and mobile media for some time (McCreanor et al., 2013). Contemporary shifts in alcohol advertising and promotion reflect and reinforce the changes described in this chapter. As Carah and Shaul (2016) argue, 'brands are a critical part of the ongoing experimentation that underpins the development of mobile social media platforms like Instagram' (p. 69). They use the vodka brand Smirnoff (owned by Diageo) to highlight how Instagram 'expands the terrain upon which brands operate by dispersing the work of creating and engaging with [branded] images into consumers' everyday lives' (p. 69). Smirnoff creates purpose-built bars at cultural events like music festivals, replete with branding, and invites celebrities and musicians to party with consumers while there (Carah & Shaul, 2016). Photography via smartphones is encouraged, and hashtags promoted at the venue for coordinating the subsequent flow of images as they are uploaded by party-goers to Instagram. This attracts the attention of their followers, who then spread the content across the platform in ways mediated by Instagram's algorithms (algorithms that, over time, can be fine-tuned to aid this process). The reach of the 'brand activation' (p. 74) at the festival can then be assessed by Diageo using various forms of user-generated data made available by the platform. As these interactive real-time campaigns develop, Diageo can learn about individual consumer lifestyles and preferences, and subsequently increasingly target those who are most likely to consume alcohol with further marketing.

These sophisticated commercial activities explicitly measure, access and make use of the kind of communicative visuality we have highlighted as increasingly prevalent on mobile social media. Moreover, the form of glamorous partying Smirnoff encourages fits well with the specific 'repertoire' user's associate with Instagram as 'an environment for stylized self-presentation' (Boczkowski et al., 2018: 1). Smirnoff does not simply target the 'audience' on Instagram with promotional messages, but helps to *co-produce* 'appropriate' uses of Instagram and its relative positioning within a complex social media ecology. Instagram becomes an environment where the stylised production of the self is enacted within and through specific forms of glamorous alcohol consumption, in a seamless manner. 'Appropriate' user-generated and commercial content on Instagram become mutually reinforcing and essentially indistinguishable. Elsewhere Carah and Meurk (2017) describe the changes involved in more general terms, as a shift towards a 'post-exposure paradigm' (p. 370) by alcohol brands that works across various social media. That is, platforms such as Facebook, Snapchat, WhatsApp and Instagram increasingly enable brands to 'plan and fund their marketing activities' (p. 370) based on designing branded content appropriate for the specific platform/user base, that will stimulate and maximise user *engagement*. This is a shift away from advertising that works by simply exposing the most people possible to commercial messages. The creation of branded content 'woven into the everyday mediation of drinking culture' (p. 370) becomes the key goal. Quality time spent engaging with brands becomes the focus, because it is the quality of engagement that is most useful as data for the algorithmic sorting and prioritising of marketing content.

Such 'post-exposure', engagement-driven uses of mobile social media by alcohol corporations increasingly permeate the design and use of various urban spaces such as bars, clubs and nightlife precincts more generally. These are more covert than traditional, 'exposure-driven' marketing practices. They mimic the user cultures developing on social media, draw directly on users' everyday identity-making processes and sociality and recruit users to do free work for alcohol brands (Carah et al., 2014; Niland et al., 2017). They are supplemented by alcohol companies' own developments in cutting-edge mobile technologies including augmented reality and immersive, interactive apps (Zaitsev, 2017). For example, *Heineken Live* is a Pokemon Go-style geolocative app based on gamification techniques that entices drinkers to obtain points towards drink/venue rewards during real-time socialising in the NTE. The effectiveness of such apps as marketing devices is currently unclear. Nevertheless, it does seem clear that they become co-constitutive of the new forms of drinking culture that we now need to understand.

Conclusions: Rethinking Young Adult Drinking in a Mobile Social Media Ecology

We have come a long way, in a relatively short period, in our understandings of the complex interrelationships between young adults, drinking and SNS. Established issues, such as the careful and considered curation of drinking identities on sites like Facebook, will continue to remain important and will continue to have cultural and health consequences. However, social media multiplicity and mobility produce a range of developments that are poorly understood at present. A more dynamic, real-time social media ecology is emerging that needs to be investigated more holistically, and in terms of its implications for new forms of identity work, sociality and social practices that occur while drinking is taking place in the NTE. This will help drinking-related SNS research develop a focus on new dimensions of young adults' social worlds and leisure practices. Taking account of how 'post-exposure' alcohol marketing and promotion work to co-constitute drinking cultures on mobile SNS will need to form a key part of this endeavour. Importantly, there are also methodological implications for any research seeking to understand new forms of young adult drinking in a mobile social media ecology. If we are to understand evolving forms of young adult drinking culture and their relationships to mobile SNS, we will need to continue to seek innovative ways of capturing and modelling the complexities involved, including young people's own practices and meaning-making (see Lyons, Goodwin, McCreanor, & Griffin, 2015).

References

Alhabash, S., VanDam, C., Tan, P. N., Smith, S. W., Viken, G., Kanver, D., … Figueira, L. (2018). 140 characters of intoxication: Exploring the prevalence of alcohol-related tweets and predicting their virality. *Sage Open, 8*, 1–15.

Atkinson, A. M., & Sumnall, H. R. (2016). 'If I don't look good, it just doesn't go up': A qualitative study of young women's drinking cultures and practices on Social Network Sites. *International Journal of Drug Policy, 38*, 50–62.

Bayer, J., Ellison, N., Schoenebeck, S., & Falk, E. (2016). Sharing the small moments: Ephemeral social interaction on Snapchat. *Information, Communication and Society, 19*(7), 956–977.

Bertel, T., & Ling, R. (2016). "It's just not that exciting anymore": The changing centrality of SMS in the everyday lives of young Danes. *New Media and Society, 18*(7), 1293–1309.

Beullens, K., & Schepers, A. (2013). Display of alcohol use on Facebook: A content analysis. *Cyberpsychology, Behaviour and Social Networking, 16*(7), 497–503.

Boczkowski, P., Matassi, M., & Mitchelstein, E. (2018). How young users deal with multiple platforms: The role of meaning-making in social media repertoires. *Journal of Computer Mediated Communication, 23*, 245–259.

Boyd, D. (2007). Why youth (heart) social network sites: The role of networked publics in teenage social life. In D. Buckingham (Ed.), *McArthur foundation series on digital learning: Youth, identity and digital media volume* (pp. 119–142). Cambridge, MA: MIT Press.

Boyle, S., Earle, A., LaBrie, J., & Ballou, K. (2017). Facebook dethroned: Revealing the more likely social media destinations for college students' depiction of underage drinking. *Addictive Behaviours, 65*, 63–67.

Bucher, T. (2018). *If… then: Algorithmic culture and politics.* Oxford, UK: Oxford University Press.

Bucher, T., & Helmond, A. (2017). The affordances of social media platforms. In J. Burgess, T. Poell, & A. Marwick (Eds.), *Sage handbook of social media* (pp. 233–253). New York: Sage.

Buehler, E. (2017). "You shouldn't use Facebook for that". Navigating norm violations while seeking emotional support on Facebook. *Social Media+ Society, 3*(3), 1–11.

Carah, N., Brodmerkel, S., & Hernandez, L. (2014). Brands and sociality: Alcohol branding, drinking culture and Facebook. *Convergence, 20*(3), 259–275.

Carah, N., & Meurk, C. (2017). We need a media platform perspective on alcohol marketing: A reply to Lobstein et al. *Addiction, 12*, 370–373.

Carah, N., & Shaul, M. (2016). Brands and Instagram: Point, tap, swipe, glance. *Mobile Media and Communication, 4*(1), 69–84.

Cavazos-Rehg, P., Krauss, M., Sowles, S., & Bierut, L. (2015). "Hey everyone, I'm drunk". An evaluation of drinking-related Twitter chatter. *Journal of Studies on Alcohol and Drugs, 76*(4), 635–643.

Cherrier, H., Carah, N., & Meurk, C. (2017). Social media affordances for curbing alcohol consumption. In A. C. Lyons, T. McCreanor, I. Goodwin, & H. Moewaka Barnes (Eds.), *Youth drinking cultures in a digital world* (pp. 167–184). London: Routledge.

Demant, J., & Landholt, S. (2014). Youth drinking in public places: The production of drinking spaces in and outside of nightlife areas. *Urban Studies, 51*(1), 170–184.

Egan, K. G., & Moreno, M. A. (2011). Alcohol references on undergraduate males' Facebook profiles. *American Journal of Men's Health, 5*(5), 413–420.

Frith, J. (2013). Turning life in to a game: Foursquare, gamification, and personal mobility. *Mobile Media and Communication, 1*(2), 248–262.

Goggin, G. (2012). The iPhone and communication. In L. Hjorth, J. Burgess, & I. Richardson (Eds.), *Studying mobile media* (pp. 11–27). London: Routledge.

Goodwin, I., & Griffin, C. (2017). Neoliberalism, alcohol, and identity. In A. C. Lyons, T. McCreanor, I. Goodwin, & H. Moewaka Barnes (Eds.), *Youth drinking cultures in a digital world* (pp. 15–30). London: Routledge.

Goodwin, I., Griffin, C., Lyons, A. C., McCreanor, T., & Moewaka Barnes, H. (2016). Precarious popularity: Facebook drinking photos, the attention economy, and the regime of the branded self. *Social Media+ Society, 2*(1), 1–13.

Griffin, C., Bengry-Howell, A., Hackley, C., Mistral, W., & Szmigin, I. (2009). 'Everytime I do it I absolutely annihilate myself': Loss of (self-) consciousness and loss of memory in young people's drinking narratives. *Sociology, 43*(3), 457–467.

Griffiths, R., & Casswell, S. (2010, September). Intoxigenic digital spaces? Youth, social networking sites and alcohol marketing. *Drug and Alcohol Review, 29*, 525–530.

Helmond, A. (2015). The platformization of the web: Making web data platform ready. *Social Media+ Society, 1*(2), 1–11.

Hendriks, H., den Putte, B., Winifed, A., & Moreno, M. (2018). Social drinking on social media: Content analysis of the social aspects of alcohol-related posts on Facebook and Instagram. *Journal of Medical Internet Research, 20*(6), 1–12.

Highfield, T., & Leaver, T. (2016). Instagrammatics and digital methods: Studying visual social media, from selfies and GIFs to memes and emoji. *Communication Research and Practice, 2*(1), 47–62.

Hutton, F., Griffin, C., Lyons, A. C., Niland, P., & McCreanot, T. (2016). "Tragic girls" and "crack whores": Alcohol, femininity and Facebook. *Feminism and Psychology, 26*(1), 73–93.

Ito, M., & Okabe, D. (2005). Technosocial situations: Emergent structuring of mobile e-mail use. In M. Ito, D. Okabe, & M. Matsuda (Eds.), *Personal, portable, pedestrian: Mobile phones in Japanese life* (pp. 257–276). Cambridge, MA: MIT Press.

Katz, J., & Aakhus, M. (2002). *Perpetual contact: Mobile communication, private talk, public performance.* Cambridge, UK: Cambridge University Press.

Lindsay, J., & Supski, S. (2017). Curating identity: Drinking, young women, femininities and social media practices. In A. C. Lyons, T. McCreanor, I. Goodwin, & H. Moewaka Barnes (Eds.), *Youth drinking cultures in a digital world* (pp. 49–65). London: Routledge.

Lobstein, T., Landon, J., Thornton, N., & Jernigan, D. (2017). The commercial use of digital media to market alcohol products: A narrative review. *Addiction, 112*(1), 21–27.

Lyons, A., & Willot, S. (2008). Alcohol consumption, gender identities and women's changing social positions. *Sex Roles, 59*(9–10), 694–715.

Lyons, A. C., Goodwin, I., McCreanor, T., & Griffin, C. (2015). Social networking and young adults' drinking practices: Innovative qualitative methods for health behavior research. *Health Psychology, 34*(4), 293–302.

Mackey, A. (2016). Sticky e/motional connections: Young people, social media, and the re-orientation of affect. *Safundi, 17*(2), 156–173.

Mart, S. (2017). New marketing, new policy? Emerging debates over regulating alcohol campaigns on social media. In A. C. Lyons, T. McCreanor, I. Goodwin, & H. Moewaka Barnes (Eds.), *Youth drinking cultures in a digital world* (pp. 218–219). London: Routledge.

McCreanor, T., Lyons, A. C., Griffin, C., Goodwin, I., Moewaka Barnes, H., & Hutton, F. (2013). Youth drinking cultures, social networking and alcohol marketing: Implications for public health. *Critical Public Health, 23*, 110–120.

Moewaka Barnes, H., Niland, P., Samu, L., Sciasia, A. D., & McCreanor, T. (2017). Ethnicity/culture, alcohol and social media. In A. C. Lyons, T. McCreanor, I. Goodwin, & H. Moewaka Barnes (Eds.), *Youth drinking cultures in a digital world* (pp. 80–98). London: Routledge.

Nicholls, J. (2012). Everyday, everywhere: Alcohol marketing and social media—Current trends. *Alcohol and Alcoholism, 47*(4), 486–493.

Niland, P., Lyons, A. C., Goodwin, I., & Hutton, F. (2013). "Everyone can loosen up and get a bit of a buzz on": Young adults, alcohol and friendship practices. *International Journal of Drug Policy, 24*(6), 530–537.

Niland, P., Lyons, A. C., Goodwin, I., & Hutton, F. (2014). 'See it doesn't look pretty does it?' Young adults' airbrushed drinking practices on Facebook. *Psychology and Health, 29*(8), 877–895.

Niland, P., Lyons, A. C., Goodwin, I., & Hutton, F. (2015). Friendship work on Facebook: Young adults' understandings and practices of friendship. *Journal of Community and Applied Social Psychology, 25*(2), 123–137.

Niland, P., McCreanor, T., Lyons, A. C., & Griffin, C. (2017). Alcohol marketing on social media: Young adults engage with alcohol marketing on Facebook. *Addiction Research & Theory, 25*(4), 273–284.

Rettie, R. (2009). Mobile phone communication: Extending Goffman to mediated interaction. *Sociology, 43*(3), 421–438.

Rose, G. (2014). On the relationship between 'visual research' and contemporary visual culture. *The Sociological Review, 62,* 24–46.

Stoddard, S. A., Bauermeister, J. A., Gordon-Messer, D., Johns, M., & Zimmerman, M. A. (2012). Permissive norms and young adults' alcohol and marijuana use: The role of online communities. *Journal of Studies on Alcohol and Drugs, 73,* 968–975.

Sujon, Z., Viney, L., & Toker-Turnalar, E. (2018). Domesticating Facebook: The shift from compulsive connection to personal service platform. *Social Media + Society, 4*(4), 1–12.

Thulin, E. (2017). Always on my mind: How Smartphones are transforming social contact among young Swedes. *Young, 26*(5), 1–19.

Truong, J. (2018). Attending to others: How digital technologies direct young people's nightlife. *Geographica Helvetica, 73,* 193–201.

van Dijck, J. (2013). *The culture of connectivity: A critical history of social media.* Oxford: Oxford University Press.

Wahl-Jorgensen, K. (2018). The emotional architecture of social media. In Z. Papacharissi (Ed.), *A networked self and platforms, stories, connections* (pp. 77–93). New York: Routledge.

Wilkinson, S. (2017). Drinking in the dark: Shedding light on young people's alcohol consumption experiences. *Social and Cultural Geography, 18*(6), 739–757.

Zaitsev, D. (2017, June 17). *It's not just the booze talking: How augmented reality brought wine and spirits to life.* Retrieved from https://blog.theroar.io/its-not-just-the-booze-talking-how-augmented-reality-brought-wine-and-spirits-to-life-dc256905ac7f.

Zhao, X., Lampe, C., & Ellison, N. B. (2016). The social media ecology: User perceptions, strategies and challenges. In *Proceedings of the 2016 CHI Conference on Human Factors in Computing Systems* (pp. 89–100). New York, NY: Association for Computing Machinery.

8

Friendship and Alcohol Use Among Young Adults: A Cross-Disciplinary Literature Review

Dominic Conroy and Sarah MacLean

Links between friendships and friendship groups, and drinking patterns and practices among young adults have emerged in recent years as a growing area of interest for social scientists from many disciplinary backgrounds. From a broader cultural perspective, and perhaps intuitively, friendship and alcohol use among young adults seem to be closely paired in that both evoke associations with intimacy, liberation, transition and collective identity. Drawing together the diverse body of theoretical and empirical published work in this area presents difficulties, partly given the varied ways in which the relationship between friendship and alcohol use/practice has been formulated and explored. This chapter adopts a cross-disciplinary, methodologically plural approach to synthesise findings and themes that have emerged from more recent work.

D. Conroy (✉)
School of Psychology, University of East London, London, UK
e-mail: D.Conroy@uel.ac.uk

S. MacLean
La Trobe University, Melbourne, VIC, Australia

© The Author(s) 2019
D. Conroy and F. Measham (eds.), *Young Adult Drinking Styles*,
https://doi.org/10.1007/978-3-030-28607-1_8

In the discipline of psychology, this relationship has typically been explored from a social-cognitive perspective in which the influence of friendship has been operationalised as 'normative influence' of peer members on young adult drinking patterns. For psychology researchers, friendship has traditionally been conceptualised as something measurable at an intra-individual level. More recently, psychological research concerning friendship has attempted to break free from disciplinary divisions and to explore friendship using a more contextualised framework for considering how features of friendship might be linked to young adult drinking practices. Meanwhile, focusing on the influence of broader social change on young people's sociable alcohol use, sociologists have traced how new patterns of binge drinking among groups of young people have emerged in the context of a burgeoning night-time economy in Western countries. In this context, heavy alcohol use has become part of how young women as well as young men engage with their friends. Thus, sociological (and also anthropological) writing on friendship in the context of alcohol consumption has focused on how alcohol use is knitted into young adult lives through the activities friends engage in together and as part of the social practices that make up friendship.

In this chapter, we provide a summary and discussion of literature concerning links between friendship and alcohol use among young adults from a cross-disciplinary perspective. We focus on research concerning friendships between young adults, defined here as individuals aged between 18 and 30 years. Rather than systematically reviewing the literature, we draw here on research and theory primarily from the disciplines of psychology and sociology which offer key illustrative insights into the complex connections between alcohol and friendship. Our approach was iterative; progressively defining parameters for the most meaningfully relevant empirical work. For example, research concerning the broader peer influence on drinking practices was understood as different and less relevant to exploring links between alcohol use within (or in the context of) established or emerging friendships and was, therefore, not included in our literature review. Excluded too were studies which focused on friendships in the context of particular subcultures (e.g. sports societies) on the basis that the main unit of focus in such studies tended to the subculture itself rather friendship stemming from subculture participation.

We first define friendship for the current purposes. We then present our review under two headings: 'How do friendships influence young adults' alcohol use?' and 'How does alcohol use shape friendships?' These headings are inevitably coarse in terms of how they group relevant studies, but the headings provide a meaningful, coherent way to disentangle key themes involved in research and discussion concerning friendship and alcohol use. Finally, we consider future areas for study and how research on alcohol use and friendship among young adults might be harnessed by practitioners, policymakers and researchers to promote sustained safe and moderate alcohol consumption among young adults as a demographic group.

Defining Friendship Among Young Adults

Friendship represents one type of intimate relationship between people but is difficult to define. Rawlins (2008) usefully defines friendship as a relationship that is voluntary (the relationship cannot be forced), mutual, personal (people are interested in each other because of who they uniquely are), affectionate (we care about the person), and likely to be equal (possibility of interacting as equals). Unlike relationships with family members or spouses, friendship is not based on blood ties and is unlikely to be characterised by formal agreements which indicate how we should behave or specify how long the relationship should endure (O'Connor, 1998). Although cultural norms regarding the behaviour of friends do exist (Badhwar, 2008; Bryant and Marmo, 2012), friends need to negotiate the parameters of a friendship, for example, to establish the degrees of care and trust that are expected or acceptable (Rawlins, 1992).

Friendships arguably hold particular value and meaning for young adults during a period that may include several key life stage transitions such as living independently, developing first sexual/romantic relationships, starting paid work and perhaps engaging in further education. It has been suggested that young adults are more likely to feel close to individuals they identity as close friends than to family members with whom the individual has close ties (Pulakos, 1989). Beyond these particular transitions, young adults may also be understood as working through issues relating to identity, values and position in the world (see Arnett 2000 for discussion of 'emerging adulthood'). Friendship may therefore have a distinctive role to play during young adulthood. Because of this, understanding interactions between friendships and practices like alcohol use are important for both theoretical reasons (to explain relationships between friendship and alcohol consumption) and practical reasons (to encourage moderate alcohol consumption among those who drink excessively).

'How Do Friendships Influence Young Adults' Alcohol Use?'

Sociologists and anthropologists have shown that attitudes and practices concerning alcohol and other drug use are often shared and reproduced within friendship groups (Mayock, 2002; Pilkington, 2007; Rúdólfsdóttir & Morgan, 2009). Quantitative studies identify relationships between drinking levels of individuals and those of friends and peers, both for teenagers (Ferguson and Meehan, 2010; Fujimoto & Valente, 2012a) and young adults (Overbeek et al., 2011). In this research, friends can be typically conceptualised as potential risk or protective factors for harmful drinking (Louis-Jacques, Knight, Sherrit, Van Hook, & Harris, 2012).

Psychological research conducted in a social-cognitive tradition has tended to involve the modelling and examination of characteristics of particular types of friendship as a moderating influence over alcohol and other drug use among young adults. For example, Boman, Stogner, and Miller (2013) explored the relationship between concordance in binge drinking within friendship dyads and friendship quality. Findings from this correlational research revealed that higher friendship quality, yet simultaneously higher levels of conflict, was evident among within friendship pairs of individuals who had relatively similar levels of binge drinking. Other studies have explored moderating effects of friendship on alcohol consumption in terms of whether individuals' ratings of how intimate their friendships are influences patterns of drinking behaviour. For example, Giese, Stok, and Renner (2017) found that how frequently students consumed alcohol was linked to whether or not peers reciprocated friendships: consumption frequency was similar between student and peer when friendship was reciprocated but was dissimilar when friendship was not reciprocated. Binge drinking, by contrast, was similar only in situations where friendship was not reciprocated. The authors concluded that young adults appear to use alcohol more strategically than can sometimes be assumed in conventional thinking and that heavy drinking practices may not be dependent on the perceived intimacy of the friendship. The studies summarised above help to illustrate the social-cognitive approach to exploring how friendship influences drinking behaviour. It is notable here that the social-cognitive approach to alcohol use within friendship groups has parallels with a broader tradition in psychological research of modelling the influence that peer and friendship groups have on individual behaviour. This is evident in terms like 'social contagion' (Fujimoto & Valente, 2012b), which often frame understanding in terms of the disruptive or pathological effect of groups/crowds on otherwise rational decision making on the part of the individual.

Relatively few studies explicitly explore the influence of friendship on alcohol use among young adults. This stands in contrast to the large number of studies of friendship influences over drinking behaviour in the context of early and middle adolescence. Such studies have described different aspects of friendship influence over alcohol use among adolescents. These studies include comparisons of alcohol consumption in established and newer friendships (Cheadle, Stevens, Williams, & Goosby, 2013); how friendship quality might have implications for drinking practices within mid-late adolescent friendships (Boman et al., 2013); studies of how offline and online friendships influence alcohol use among 15–16-year olds (Huang, Soto, Fujimoto, & Valente, 2014; Huang, Unger, et al., 2014), and explorations of how friendship characteristics moderate drinking behaviour among 12–14-year olds (Bot, Engels, Knibbe, & Meeus, 2005). Exploring these myriad factors in the context of drinking practices within friendships and friendship groups would be valuable in future research to understand how friendships might sustain and/or impinge on different drinking styles, habits and practices among young adults.

Considering associations between various characteristics of sociability and drinking patterns presents another way that the influence of friendship over drinking patterns can be considered. Leifman, Kühlhorn, Allebeck, Andreasson, and Romelsjø (1995) operationalised sociability using four measures: (in)security in others' company, number of close friends, extent to which an individual has intimate conversations with friends and an individual's relative popularity in their place of education. Measured in this way, lower levels of sociability have been demonstrated among Swedish 18–19-year-old alcohol abstainers relative to sociability among alcohol consumers of the same age (Leifman et al., 1995). Higher levels of dispositional sociability have been found to predict increased and decreased substance use among US and Canadian undergraduate students, respectively (Santesso, Schmidt, & Fox, 2004). This presents a contradictory picture in terms of how 'being sociable' (and hence, potentially, having a larger friendship group) might relate to drinking practices. Decisions around styles of drinking behaviour (e.g. whether to *not* drinking during a social occasion) may be conditional on the extent to which they open or close opportunities to initiate or deepen friendship bonds among young adults. For example, discursive research conducted among UK university students has suggested that student non-drinkers may be viewed as 'not joining in' with friends and that, relatedly, the possibility of not drinking might be rejected for fear of being understood as rejecting shared values when socialising with friends (Conroy & de Visser, 2013). Qualitative research can guide understanding of how friendship-linked qualities like sociability might underpin but also be contested within young adult drinking practices. Young adults aged 18–24 in MacLean (2016) discussed drinking at a similar pace to friends to 'keep up' and maintain a similar level of intoxication, suggesting that they would drink more in order to maintain a sense of connection with friends (an example of friendship influencing alcohol use). At the same time, the bodily effects of alcohol made them able to engage with friends and generate a sense of intimacy. These findings suggest that research attention needs to explore not just the mere presence of friends (or particular types of friend) that may be important to alcohol practices, but also to attend to temporal and embodied aspects of drinking practices which may permit or accelerate a particular type of intimacy or bonding experience. This is an example of alcohol's influence on friendship, which we explore in the next chapter section.

'How Does Alcohol Use Shape Friendships?'

To this point, we have largely considered how friendships might, in different ways, 'effect' distinct features of drinking practice among young adults including the overall quantity of alcohol consumed over time or the quantity of alcohol consumed during specific occasions. Models of cause and effect in psychological research can privilege one-way relationships in which intra-individual properties are understood to causally influence subsequent behaviour. Such accounts hold clear advantages, but risk losing much detail about social phenomena. Arguably, this is particularly true in the case of understanding alcohol-friendship relationships, where a growing body of evidence (both qualitative and quantitative) points to complex and, as discussed in the previous section, reciprocal or co-constituted 'effects' between friendship characteristics and dynamics and alcohol practices and patterns of consumption. Qualitative research exploring alcohol use in the context of friendship can partly be understood as a response to the sometimes crude approach taken by alcohol harm reduction strategies and scepticism about the extent to which such approaches offer the possibility of real-world change in alcohol consumption practices among young adults.

Social scientists have long been interested in identifying norms that guide people's actions. For example, MacArthur, Jacob, Pound, Hickman, and Campbell (2017) show how an expectation to drink heavily can be policed within friendship groups. Normative expectations of gendered behaviour also strongly influence how young people drink with friends, with particular kinds of toxic or hyper-masculinity associated with aggression and violence (Peralta, 2007). Researchers have shown how wider social and economic structures frame both alcohol consumption and friendships. Groups of friends enact gendered and classed subjectivities through drinking (Griffin, Bengry-Howell, Hackley, Mistral, & Szmigin, 2009; Measham, 2002; Measham & Brain, 2005) with the alcohol-dominated night-time economy providing the setting for many young adults' leisure. Alcohol and its availability and price influence how young people socialise with their friends. UK millennials may structure a night out to enable the consumption of relatively cheaper off-licensed sales of alcohol at someone's house before they visit a licensed venue (termed 'preloading' or 'predrinking'). We note here that the growth of predrinking is historically and culturally very context specific. From a UK perspective, the price difference between licensed and off-licensed sales was negligible in the twentieth century, but predrinking (i.e. consuming alcohol drinks purchased in off-licensed settings at home) might be explained as a twenty-first-century phenomenon in the context of increasingly and relatively cheaper off-licensed sales compared to licensed sales (Institute of Alcohol Studies, 2017). While saving money appears to have emerged as one important driver for predrinking in the UK, the opportunity to spend time with friends before going out is also important. This close relationship between the availability and pricing of alcohol and young adult's engagements with friends has been evidenced in a range of international settings including Australia (MacLean & Callinan, 2013).

Research has also demonstrated the opportunities and pleasures experienced among young adults when drinking with friends and within friendship groups. For example, studies have shown how alcohol helps people generate and enjoy a sense of connection with others (e.g., Brain et al., 2000; Peralta, 2007; Törrönen & Maunu, 2007). Drinking practices have been recognised as an important catalyst for particular kinds of emotional connection that can emerge between young adults while socialising, and such connections can be closely linked with the quality of their relationships and interactions. Törrönen and Maunu (2011) explore how pride (a sense of attachment to friends) and shame (feeling excluded) experienced in relation to drinking can reinforce or undermine friendships and also serve to promote particular models and ways of talking about friendship. Friendships can be damaged or destroyed when people behave inappropriately when drunk; for example, requiring excessive levels of care, or demonstrating too much intimacy (MacLean, 2016; MacLean, Pennay, & Room, 2018).

Other research has helped develop understanding of how friendship contexts beyond the immediate boundaries of a particular drinking occasion warrant greater understanding and exploration. For example, accounts of hangovers experienced among Norwegian young adults aged 18–23 drew attention to how hangovers act as a narrative form of closure to the experience of a party which may hold implications for the emotional and social bonds that are forged within friendship groups (Fjær, 2012).

This may be manifest in collective activities (e.g. all going out for breakfast together), which involve recollections, and evidence of teasing which has been discussed as a way of 'practicing intimacy' within friendships (Keltner, Capps, Kring, Young, & Heerey, 2001: 236). Others describe how this narrating drinking events through social media such as Facebook and Instagram reinforces friendship ties (Brown & Gregg, 2012; Griffin et al., 2009; Tutenges & Sandberg, 2013). Thus, young adults use social media to disseminate a record of their friendships to others, with alcohol signifying the pleasure, intimacy and sociability they shared.

Articulating how alcohol consumption is embedded in 'friendship practices' enables researchers to consider alcohol consumption and friendship-making as co-constitutive in the production of social relationships and identities. For example, focus group research from New Zealand highlights the pleasures and sociability made possible by alcohol consumption among young adults, showing how discourses about the effects of alcohol and how alcohol should be consumed enable young adults to 'do' friendship (Niland, Lyons, Goodwin, & Hutton, 2013). This discursive research suggested that positive features of drinking (e.g. enjoying friendships, supporting each other) were invoked rhetorically to offset negative aspects of drinking experiences. Such findings hold important implications for how health promotion/harm reduction messages are conceived and delivered, suggesting that messages focused purely on risk reduction are unlikely to strike a chord with young adults able to neutralise and reject such messages.

Building on this argument, MacLean (2016) argues that drinking alcohol together is a key means by which young people in the contemporary West produce and reproduce, friendships; or in other words that alcohol use is a crucible though which friendships are forged. Drawing on the sociological argument that friendships must be continually reproduced through sets of practices (Pahl, 2000)—she proposes that drinking enables young adults to generate a sense of intimacy and demonstrate trust in each other, both of which are hallmarks of contemporary friendship relationships. Young people are also able to negotiate the unclear parameters of friendship though alcohol use—by providing care for friends when they are out, with men and women sometimes holding different expectations about what this entails. The critical role of alcohol in constituting young adults' friendships may go some way towards explaining the persistence of heavy drinking within this demographic.

Research concerning alcohol abstinence has provided important insights into the status and symbolic power of alcohol as an often-present device relevant to contexts where young adults have opportunities to make friends or where there are opportunities to consolidate intimacy within established friendships or groups of friends. Interview research with UK undergraduates has suggested that not drinking can limit opportunities to forge new friendships during socially intense periods like 'Fresher's week' (Jacobs, Conroy, & Parke, 2018), but may also play a role in 'knowing which friends care about you' and therefore guide recognition of which friendships are worth pursuing (Conroy & de Visser, 2014). Discerning the genuineness of emerging friendships has been reported as a key concern for non-/light-drinking young adults when interacting with alcohol-consuming peers in several qualitative studies involving university students (Conroy & de Visser, 2015; Jacobs et al., 2018). Non-drinking therefore provided a range of issues for young adults in terms of diminished opportunities to make friends or sustain friendships; but also in providing a basis for new standards or criteria about the kinds of friendship that might be desirable.

While it is possible to trace unidirectional relationships between alcohol and friendship, with heavier drinkers engaged in different friendship practices (MacLean, Pennay, Room, 2018) and friendships with heavier drinkers producing higher consumption levels in individuals, these relationships are inevitably complex and interactional. Alcohol and friendship-making have emerged in recent sociological research as part of a configuration of factors—including the night-time economy, work, family, education and discourses of selfhood, that inform young adult's contemporary experiences, understandings and actions. One ongoing commitment for future qualitative research seems likely to involve maintaining an explicit acknowledgement of the inherent tension involved in producing a narrative account that successfully articulates these 'pros' and 'cons' that different kinds of drinking practice hold for young adult friendships.

Areas for Future Research and Application

Empirical work discussed in this chapter draws attention to scope for more, and more diverse, research concerning alcohol use and friendships. The literature reviewed here is overwhelmingly located in Western countries, and even here mostly in English speaking or Scandinavian contexts. Friendships are historically and culturally variable but also vary within cultural settings—for example, drinking together and drunkenness among Icelandic young adults were found to signify diverse types of connection between people (Pinson, 1985). We need to understanding how dynamics between alcohol and friendships operate within groups of young adults from diverse cultural backgrounds living in developed countries. Investigation of the relationship between alcohol and contemporary patterns of sociality in low- and middle-income countries is sorely needed, particularly as some alcohol companies aggressively market their products to emerging markets. Future research could further explore whether alcohol's role in initiating and maintaining friendships differs for young men and women and sexual minority young people.

Growing numbers of young people now drink less than previous age cohorts (e.g. Pennay, Livingston, & MacLean, 2015 and see also Chapters 2 and 3 in this collection). Further research designed to explore how contemporary friendship operates among friendship groups reflecting heterogeneous styles of drinking practice (e.g. lighter drinkers; heavier drinkers; people who do not drink) presents another route for extending the present literature. For example, in light of some suggestion that drinkers may experience non-drinkers present during a social occasion as judgmental (Conroy & de Visser, 2013), future research might usefully investigate the degree of consensus and conflict that different drinking styles may pose for established/emerging friendships or within friendship groups. Seffrin (2012) usefully explored how members of ethnic groups, where heavy drinking is less culturally prevalent, frame friendships or resist the imperative to drink with friends. New studies drawing on experiences of these individuals would be useful. The relationships between friendship, friendship groups and alcohol practices are increasingly recognised as complex and multifaceted. Exploring clearly defined causal pathways between aspects of friendship and alcohol practices may therefore by misjudged. With that caveat acknowledged, there is scope for more advanced quantitative designs to explore reciprocal pathways between characteristics of friendship (e.g. historical length of friendship; perceived quality of friendship) and different features of drinking belief and drinking practice. Such work might draw on relatively ambitious quantitative designs adopted in previous research modelling reciprocal effects of alcohol use and friendship among 12–14 year olds (Sieving, Perry, & Williams, 2000).

Many studies explore friendship dynamics in relation to alcohol use among youth (e.g. aged 11–17 years). Given the links identified in the extant literature between alcohol practices and accessing friendship intimacy, expanding friendship groups and as a resource for managing life stress within close friendships, greater efforts to understand synergies between alcohol use and friendships among young adults are important in the interests of producing effective and realistic harm reduction strategies designed to promote sustainable moderate alcohol practices. Future research concerning alcohol use over the lifespan might involve exploring alcohol's differential and/or similar role in friendships for individuals at different life stages. Recent qualitative research concerning alcohol use among middle-aged Scots women and men has underscored alcohol's multifaceted role in producing and consolidating friendships (Emslie, Hunt, & Lyons, 2013, 2015). Such work provides an important reference point to guide the development of research which can link alcohol practices among young adults to alcohol practices at later points in life. For example, members of sexual minority groups maintain a higher average alcohol consumption as they move into middle age (MacLean et al., 2018). One specific future research focus is to explore opportunities and impediments that might be found among gay, lesbian or bisexual young adults for making connections within their communities with reduced reliance on alcohol.

Health promotion messages and interventions should place greater emphasis on the important role of alcohol within friendships to promote more moderate alcohol consumption among young people and young adults. In a policy environment that relies heavily on promoting individual self-management of drinking, measures to support people to look after friends at social occasions involving alcohol have potential to make an important contribution to reducing alcohol-related harms. This seems to be particularly needed for young men, who may, for wide-ranging reasons, be more constrained in providing care to their friends when drinking together than are young women (MacLean, 2016; MacArthur et al., 2017). Research reviewed above has shown how health promotion messages can be digested or processed within friendship groups. Research has suggested that friendships may act as effective micro-climates for fostering resistance to health promotion messages concerning dangers of harmful drinking or the importance of moderate drinking. For example, one study has pointed to displays of skill and resourcefulness within young adult friendship groups in terms of how they manage to ignore and reject health promotion messages concerning the dangers of high levels of alcohol consumption (de Visser, Wheeler, Abraham, & Smith, 2013; Niland et al., 2013). From a risk-based model of young adult drinking, developing understanding of how the unique properties of friendship groups might serve to moderate the effectiveness or visibility of alcohol-related health promotion messages and should be another important focus for future research. From a pleasure-based model of young adult drinking, further research can help provide new and contemporary insights into sociable and celebratory drinking too.

The intersection between social media use, drinking practices and friendship is a growing field of research that warrants more research attention (please consult Chapters 6 and 7 of this collection for discussion of themes in this emergent subfield of alcohol research). In advocating more research in this area, we should briefly acknowledge that the alcohol industry is quick to capitalise on the importance of alcohol in friendship practices, for example, by inserting alcohol advertising into social media outlets typically used by young adults to interact (McCreanor, Barnes, Gregory, Kaiwai, & Borell, 2005). Rather than simply using social media as a host for advertisements, alcohol companies harness the interactive potential of platforms such as Facebook to engage young adults by sharing images of people drinking together and encouraging comments that reinforce the centrality of alcohol to social life. Young people who identify with images and identities spread in this way may go onto share content with friends, effectively becoming collaborators in alcohol promotions. Thus, social media allows alcohol producers to engage 'young drinkers in a continuous incorporation of the brand into their everyday life, peer networks, identity and cultural experiences' (Brodmerkel & Carah, 2013, p. 277). More stringent regulation of alcohol industry use of social media is imperative to a comprehensive response to the embedding of alcohol into friendship practices.

Conclusion

In this chapter, we have reviewed empirical work concerning friendships and alcohol practices/use among young adults. Adopting a cross-disciplinary, methodologically inclusive approach has allowed us to consider a wide range of interweaving issues involved in alcohol consumption in the context of current or emerging friendships among young adults. Many (but not all) psychological studies exploring links between friendship and alcohol practices have involved quantitative methods designed to test causal pathways or associations. This has helped us to refine understanding of the close nexus between friendships and individual drinking patterns. Sociological studies, many of which entail qualitative explorations, highlight the complex embeddedness of alcohol in social life and relationships in the contemporary era. Together, both approaches reinforce the importance of considering the impact of friendships on the reception and uptake of health promotion and the efficacy of other interventions such as restrictions on advertising and alcohol availability. We hope that this initial literature review will help to generate further work in this important but poorly integrated area of social science research.

References

Arnett, J. J. (2000). Emerging adulthood: A theory of development from the late teens through the twenties. *American Psychologist, 55*(5), 469–480.

Badhwar, N. K. (2008). Friendship and commercial societies. *Politics, Philosophy & Economics, 7*(3), 301–326.

Boman, J. H., Stogner, J., & Miller, B. L. (2013). Binge drinking, marijuana use, and friendships: The relationship between similar and dissimilar usage and friendship quality. *Journal of Psychoactive Drugs, 45*(3), 218–226.

Bot, S. M., Engels, R. E., Knibbe, R. A., & Meeus, W. J. (2005). Friend's drinking behaviour and adolescent alcohol consumption: The moderating role of friendship characteristics. *Addictive Behaviors, 30*(5), 929–947.

Brain, K., Parker, H., & Carnwath, T. (2000). Drinking with design: Young drinkers as psychoactive consumers. *Drugs: Education, Prevention and Policy, 7*(1), 5–20.

Brodmerkel, S., & Carah, N. (2013). Alcohol brands on Facebook: The challenges of regulating brands on social media. *Journal of Public Affairs, 13*(3), 272–281.

Brown, R., & Gregg, M. (2012). The pedagogy of regret: Facebook, binge drinking and young women. *Continuum: Journal of Media & Cultural Studies, 26*(3), 357–369.

Bryant, E. M., & Marmo, J. (2012). The rules of Facebook friendship: A two-stage examination of interaction rules in close, casual, and acquaintance friendships. *Journal of Social & Personal Relationships, 29*(8), 1013–1035.

Cheadle, J. E., Stevens, M., Williams, D. T., & Goosby, B. J. (2013). The differential contributions of teen drinking homophily to new and existing friendships: An empirical assessment of assortative and proximity selection mechanisms. *Social Science Research, 42*(5), 1297–1310.

Conroy, D., & de Visser, R. O. (2013). 'Man up!': Discursive constructions of non-drinkers among UK undergraduates. *Journal of Health Psychology, 18*(11), 1432–1444.

Conroy, D., & de Visser, R. O. (2014). Being a non-drinking student: An interpretative phenomenological analysis. *Psychology & Health, 29*(5), 536–551.

Conroy, D., & de Visser, R. O. (2015). The importance of authenticity for student non-drinkers: An interpretative phenomenological analysis. *Journal of Health Psychology, 20*(11), 1483–1493.

de Visser, R. O., Wheeler, Z., Abraham, C., & Smith, J. A. (2013). 'Drinking is our modern way of bonding' Young people's beliefs about interventions to encourage moderate drinking. *Psychology & Health, 28*(12), 1460–1480.

Emslie, C., Hunt, K., & Lyons, A. (2013). The role of alcohol in forging and maintaining friendships amongst Scottish men in midlife. *Health Psychology, 32*(1), 33–41.

Emslie, C., Hunt, K., & Lyons, A. (2015). Transformation and time-out: The role of alcohol in identity construction among Scottish women in early midlife. *International Journal of Drug Policy, 26*(5), 437–445.

Ferguson, C. J., & Meehan, D. C. (2010). Original article: With friends like these…: Peer delinquency influences across age cohorts on smoking, alcohol and illegal substance use. *European Psychiatry, 26*, 6–12.

Fjær, E. G. (2012). The day after drinking: Interaction during hangovers among young Norwegian adults. *Journal of Youth Studies, 15*(8), 995–1010.

Fujimoto, K., & Valente, T. W. (2012a). Decomposing the components of friendship and friends' influence on adolescent drinking and smoking. *Journal of Adolescent Health, 51*(2), 136–143.

Fujimoto, K., & Valente, T. W. (2012b). Social network influences on adolescent substance use: Disentangling structural equivalence from cohesion. *Social Science and Medicine, 74*(12), 1952–1960.

Giese, H., Stok, F. M., & Renner, B. (2017). The role of friendship reciprocity in university freshmen's alcohol consumption. *Applied Psychology: Health and Well-Being, 9*(2), 228–241.

Griffin, C., Bengry-Howell, A., Hackley, C., Mistral, W., & Szmigin, I. (2009). 'Every time I do it I absolutely annihilate myself': Loss of (self-)consciousness and loss of memory in young people's drinking narratives. *Sociology, 43*(3), 457–476.

Huang, G. C., Soto, D., Fujimoto, K., & Valente, T. W. (2014). The interplay of friendship networks and social networking sites: Longitudinal analysis of selection and influence effects on adolescent smoking and alcohol use. *American Journal of Public Health, 104*(8), e51–e59.

Huang, G. C., Unger, J. B., Soto, D., Fujimoto, K., Pentz, M. A., Jordan-Marsh, M., & Valente, T. W. (2014). Peer influences: The impact of online and offline friendship networks on adolescent smoking and alcohol use. *Journal of Adolescent Health, 54*(5), 508–514.

Institute of Alcohol Studies. (2017). *How has the cost of alcohol changed over time?* Retrieved 5 June 2019 http://www.ias.org.uk/Alcohol-knowledge-centre/Price/Factsheets/How-has-the-cost-of-alcohol-changed-over-time.aspx.

Jacobs, L., Conroy, D., & Parke, A. (2018). Negative experiences of non-drinking college students in Great Britain: An interpretative phenomenological analysis. *International Journal of Mental Health and Addiction, 16*, 737–750.

Keltner, D., Capps, L., Kring, A. M., Young, R. C., & Heerey (2001). Just teasing: A conceptual analysis and empirical review. *Psychological Bulletin, 127*(2), 229–248.

Leifman, H., Kühlhorn, E., Allebeck, P., Andreasson, S., & Romelsjø, A. (1995). Abstinence in late adolescence: Antecedents to and covariates of a sober lifestyle and its consequences. *Social Science and Medicine, 41*(1), 113–121.

Louis-Jacques, J., Knight, J., Sherrit, L., Van Hook, S., & Harris, S. (2012). Do risky friends matter? Comparing the effect of a primary care alcohol intervention by whether friends drink. *Journal of Adolescent Health, 50*(2, Suppl.), S13–S14.

MacArthur, G. J., Jacob, N., Pound, P., Hickman, M., & Campbell, R. (2017). Among friends a qualitative exploration of the role of peers in young people's alcohol use using Bourdieu's concepts of habitus, field and capital. *Sociology of Health & Illness, 39*(1), 30–46.

MacLean, S. (2016). Alcohol and the constitution of friendship for young adults. *Sociology, 50*(1), 93–108.

MacLean, S., & Callinan, S. (2013). "Fourteen dollars for one beer!" Pre-drinking is associated with high-risk drinking among Victorian young adults. *Australian and New Zealand Journal of Public Health, 37*(6), 579–585.

MacLean, S., Pennay, A., & Room, R. (2018). 'You're repulsive': Limits to acceptable drunken comportment for young adults. *The International Journal of Drug Policy, 53*, 106–112.

MacLean, S., Savic, M., Pennay, A., Dwyer, R., Stanesby, O., & Wilkinson, C. (2018). Middle-aged same-sex attracted women and the social practice of drinking. *Critical Public Health*, 1–12.

Mayock, P. (2002). Drug pathways, transitions and decisions: The experiences of young people in an inner-city Dublin community. *Contemporary Drug Problems, 29*(Spring), 117–156.

McCreanor, T., Barnes, H. M., Gregory, M., Kaiwai, H., & Borell, S. (2005). Consuming identities: Alcohol marketing and the commodification of youth experience. *Addiction Research & Theory, 13*(6), 579–590.

Measham, F. (2002). "Doing gender"—"Doing drugs": Conceptualizing the gendering of drugs cultures. *Contemporary Drug Problems, 29*(2), 335–373.

Measham, F., & Brain, K. (2005). 'Binge' drinking, British alcohol policy and the new culture of intoxication. *Crime Media Culture, 1*(3), 262–283.

Niland, P., Lyons, A. C., Goodwin, I., & Hutton, F. (2013). 'Everyone can loosen up and get a bit of a buzz on': Young adults, alcohol and friendship practices. *International Journal of Drug Policy, 24*(6), 530–537.

O'Connor, P. (1998). Women's friendships in a post-modern world. In R. G. Adams & G. Allan (Eds.), *Placing friendship in context* (pp. 117–135). Cambridge: Cambridge University Press.

Overbeek, G., Bot, S. M., Meeus, W. H. J., Sentse, M., Knibbe, R. A., & Engels, R. (2011). Where it's at! The role of best friends and peer group members in young adults' alcohol use. *Journal of Research on Adolescence (Blackwell Publishing Limited), 21*(3), 631–638.

Pahl, R. (2000). *On Friendship*. Cambridge: Polity Press.

Pennay, A., Livingston, M., & MacLean, S. (2015). Young people are drinking less: It is time to find out why. *Drug and Alcohol Review, 34*(2), 115–118.

Peralta, R. (2007). College alcohol use and the embodiment of hegemonic masculinity among European American men. *Sex Roles, 56*(11/12), 741–756.

Pilkington, H. (2007). In good company: Risk, security and choice in young people's drug decisions. *The Sociological Review, 55*(2), 373–392.

Pinson, A. (1985). The institution of friendship and drinking patterns in Iceland. *Anthropological Quarterly, 58*, 75–82.

Pulakos, J. (1989). Young adult relationships: Siblings and friends. *The Journal of Psychology, 123*(3), 237–244.

Rawlins, W. K. (1992). *Friendship matters: Communication, dialectics, and the life course.* New York: Aldine de Gruyter.

Rawlins, W. K. (2008). *The compass of friendship: Narratives, identities, and dialogues.* Thousand Oaks: Sage.

Rúdólfsdóttir, A. G., & Morgan, P. (2009). 'Alcohol is my friend': Young middle class women discuss their relationship with alcohol. *Journal of Community & Applied Social Psychology, 19*(6), 492–505.

Santesso, D. L., Schmidt, L. A., & Fox, N. A. (2004). Are shyness and sociability still a dangerous combination for substance use? Evidence from a US and Canadian sample. *Personality and Individual Differences, 37*(1), 5–17.

Seffrin, P. (2012). Alcohol use among black and white adolescents: Exploring the influence of interracial friendship, the racial composition of peer groups, and communities. *The Sociological Quarterly, 53*(4), 610–635.

Sieving, R., Perry, C., & Williams, C. (2000). Do friendships change behaviors, or do behaviors change friendships? Examining paths of influence in young adolescents' alcohol use. *Journal of Adolescent Health, 26*(1), 27–35.

Törrönen, J., & Maunu, A. (2007). Light transgression and heavy sociability: Alcohol in young adult Finns' narratives of a night out. *Addiction Research & Theory, 15*(4), 365–381.

Törrönen, J., & Maunu, A. (2011). Friendship and social emotions in young adult Finns' drinking diaries. *Sociological Research Online, 16*(1), 4.

Tutenges, S., & Sandberg, S. (2013). Intoxicating stories: The characteristics, contexts and implications of drinking stories among Danish youth. *International Journal of Drug Policy, 24*(6), 538–544.

9

Gender in Young Adult's Discourses of Drinking and Drunkenness

Alexandra Bogren

Introduction

In many parts of the world, alcohol has been assigned gendered meanings throughout the twentieth century. For example, it has been considered a threat to femininity but central and even essential to masculinity. However, societal shifts during the last 30–40 years have introduced further layers of complexity to these meanings. The emergence and further development of consumer society and third-wave feminism and an ongoing health policy interest in risk groups seem to have affected the forms and patterns of drinking that are now seen as socially acceptable. Using examples from Sweden, this chapter presents and discusses current international research on the gendered discourses of young adults' drinking in the context of some of these shifts. Broadly defined, discourses are culturally and historically specific ways of signifying the world or particular aspects of it. Thus, discourses identified as dominant in Sweden in the 1990s may not be

---

A. Bogren (✉)
School of Social Sciences, Södertörn University, Stockholm, Sweden
e-mail: alexandra.bogren@sh.se

© The Author(s) 2019
D. Conroy and F. Measham (eds.), *Young Adult Drinking Styles*,
https://doi.org/10.1007/978-3-030-28607-1_9

173

dominant in other parts of the world or other times. Since they are not inherently fixed or stable, discourses also shift over time within specific domains and contexts.

In general, historical research shows that the forms and patterns of drinking considered socially acceptable for women and men vary over time and according to social class. For example, in England, Warner (1997) traces the emergence of "temperance as a feminine virtue" back to the early sixteenth century, while in Sweden a similar ideal seems to have appeared around the nineteenth century (Enefalk, 2015). This feminine low or non-drinking style gradually came to be linked with respectable, bourgeois femininity, a doctrine embraced by the higher strata of society (Enefalk, 2015; Warner, 1997). In this way, drinking served as a symbol of the moral status and respectability of an actor or social group. In contemporary societies, this normative aspect of alcohol consumption is articulated both in social interaction (face-to-face and in various forms of communication using digital technologies) and in cultural representations aimed at larger audiences, such as official documents, advertising, and media texts. Stories and images that reach large audiences have a specific position when it comes to the diffusion and negotiation of social norms because, unlike direct interaction with peers, they allow people access to information about the actions of large numbers of spatially and temporally dispersed others. In communicating such information, stories and images contribute to shaping our views of drinking among young adults.

This chapter is designed to present an overview of literature concerning the gendering of drinking and drunkenness in discourse. This includes discussion of research that has revealed drinking discourses that problematize and celebrate drinking in relation to femininity and masculinity among young adults. Future research suggestions are included in the final chapter section.

Studying Gendered Discourses of Drinking and Drunkenness

Discourse is a complex and contested concept. It may refer to speech and discussion in general, as well as to a specific verbal presentation of a topic

9 Gender in Young Adult's Discourses of Drinking and Drunkenness 175

but may also refer specifically to spoken language in contrast to written texts. Foucault understands discourse to refer to a historically contingent social system that produces ways of naming, understanding, and acting in relation to a phenomenon (e.g. addiction) within a certain type of institutionalized practice (e.g. biomedical science) (Titscher, Meyer, Wodak, & Vetter, 2000). Discursive research can involve the study of how discourse unfolds in naturally occurring talk but also how broader patterns of societal or political discourse can be revealed from analysing other kinds of textual data such as official documents, media representations, and organizational minutes (Howarth, 2000). These different approaches tend to either see social actors as *users* of discourse, or to see subjectivity—and by way of extension, agency—as *constituted* in discourse (Bacchi, 2005). In this chapter, I adopt a synthetic approach that draws on both discursive psychology (e.g. Potter & Wetherell, 1987) and critical discourse analysis (e.g. Carvalho, 2008). In doing so, I am acknowledging that actors can use discourses and sometimes do so strategically, but that use is constrained both by the cultural resources available to them and by the social context in which they are situated.

A gendered discourse refers to a discourse that in one way or another emphasizes gender difference or relies on gender as a category that is central to understanding drinking practices. Textual examples include repeated patterns of address (e.g. specifically addressing women or men, or using gendered personal pronouns) or repeated mention of gender differences. In this chapter, I adopt the position that alcohol norms and discourses on alcohol can become more or less gendered over time.

Four Key Emergent Gendered Discourses from a Swedish Perspective

Despite the common perception of Swedish gender equality, researchers have questioned the extent to which gender equality permeates all sectors of society. For example, the Swedish labour market is comparatively gender-segregated, and men are clearly over-represented in top wage positions in the business elite (Bihagen, Nermo, & Stern, 2014). Researchers have also identified differences in gender equality discourses between

Nordic countries. In a study of elite perceptions, Teigen and Wängnerud (2009: 29) found that radical feminism—which sees "gender differences as caused by patriarchal structures, where men as a group dominate women as a group"—was more dominant in Sweden, while liberal feminism—"an individualist-centred perspective, based on claims for equal rights"—was more dominant in Norway. By contrast, public debate about alcohol has been preoccupied with the idea that gender equality has "gone too far". From the 1990s to the 2010s, discourses of drinking in Sweden and elsewhere in northern Europe have been shaped by this criticism of gender equality and by the notion of post-feminism—the idea that gender equality is already achieved and therefore feminism is outdated (Månsson & Bogren, 2014). Within post-feminist discourse, agency and choice are central, for example in the sense that an interest in beauty and fashion is a sign of empowerment and independence rather than symptomatic of patriarchal oppression. This period has also seen a general cultural and political shift towards consumer culture and market liberalism (Measham & Brain, 2005) and a health policy interest in risk groups, especially young people and women. In the alcohol and drugs field, a growing body of evidence has supported more nuanced and situated understandings of public discourses around women's drug use, for example how discourses can position women's drinking as risky, pleasurable, or post-feminist (Campbell & Ettorre, 2011; Henderson, 1999; Månsson & Bogren, 2014; Measham, 2002).

What follows in the remainder of this chapter are four key discourses that emerge from the literature: a problematizing discourse of risky drinking; a celebratory discourse of pleasurable drinking; a discourse of drinking, assertiveness, and aggression; and a discourse of drinking, respectability, and class.

Risky Drinking: Gender and Risk in Discourses of Young Adults' Alcohol Consumption

Governmental reports, policy guidelines, and news reports tend to emphasize the risks of drinking. A common objective is often to educate or warn the public about the downsides and dangers of alcohol. When gender is

9 Gender in Young Adult's Discourses of Drinking and Drunkenness

brought to the fore in these materials, it is often equated with women. This is visible in several ways. Firstly, official documents, policy guidelines, and news reports frequently describe girls and women, but not boys and men, as groups at risk of high levels of alcohol consumption, excessive in-occasion drinking, and/or adverse consequences of drinking (Abrahamsson & Heimdahl, 2010; Bogren, 2011a; Day, Gough, & McFadden, 2004; Månsson & Bogren, 2014). This happens even though there are good reasons to consider men's drinking risky; e.g., men binge drink more than women (Wilsnack, Wilsnack, Gmel, & Wolfgang Kantor, 2018) and are at a higher risk of alcohol-related mortality (Rosén & Haglund, 2018). Secondly, newspapers explicitly address women using gendered personal pronouns, but much more seldom address men this way (Månsson & Bogren, 2014). Thirdly, information and news reporting often describe women as more biologically vulnerable to alcohol than men (Bogren, 2011b; Keane, 2017). For example, alcohol's effects on ovulation, menstruation, pregnancy, and levels of oestrogen in female bodies are described, but only very rarely are similar references made to alcohol's effect on gonadal hormones and reproductive capacity among men.

Drinking and intoxication are presented as risky for women in multiple ways. In summary, alcohol is constructed as a reproductive risk; a risk to one's physical appearance; a sexual risk; a social risk (the risk of losing one's status and reputation); and a health risk. Research shows that the media discusses all these risks in reporting on young adult women's drinking and that health, reproduction, and sexual risks (e.g. sexually transmitted diseases and sexual victimization) are recurrent themes in policy documents as well (Abrahamsson & Heimdahl, 2010; Bogren, 2011a; Day et al., 2004; Keane, 2013; Lyons, Dalton, & Hoy, 2006). Central to these portrayals are discourses of gender difference, gender equality, and health understood as a biological phenomenon (Månsson & Bogren, 2014). Media debaters in particular argue that young women's alcohol consumption is a sign of the problems of gender equality. They claim that young women "drink like men" because gender equality discourse has led them to believe that they can do so. On the contrary, according to these debaters, women must accept biological sex differences in alcohol tolerance in order to stay healthy.

In the UK, media debate about millennial young women's alcohol consumption was particularly persecutory towards women who presumably "drink like men". Labelled "ladettes", they were described as "crude", "aggressive", and "sexually loose" (e.g. Day et al., 2004; Griffin, Szmigin, Bengry-Howell, Hackley, & Mistral, 2013; Lyons et al., 2006; Skeggs, 2005). These debates in the Swedish media have not been as openly critical and condemning as in the British media. However, there is evidence of moralizing criticism in journalist accounts of women's drinking behaviour in Sweden too, often taking an assuming position that "party girls" or women who "drink like men" put themselves at risk of sexual assault (Bernhardsson & Bogren, 2012; Bogren, 2011a).

Celebratory Discourses of Pleasurable Drinking Among Young Adult Women

In advertising and women's magazines, drinking is primarily constructed as a project of pleasure, liberation, and freedom of choice for women rather than as a gendered risk (Beccaria, Rolando, Törrönen, & Scavarda, 2018; Lyons et al., 2006; Månsson, 2014). In the 1990s and early 2000s, these media outlets depict women's drinking as trendy, cool, and professional, addressing the audience primarily as potential consumers (Lyons et al., 2006; Månsson, 2014).

Discourses that conceptualize women's drinking as pleasurable do this in several ways. One aspect is the portrayal of drinking as a form of pleasuring the self in accounts of women's drinking. Visual and linguistic images are key to producing this effect. Especially in commercial media, the glass of alcohol is depicted as a key ingredient in relaxing, self-indulgent, and self-pampering practices (e.g. in photos of a colourful drink beside a bathtub filled with bubbles) (Månsson, 2014), images that echo the advertising of chocolate to female consumers. In this context, fashion reports and advertising images of women who drink convey both sensuality (Månsson, 2014) and sexualizing of women (Törrönen & Juslin, 2013). Apart from enjoyment and pleasure, drinking is also associated with women having time for themselves and depicted as an escape from, or reward for, a hectic lifestyle (Törrönen & Juslin, 2013). Secondly, in Swedish women's magazines, drinking appears as a pleasurable aspect of close friendships between women. In these situations, a small group of women are portrayed as relaxing in an intimate and private sphere while sipping on wine or drinks. Again, alcohol is shown as a key ingredient in creating a gendered private space among a smaller group of "girlfriends" (Månsson, 2014). Thirdly, drinking is portrayed as pleasurable in the context of partying (Lyons et al., 2006; Månsson, 2014; Törrönen & Juslin, 2013). In Swedish women's magazines, intoxication and wild partying are glorified and celebrated as fun and popular activities where drinking represents an instrument for successfully becoming a fashionable and social person (Månsson, 2014). Similarly, UK women's magazines directed at the 18–25 age group repeatedly describe the "goodtime girl" as a category that is professional, glamourous, and likes to party (Lyons et al., 2006).

Women's magazines seldom discuss gender differences in text or portray differences as biological. Instead, they rely on the visual representation of women who exhibit a "girly", sensual, or eroticized femininity in clothing, style, and posture (Månsson, 2014; Månsson & Bogren, 2014; Törrönen & Juslin, 2013). Rather than stressing biological differences between the male and female body, these representations emphasize femininity in behaviour and appearance. Via the portrayal of drinking as fashionable, cool, and professional, alcohol consumption is articulated as a sign of empowerment, entitlement, and choice (Månsson & Bogren, 2014). Empowerment, choice, style, and beauty are all central in both the post-feminist and the consumerist discourse of the time. Thus, in line with both post-feminist and consumerist discourse, adverts and women's magazines represent femininity as an identity display and a lifestyle choice for young adult women, a position they can cultivate through alcohol consumption.

Interview studies consistently show that the opposing discourses of risky and pleasurable drinking reappear in young women's narratives of alcohol, shaping their self-presentations and identity formation. For young women, drinking is a normal and pleasurable part of everyday life, and essential to partying, but it also involves the risk of being positioned as "unfeminine" or "slutty" (e.g. Griffin et al., 2013; Kobin, 2013; Measham, 2002; Watts, Linke, Murray, & Barker, 2015). Moreover, an American study shows that many college women think that "to drink like a guy" is something *other* women do, not because they are striving for gender equality, but because they want to be attractive to men (Young, Morales, McCabe, Boyd, & D'Arcy, 2005). Taken together, these studies imply that young adult women are active in managing self-positioning and attempt to orient towards preferred positions, but also that their drinking is constrained by others' reactions and by the widespread official discourses that problematize their drinking. The studies also indicate that media debaters' views of the motives behind women's drinking are too narrowly conceived.

Assertiveness, Aggression, and Alcohol: Problematizing and Positive Discourses of Young Adult Men's Drinking

Research suggests that governmental reports, policy guidelines, and news reports on alcohol seldom treat men as a gendered risk group or address men as a gender category in headlines and text (Månsson & Bogren, 2014). For example, unlike for young women, Swedish newspapers do not exhort young men to stop drinking "like lads" or claim that heavy drinking among men is due to a misunderstanding of gender equality (Bogren 2011a, 2011b). In Australia, by contrast, Keane (2013) notes a discursive shift in the gendering of drinking occurred in the 2009 national alcohol policy guidelines. Instead of claiming that women are more vulnerable to alcohol because of their biology—an argument that had been central to previous policy guidelines—the 2009 guidelines reduced the safe drinking amount for men to the women's level, arguing that the risk of injury increases more rapidly for men at high levels of alcohol consumption (Keane, 2013). Thus, in the 2009 guidelines, risk was conceptualized within a public health discourse that includes both individual health risk (e.g. physical disease) and also wider risks of injury associated with alcohol (e.g. traffic accidents, interpersonal violence). An article from the newspaper *Svenska Dagbladet* (Asker, 2017) is a sign that a similar shift may be underway in Swedish alcohol policy discourse, only eight years later. Along similar lines, research shows that when the Swedish media *do* address men as a gender category, their drinking is portrayed as linked to aggression and violence and as associated with "laddish" masculinity.

9 Gender in Young Adult's Discourses of Drinking and Drunkenness   181

News portrayals take on a problematizing approach to drinking behaviour and drinking practices among men. In Swedish newspapers in the early 2000s, men's drinking was primarily discussed as related to violence in intimate relationships and to "macho behaviour" in the sports world (Bogren, 2011a). Although the concept of hegemonic masculinity (Connell, 1995) was introduced to a wider audience just prior to this period, the notion of multiple and oppositional masculinities did not appear in Swedish news reporting about men's drinking at this time. Instead, representatives from temperance organizations drew on a radical feminist discourse in arguing that men's drinking leads to physical violence against women. Similarly, sports journalists accused sports coaches of ignoring the "laddish" locker-room mentality that was said to encourage both alcohol consumption and "macho behaviour" among young men (Bogren, 2011a). Yet despite these attempts at focussing on men's drinking as a gendered problem, a large majority of the news articles that discussed gender and alcohol in the period between 2000 and 2008 were about women (Bogren, 2011a). Thus, newspapers still often equated "the gendered problems of drinking" with "the problems of women's drinking".

By contrast, UK men's magazines directed at the 18–25 age group depicted men's nights out drinking as battles or adventures. In nightlife contexts, masculine assertiveness and aggression were either condoned or valued positively (Lyons et al., 2006). Moreover, in popular culture, drinking and assertiveness are sometimes linked with "playboy" masculinity. Studying a smaller number of mainstream music videos, Lindsay and Lyons (2017) found that "playboys" were portrayed as "having the 'freedom' to consume alcohol and sex excessively and without repercussion" (Lindsay & Lyons, 2017: 9). At the same time, women were portrayed as actively choosing and enjoying their characterization as "sex objects" who like to drink and party. In post-feminist discourse, self-objectification is construed as a choice that women make or, alternatively, as a representation drawing on irony and pastiche (Lindsay & Lyons, 2017). Thus, in this discourse and in the music videos, women's bestowed identities as "sex objects" were framed positively as a source of power and agency. When considered from a micro-oriented discursive perspective, the playboy and sex object identities can be understood as part of a broader repertoire of identities made available through media portrayals of drinking. This repertoire allows young adults the opportunity to select from shifting available identities across contexts and in response to others' reactions, including the option to withdraw from a playboy identity if criticized and the option to adopt a sex object identity to facilitate transgression of gendered drinking norms (cf. Peralta, 2008). However, the post-feminist discourse also allows a shift in responsibility to take place, where men are positioned as less responsible for their own excessive drinking and behaviour towards women, while women are positioned as complicit. In this sense, the identity of sex object is restrictive, and adopting it might make it more difficult for women to speak openly about sexual victimization.

Interview studies suggest that drinking identities are contradictory for men as well. Some groups embrace a "laddish" or "playboy" identity in drinking situations, where high levels of alcohol consumption and drunkenness symbolize "toughness" (Dempster, 2011; Törrönen & Roumeliotis, 2014). Others see heavy "laddish" drinking as an inauthentic front or adopt more egalitarian identities centred around moderate drinking (Dempster, 2011; de Visser & McDonnell, 2012; Peralta, 2008; Törrönen & Roumeliotis, 2014). Research further shows that the construction of certain drinks or drinking practices as "unmanly" shapes young adult's views of drinking. For example, both young men and women can be sceptical of men who do not drink and evidence from UK interview research has suggested that male non-drinkers may encounter pressure for them to "man up" (Conroy & de Visser, 2013). However, being viewed as "unmanly" in drinking contexts could also be counterbalanced by investing in masculine capital in other domains (e.g. having a muscular physique) (Conroy & de Visser, 2013; de Visser & McDonnell, 2013). In addition, another study found that the excuse value of alcohol allowed some young heterosexual men to do things they wouldn't do when sober because it would be considered unmanly, such as expressing emotions of vulnerability or thoughts about religion and existence (Peralta, 2008). Taken together, these studies imply that young adult men too are active in managing self-positioning, that they attempt to orient towards preferred positions, and that their actions are constrained by others' reactions.

9 Gender in Young Adult's Discourses of Drinking and Drunkenness

Drinking, Respectability, and Class

In discussing drinking, young adults assign problematic positions to others whose drinking they perceive as inappropriate (Dempster, 2011; Griffin et al., 2013; Rudolfsdottir & Morgan, 2009). Such conceptions of proper and respectable drinking are also related to class. Notably, the ladette is discursively constituted through a series of derogatory labels ("chavvy", "lairy") and descriptions of clothing (low-necked blouses, short skirts, bleached hair) used to signify working-class status (Bernhardsson & Bogren, 2012; Day et al., 2004; Griffin et al., 2013; Lyons et al., 2006; Skeggs, 2005). Interview findings suggest that young adult women manage the risk of being subject to such derogatory labels via the tactical use of middle-class femininity as capital. Aware of the problems of being positioned as "unfeminine" or "slutty" when drinking, middle-class women use the power available to them via gendered and classed discourses to construct working-class women's drinking as more problematic than their own (Griffin et al., 2013; Rudolfsdottir & Morgan, 2009). This can be described as a case of othering where the middle-class women assign group-based shame to working-class women in a defensive manner, to protect themselves from shaming and to assert class advantage (cf. Skeggs, 1997). By implication, idealizing media portrayals of middle-class women who drink may serve to strengthen the positive self-image of that social group, while problematizing portrayals of working-class "ladettes" may affect the group-image of working-class women negatively through shaming.

With regard to masculinity and class, a recent study suggests that men from different educational backgrounds adopt different positions vis-à-vis drinking (Törrönen, Rolando, & Beccaria, 2017). Educated middle-class men "unlink their masculinity from traditional drinking styles or [...] mix into it new, traditionally feminine elements" such as wine drinking, while less educated men "are inclined to emphasize traditional features of masculinity" and exclude what they perceive as feminine practices from their repertoire (Törrönen et al., 2017: 139). The study describes working and middle-class men's self-positioning less as a tactical use of masculinity vis-à-vis other men and more as positive identification with class-specific masculinities. On the other hand, research on working-class men's health behaviours suggests that heavy drinking can also be understood as release or escape from hard work or a difficult life situation (Dolan, 2011).

Discussion and Future Research Agenda

The idea that drinking is unfeminine and the idea that young women today "drink like men" are recurrent in alcohol discourse in the twentieth century. These ideas are partly in opposition. If young adult women currently "drink like men", the idea of "drinking as unfeminine" would be expected to disappear. Some research findings suggest that young adult women binge drink more than before, implying that the notion that drinking is unfeminine is set on a trajectory to become outdated. However, men still binge drink more than women and gendered drinking patterns vary in a complex way across countries and age groups (see, e.g., Wilsnack et al., 2018 for an overview). Moreover, research based on the analysis of official documents, media representations, and narratives of people's everyday experiences shows that so far, the idea that young adult women "drink like men" persists in public debate. Advocates of post-feminism argue that people no longer feel a need to classify behaviour according to gender, but the enduring presence of the figure of the young woman who "drinks like a man" in media debates from the 1970s until today implies that this is only partly true. Whereas important advances in gender equality have been made in the decades from the 1970s until today (Deutsch, 2007), gender stereotypes continue to influence contemporary debate on drinking patterns. Thus, there appears to be a disconnect between drinking patterns, on the one hand, and cultural representations, discourses, and norms of drinking, on the other.

The ambiguous representations of young adult women's drinking across media outlets tell us that young women today are perceived as strong and independent consumers, but also as potentially passive victims of gender equality ideology. To avoid such undersocialized and oversocialized conceptions of agency, research on alcohol (as on drugs cf. Ettorre, 2007; Measham, 2002) needs to avoid simply siding with either pleasure or risk-based discourses and instead develop a more complex understanding of young women's drinking. On a broader note, it is possible that polarized

9 Gender in Young Adult's Discourses of Drinking and Drunkenness

media representations such as those of women's drinking will continue to exist. Following economic change and competition from digital and social media platforms, media publishing houses are now under greater pressure to sell and lifestyle reporting has become increasingly important (Fairclough, 2010). On the one hand, this means an increasing pressure to publish controversial content. On the other hand, because audiences have a greater variety of media to choose from, the opportunity to ignore media outlets that publish controversial or unpopular content is greater. To the extent that polarized media representations are increasingly directed at different audience groups, they may continue to co-exist side by side.

When it comes to young men's drinking, research indicates that masculinities are formed in a field of tensions between a "laddish" position where alcohol is associated—positively or negatively—with "toughness", aggression, and violence and positions centred around moderate and egalitarian drinking styles. However, we still do not know enough about the relation between these practices and ideals and wider social change in men's lives. In addition, given gender differences in access to power and opportunity in wider society, as well as in many substance use contexts (Miller & Carbone-Lopez, 2015), the social processes of identity formation are likely to be different for women and men, as well as to be shaped by other intersecting forms of social categorization, such as class, ethnicity/racialization, and sexuality. Although research on masculinities and drinking is growing, many issues are still unexplored. For example, future studies might examine whether there is something specific to the construction of masculine identities in drinking contexts as compared to other social contexts. Are the social and material characteristics of alcohol itself important in the construction of different masculinities, and if so, how? The media portrayal of laddish drinking, assertiveness, and aggression is only one aspect of the broader cultural depiction of masculinity. Although men's magazines often include elements of "laddish" masculinity (e.g. photos of semi-clothed and topless women; stories of bravery, danger, drunkenness, and hangovers), they also include advice on fashion and grooming; on how to manage problems of drinking and gambling; and on how to succeed at work and as a father (Gauntlett, 2008). To better understand the relation between such media portrayals and young adults' views of drinking, research should address how men and women interpret, relate to, and resist the variety of portrayals of drinking and intoxication that appear in different media outlets.

Greater attention should be paid to intersectionality in relation to gendered discourses of drinking in future research. For example, future research could explore women's self and other positioning in drinking situations from the perspective of social class. Future research could also focus on when and how men assign group-based shame to other men in drinking situations and the potential relation between drinking, masculinity, shaming, and social class. It is especially important to examine relations of power in these studies, since media representations of drinking may contribute to perpetuating class and racial stereotypes and racism. For example, in Sweden, ethnicity was brought to the fore in the news reporting of some highly publicized rape cases involving alcohol where commentators described "immigrant men" as particularly problematic (Bernhardsson & Bogren, 2012). Other research could usefully explore drinking and drug use in relation to place (regional, local, and social context, rural, or urban setting) to guide understanding of why "particular narratives of gender or particular ways of performing or 'doing' gender [are] more or less available within the life situations" of different groups of individuals (Miller & Carbone-Lopez, 2015: 698). In addition, a better understanding of the friendship and reference groups that women and men interact in and compare themselves to could be one way forward in addressing this issue. Finally, on a methodological level, scholars need to address the difficulty of producing research that does not primarily react to or mirror media and everyday accounts of gendered drinking practices. An important tension for researchers here is to decide whether, and to what extent, this difficulty can or should be resisted or accommodated. Indeed, addressing this tension may help guide understanding of why gendered representations, norms, and discourses of drinking may change at different rates and in different ways to ongoing patterns of change in young adult drinking practices.

References

Abrahamsson, M., & Heimdahl, K. (2010). Gendered discourse in Swedish national alcohol policy action plans 1965–2007: Invisible men and problematic women. *Nordic Studies on Alcohol and Drugs, 27*(1), 63–86.

Asker, A. (2017, March 6). False image that men can drink more than women. *Svenska Dagbladet.* https://www.svd.se/falsk-bild-att-man-kan-dricka-mer-an-kvinnor.

Bacchi, C. (2005). Discourse, discourse everywhere: Subject agency in feminist discourse methodology. *Nordic Journal of Women's Studies, 13*(3), 198–209.

Beccaria, F., Rolando, S., Törrönen, J., & Scavarda, A. (2018). From housekeeper to status-oriented consumer and hyper-sexual imagery: Images of alcohol targeted to Italian women from the 1960s to the 2000s. *Feminist Media Studies, 18*(6), 1012–1039.

Bernhardsson, J., & Bogren, A. (2012). Drink sluts, brats, and immigrants as others: An analysis of Swedish media discourse on gender, alcohol and rape. *Feminist Media Studies, 12*(1), 1–16.

Bihagen, E., Nermo, M., & Stern, C. (2014). The gender gap in the business elite: Stability and change in characteristics of Swedish top wage earners in large private companies, 1993–2007. *Acta Sociologica, 57*(2), 119–133.

Bogren, A. (2011a). Gender and alcohol: The Swedish press debate. *Journal of Gender Studies, 20*(2), 155–169.

Bogren, A. (2011b). Biologically responsible mothers and girls who act like men: Shifting discourses of biological sex difference in Swedish newspaper debate on alcohol in 1979 and 1995. *Feminist Media Studies, 11*(2), 197–213.

Campbell, N., & Ettorre, E. (2011). *Gendering addiction: The politics of drug treatment in a neurochemical world.* London: Palgrave Macmillan.

Carvalho, A. (2008). Media(ted) discourse and society. *Journalism Studies, 9*(2), 161–177.

Connell, R. (1995). *Masculinities.* Cambridge: Polity Press.

Conroy, D., & de Visser, R. (2013). Man up! Discursive constructions of non-drinkers among UK undergraduates. *Journal of Health Psychology, 18*(11), 1432–1444.

Day, K., Gough, B., & McFadden, M. (2004). Warning! Alcohol can seriously damage your feminine health. *Feminist Media Studies, 4*(2), 165–183.

Dempster, S. (2011). I drink, therefore I'm man: Gender discourses, alcohol and the construction of British undergraduate masculinities. *Gender and Education, 23*(5), 635–653.

Deutsch, F. (2007). Undoing gender. *Gender & Society, 21*(1), 106–127.

de Visser, R., & McDonnell, E. (2012). That's OK. He's a guy: A mixed-methods study of gender double-standards for alcohol use. *Psychology & Health, 27*(5), 618–639.

de Visser, R., & McDonnell, E. (2013). Man points: Masculine capital and young men's health. *Health Psychology, 32*(1), 5–14.

Dolan, A. (2011). You can't ask for a Dubonnet and lemonade! Working class masculinity and men's health practices. *Sociology of Health & Illness, 33*(4), 586–601.

Enefalk, H. (2015). Alcohol and femininity in Sweden c. 1830–1922: An investigation of the emergence of separate drinking standards for men and women. *Substance Use & Misuse, 50*(6), 736–746.

Ettorre, E. (2007). *Revisioning women and drug use.* London: Palgrave Macmillan.

Fairclough, N. (2010). *Media discourse.* London: Bloomsbury.

Gauntlett, D. (2008). *Media, gender and identity: An introduction.* London: Routledge.

Griffin, C., Szmigin, I., Bengry-Howell, A., Hackley, C., & Mistral, W. (2013). Inhabiting the contradictions: Hypersexual femininity and the culture of intoxication among young women in the UK. *Feminism & Psychology, 23*(2), 184–206.

Henderson, S. (1999). Drugs and culture: The question of gender. In N. South (Ed.), *Drugs: Culture, controls, and everyday life* (pp. 36–48). London: Sage.

Howarth, D. (2000). *Discourse.* Buckingham: Open University Press.

Keane, H. (2013). Healthy adults and maternal bodies: Reformulations of gender in Australian alcohol guidelines. *Health Sociology Review, 22*(2), 151–161.

Keane, H. (2017). Female vulnerability and susceptible brains: Gendered discourses of addiction. *Social History of Alcohol and Drugs, 31,* 126–139.

Kobin, M. (2013). Gendered drinking: Meanings and norms among young Estonian adults. *Nordic Studies on Alcohol and Drugs, 30*(4), 277–295.

Lindsay, S., & Lyons, A. (2017). Pour it up, drink it up, live it up, give it up: Masculinity and alcohol in pop music videos. *Men and Masculinities, 21*(5), 624–644.

Lyons, A., Dalton, S., & Hoy, A. (2006). Hardcore drinking: Portrayals of alcohol consumption in young women's and men's magazines. *Journal of Health Psychology, 11*(2), 223–232.

Månsson, E. (2014). Drinking as a feminine practice: Post-feminist images of women's drinking in Swedish women's magazines. *Feminist Media Studies, 14*(1), 56–72.

Månsson, E., & Bogren, A. (2014). Health, risk and pleasure: The formation of gendered discourses on women's alcohol consumption. *Addiction Research & Theory, 22*(1), 27–36.

Measham, F. (2002). "Doing gender"—"doing drugs": Conceptualizing the gendering of drugs cultures. *Contemporary drug problems, 29*(2), 335–373.

Measham, F., & Brain, K. (2005). Binge drinking, British alcohol policy and the new culture of intoxication. *Crime, Media, Culture, 1*(3), 262–283.

Miller, J., & Carbone-Lopez, C. (2015). Beyond doing gender: Incorporating race, class, place and life transitions into feminist drug research. *Substance Use & Misuse, 50*(6), 693–707.

Peralta, R. (2008). Alcohol allows you not to be yourself: Toward a structured understanding of alcohol use and gender difference among gay, lesbian, and heterosexual youth. *Journal of Drug Issues, 38*(2), 373–400.

Potter, J., & Wetherell, M. (1987). *Discourse and social psychology.* London: Sage.

Rosén, M., & Haglund, B. (2018). Follow-up of an age-period-cohort analysis on alcohol-related mortality trends in Sweden 1970–2015 with predictions to 2025. *Scandinavian Journal of Public Health, 47*(4), 446–451.

Rudolfsdottir, A., & Morgan, P. (2009). Alcohol is my friend: Young middle-class women discuss their relationship with alcohol. *Journal of Community & Applied Social Psychology, 19*(6), 492–505.

Skeggs, B. (1997). *Formations of class and gender.* London: Sage.

Skeggs, B. (2005). The making of class and gender through visualizing moral subject formation. *Sociology, 39*(5), 965–982.

Teigen, M., & Wängnerud, L. (2009). Tracing gender equality cultures: Elite perceptions of gender equality in Norway and Sweden. *Politics & Gender, 5*(1), 21–44.

Titscher, S., Meyer, M., Wodak, R., & Vetter, E. (2000). *Methods of text and discourse analysis.* London: Sage.

Törrönen, J., & Juslin, I. (2013). From genius of the home to party princess: Drinking in Finnish women's magazine advertisements from the 1960s to the 2000s. *Feminist Media Studies, 13*(3), 463–489.

Törrönen, J., & Roumeliotis, F. (2014). Masculinities of drinking as described by Swedish and Finnish age-based focus groups. *Addiction Research & Theory, 22*(2), 126–136.

Törrönen, J., Rolando, S., & Beccaria, F. (2017). Masculinities and femininities of drinking in Finland, Italy and Sweden: Doing, modifying and unlinking gender in relation to different drinking places. *Geoforum, 82,* 131–140.

Warner, J. (1997). The sanctuary of sobriety: The emergence of temperance as a feminine virtue in Tudor and Stuart England. *Addiction, 92*(1), 97–111.

Watts, R., Linke, S., Murray, E., & Barker, C. (2015). Calling the shots: Young professional women's relationship with alcohol. *Feminism & Psychology, 25*(2), 219–234.

Wilsnack, R., Wilsnack, S., Gmel, G., & Wolfgang Kantor, L. (2018). Gender differences in binge drinking: Prevalence, predictors, and consequences. *Alcohol Research Current Reviews, 39*(1), 57–76.

Young, A., Morales, M., McCabe, S., Boyd, C., & D'Arcy, H. (2005). Drinking like a guy: Frequent binge drinking among undergraduate women. *Substance Use and Misuse, 40*(2), 241–267.

10

Alcohol Consumption Among Young People in Marginalised Groups

Lana Ireland

Introduction

Alcohol use in youth has long been regarded as a rite of passage, bestowing perceptions of social permissiveness around periodic heavy drinking for those at this life stage (Crawford & Novak, 2006). It is easy, as academics or healthcare professionals, to problematise drinking among this group by focusing on physiological and behavioural harms, but for many young people, sensation-seeking through alcohol use serves as functional for their life stage in terms of becoming independent, socialising with peers and pursuing romantic endeavours (Spear, 2000; Van der Zwaluw et al., 2009). Young people often experience the physiological cues that serve to limit alcohol intake to a lesser extent than older adults. For example, young people experience reduced alcohol-related sedative effects, slighter social and motor deficiencies, and fewer hangover effects than mature adults (Spear & Varlinskaya, 2006). This youth advantage in the processing of

L. Ireland (✉)
Lecturer in Psychology, Glasgow Caledonian University, Glasgow, Scotland
e-mail: Lana.Ireland@gcu.ac.uk

© The Author(s) 2019
D. Conroy and F. Measham (eds.), *Young Adult Drinking Styles*,
https://doi.org/10.1007/978-3-030-28607-1_10

ethanol may operate as a false sense of invincibility around alcohol use, as youths create and recreate their drinking patterns into young adulthood.

Problem drinking has been associated with myriad harms for young people, especially those with additional life challenges including membership of marginalised groups. For such young people, risks around alcohol use can be heightened as they may lack the protective factors (e.g. stable family, peer and school life) that socially included young people possess. This lack of protective factors and forces that might help better guide their use of alcohol into adulthood presents as a further risk for problematic alcohol use later in life (Niño, Cai, & Ignatow, 2016).

This chapter is designed to explore some of the research literature around alcohol use among some marginalised groups of young people. It will explore the differential impacts of drinking alcohol for marginalised groups including: young offenders, lesbian, gay, bisexual and transgender (LGBT) groups, and young people who have experienced familial domestic abuse. There is obviously considerable overlap within and between these categories of young people, though heterogeneity of experiences and needs relating to these labels will be discussed. Multiple adverse childhood experiences (ACEs), such as poverty, educational exclusion, and family violence, have been associated with a greater risk of health problems (including alcohol abuse) into adulthood (Felitti et al., 1998; Lanier, Maguire-Jack, Lombardi, Frey, & Rose, 2018). These findings imply that young people's membership of more than one of these marginalised groups may be cumulative in their association with a greater risk of alcohol-related harms across the lifespan.

Interventions intended to ameliorate alcohol harms for young marginalised individuals will be explored, with focus on the success of innovative, wide-ranging and integrated approaches as adopted in the Scottish public health model over the last decade. The extent to which the implementation of effective alcohol interventions for marginalised young people can be affected by political decisions and policy directions will also be addressed. Finally, the chapter will cover the emergence of 'Generation Sensible' (Oldham, Holmes, Whitaker, Fairbrother, & Curtis, 2018), where young people are described as less likely than their parents to have problems with alcohol. This might suggest that interventionist approaches to alcohol may not be required or appropriate for all marginalised young people.

Operational Definitions

Psychological understandings of alcohol problems reference 'Alcohol Use Disorder (AUD)' which encompasses dependency indicators such as increased tolerance, negative effects on functioning in everyday life and withdrawal symptoms (DSM-V, 2013). Binge-drinking is defined as consumption of 6 units within around 2 hours (NHS, 2016), and whilst regarded as dangerous to physical health, and associated with risky behaviours, is distinct from dependent drinking.

The United Nations defines youth, for the purposes of international statistical parity, as the period after childhood dependence and before adult independence, experienced between 15 and 24 years old (UNESCO, 2017). This wide definition is utilised here, synonymously with 'young people', with the proviso that peri-adolescence (an important period covered in much of the youth alcohol research literature) can encompass younger children depending on their developmental rate.

There exists significant debate around the use of terms such as 'marginalised' or 'excluded' to describe groups who, through social processes such as discrimination, are not included (or indeed visible) in the full sphere of social life that the majority population enjoys (Ahmed & Rogers, 2016). Both terms are used interchangeably in this chapter and are not intended as pejorative (i.e. othering or homogenising individuals and their intersectional experiences). Rather, 'marginalised' and 'excluded' are used here as a means of identifying individuals who can be meaningfully understood to face additional societal challenges and tend to be underrepresented in research literature and government policy.

Poverty, Violence and Youth Drinking in Glasgow

One way that young people can find themselves marginalised is socioeconomically, through poverty and associated deprivations, e.g. in local levels of crime, drug use, barriers to education and poor housing. Intersectional understandings of such experiences permit nuance around young people's identities here, whilst being 'White' may confer general privilege, being 'poor' can confer general exclusion (Hershberg & Johnson, 2019). Thus, poor White young men are increasingly recognised as a socially excluded group. This section aims to describe some of the ways in which cheap high-strength alcohol has been marketed towards this group in central Scotland, and how aspects of the associated drinking culture have been tied up in personal and social identities.

Excessive alcohol consumption among young people in areas of high socioeconomic deprivation (as measured by the Scottish Index of Multiple Deprivation, Scottish Government, 2016), in Glasgow and surrounding areas in Scotland, has historically been associated with street violence (McKinlay, Forsyth, & Khan, 2009). Research over the last few decades has sought to understand the patterns in drinking styles for this excluded group and has implicated certain types of alcohol, vessels and poly-drug use as important variables for further study.

Purportedly 'tonic' fortified wine (i.e. *Buckfast*) and cheap white cider (e.g. *Frosty Jack's*) have been foremost among the drinks of choice for young people in these areas (Galloway, Forsyth, & Shewan, 2007), and large quantities are frequently consumed in short spaces of time. *Frosty Jack's* is sold in plastic bottles, but the binge-drinking of *Buckfast* in particular, which has a glass bottle shape (long neck) such that the vessel is often turned upside-down and used as a weapon (as an alternative to carrying knives), has, until perhaps the last decade, been implicated in a high level of violent offending by young men (Forsyth, Khan, & McKinley, 2010; McKinlay et al., 2009). For context, 40% of the inmates aged 18–24 years old, in a single Scottish prison, were found to have AUDIT (Alcohol Use Disorder Identification Test; Babor, Higgins-Biddle, Saunders, & Monteiro, 2001) scores indicating 'possible dependence' on alcohol (MacAskill et al., 2011), highlighting Scotland's problem relationship

10 Alcohol Consumption Among Young People in Marginalised Groups   195

with alcohol and violence. Longitudinal research found that a majority, 43.4% of young offenders questioned, admitting they had consumed *Buckfast* prior to their offence (McKinlay et al., 2009).

Indeed, *Buckfast* has been associated with 'Ned' (Scottish derogatory term similar to 'yob', 'chav' or hooligan) culture in Scotland. Being regarded as the drink of choice for young street drinkers who regard it as '*being symbolic of masculinity, group affiliation, class and national identity*', *Buckfast* is also simultaneously rejected as an alcohol type to imbibe by street-drinking who reject the 'Ned' label (Galloway et al., 2007: 6). Containing caffeine, and with an alcohol by volume level of 15%, *Buckfast* combines alcohol intoxication with stimulant, and when consumed in conjunction with diazepam (e.g. *Valium*), this cocktail has been associated with violent street crime in particular. Qualitative accounts from young offenders within the Scottish Prison System (SPS) explained how using this combination had led to their worst violent offending (McKinlay et al., 2009). Whilst *Buckfast* in particular has been implicated in the alcohol-aggression link for this marginalised group of young men, it must be recognised that this relationship is often heavily mediated by simultaneous use of illicit substances. Despite the fact that comparable psychopharmacological effects are found in the consumption of, e.g. vodka and *Red Bull*, or Chianti and an espresso chaser, the cultural significance of *Buckfast* drinking persists for this youth group, tied up with projection of their alcohol-related identities.

Such is the infamy of alcoholic drinks such as *Buckfast* in relation to violent offending in this cultural context that a validated measure of alcohol-related aggression specifically cites it. The Alcohol-Related Aggression Questionnaire (ARAQ; McMurran et al., 2006) asks respondents about the extent to which they agree that: '*I get aggressive when I drink strong wines e.g. sherry, Mad Dog, Buckfast*'. Following research findings around the *Buckfast*-violence link in central Scotland, evidence that the glass bottles have been used as weapons, and the resultant high proportion (54%) of glass street litter comprising the remnants of these bottles (Forsyth & Davidson, 2010), *Buckfast* started, in 2014, to produce their ware in smaller cans (whilst retaining the original bottle offering too). Given the recent historical function of *Buckfast* drinking and use of the glass vessels as a common signifier of membership of the 'Ned' subculture (Young, 2012), there is little evidence as yet that this offering of a choice of vessel (can versus bottle) has impacted positively on related binge-drinking and offending behaviours.

Instead, population-level interventions such as minimum unit pricing (MUP, introduced in 2018), in conjunction with Scotland's Violence Reduction Unit's (VRU) holistic public health approach (where violence is approached more as a problem to be treated rather than a crime to be punished) have begun to attempt to have a measurable impact on this alcohol-violence relationship.

In terms of MUP, whilst *Buckfast* price was not affected by this policy (MUP is set at 50p per unit, with a 75cl bottle of Buckfast at around £7.50 for 11 units of alcohol), there have reportedly been initial massive reductions (up to 70%) in purchases of *Frosty Jack's* (previously £3.69 for 22.5 units of alcohol in a three-litre plastic bottle and now costing around £11.25). However, these same initial assessments suggest that *Buckfast* sales have increased by 17% in Scotland in the same period (Millar, 2018). One must caution that these are reported retail figures, and that in the absence of longitudinal academic research, the ostensible displacement in young people's alcohol consumption from white cider to fortified wine must be treated as insufficiently explored. The first annual monitoring report on MUP has indicated that alcohol sales have fallen by at least 3% in Scotland, with increases in sales of tonic wine and decreases in sales of cider. For young people (under 15 years old) rates of hospitalisation for alcohol have increased from 14.9 to 20.2 per 100,000 over 3 years, suggesting that MUP may not yet be as effective at reducing consumption among all age groups. Whilst overall consumption rates seem to be decreasing (or changing) in response to MUP, further research work is planned to assess patterns around associated harms (Giles & Robinson, 2019).

The impact of the VRU has also seen reliable results, in the reduction of violence among young men in a Scottish context (Crichton, 2017), and their work has included intervention around alcohol (and wider substance) misuse. Launched in 2005 by (the then) Strathclyde Police, the VRU has moved beyond a punitive criminal justice approach to dealing with young men's violence and has adopted a public health approach in conjunction with medical practitioners, youth workers, social workers and researchers. Hospital treatment (often for victims of violence offences) has been approached as a 'reachable moment' where support workers known as 'Navigators' visit young people involved in violence, offer support for alcohol problems, employability and so forth, and aim to build human connections that can be followed up after discharge (Stewart, 2018b).

Social exclusion factors such as unemployment and poverty have been identified by the VRU as major contributory factors in alcohol problems and violent offending (particularly gang violence). Diagnosis of exclusion factors leading to the symptoms of alcohol problems and violence has been analysed, and a 'what works for whom' approach has been taken in resultant treatment of these (including diversionary activities, brief alcohol intervention and employability work). Criminal justice measures were employed at the same time (e.g. the sentence for carrying a knife increased threefold), but the person-centred approach has seen real improvements. This notion that violence is preventable and treatable has coincided with a reduction in violent crime in Scotland over the past decade—now at a 40-year low, and Glasgow has lost its label as the murder capital of Europe (Younge & Barr, 2017).

Thus, in order to make changes in problematic drinking behaviour by young people in general and violence by marginalised groups of young men in particular, the most effective intervention has been holistic and assets-based (rather than targeted and deficits-based). That is, problems were not considered in isolation, rather as part of a set of symptoms to be treated in ways that increase the agency and resilience of recipients. The potential scalability of this public health intervention approach is highlighted by the fact that the VRU is now set to be replicated in London (Stewart, 2018c), where 41% of young offenders have reported that they were using alcohol at the time of their offence (Alcohol Concern, 2016).

LGBT Young People and Drinking on 'The Gay Scene'

There is a growing body of research on alcohol use among young LGBT groups. Studies have tended to focus on particular risk and protective factors for these historically marginalised social groups, and also, recently, on 'dual diagnosis', or the concurrent experience of both mental health and substance use problems (Cortes, Fletcher, Latini, & Kauth, 2018; Newcomb, Heinz, & Mustanski, 2012). This recent research interest could be viewed as a positive means of reducing the exclusion and marginalisation from which this group has traditionally suffered, though policy and practice in terms of LGBT alcohol interventions are arguably lagging behind.

Prevalence of use of alcohol and other drugs has been found to be significantly greater (2–4 times higher) among lesbian, gay and bisexual (LGB) young people, as compared to heterosexual young people, with greatest risk for bisexuals and female LGB groups compared to heterosexual groups, reflecting the heterogeneity within the category of LGBT and more widely among young people (Marshal et al., 2008). Explanations for this state of affairs (mainly from US studies) tend to focus on this group's status as marginalised in terms of societal homophobia, discrimination and victimisation, and the contribution of these oppressive factors to 'minority stress' and mental ill-health (Marshal, Friedman, Stall, & Thompson, 2009; Meyer, 2013).

Alcohol use can thus be understood to operate as a coping mechanism for these stressful prejudicial experiences, with the age of 'coming out' functioning as an important mediating factor. Those same-sex attracted young people who adopt their sexual identities at an earlier stage (in their teens as opposed to mid-20s) tend to develop healthier alcohol-related behaviours as they transition into adulthood (Fish & Pasley, 2015). Putative reasons for this finding include the protective function of becoming aligned with a clear social identity and benefitting from the community support therein. Indeed, sociological research in this area has coined the term 'gay capital' to describe this prestige of belonging (Morris, 2018).

Whilst the notion of stigmatised LGBT young people turning to alcohol in order to cope may be valid in terms of the research evidence base, there is comparable (UK-based) research that indicates that drinking on the 'gay scene' (i.e. bars and clubs that are popular with LGBT groups) has been the main means of socialising for these groups (Emslie, Lennox, & Ireland, 2015). Alcohol and illicit drugs, used in conjunction, have also been described by gay men as both integral to their social lives and facilitative in terms of their sex lives (Keogh et al., 2009). Thus reasons for

10 Alcohol Consumption Among Young People in Marginalised Groups

higher rates of alcohol use and misuse here may be related to the historical social context of LGBT drinking, providing both a protective social support mechanism and an anxiolytic around sexual practices, but also a risk of developing unhealthy relationships with alcohol into adulthood.

There has been, however, some evidence of changes in leisure opportunities available to LGBT individuals over the last decade, with recent research work suggesting some movement away from this unitary gay scene. The advent of online, app-based social networking services (SNS) and related 'hook-up' culture has heralded a move away from the unitary 'gay scene' towards mixed venues and home drinking (Morris, 2018; Stewart, 2018a). Research into LGBT groups' alcohol use has moved beyond comparative risk measures and has started to explore aspects of alcohol and identity signalling.

The types of alcoholic drinks consumed by LGBT groups, and indeed the vessel they are contained within, have been shown to have a role in their multifaceted identity construction and projection. Scottish research indicated that gay men would be expected to conform to drinking feminised drinks such as alcopops, and lesbians 'butch' drinks such as pints of beer, in order to adequately project their sexualities on 'the scene'—a mirror image of the traditional stereotypical drinks for men and women. Interestingly, conformity to 'straight nights' (non-gay scene clubbing) would often involve lesbians changing their preferred drink to something more feminine and acceptable like a glass of vodka. Some male-to-female trans people discussed how, when in drag, they deliberately played around with these alcohol-related drink choice expectations by drinking from pint glasses, which was often met with criticism from their peers (Emslie, Lennox, & Ireland, 2017).

Beyond the utilisation of alcohol in identity work among LGBT groups, for those who do develop alcohol problems, there are various barriers that exist in trying to access health interventions. Older LGBT people have described reticence in approaching healthcare providers for alcohol misuse, often as a result of differential social norms around alcohol use (between the LGBT patients and their medics) given its historical centrality to drinking in gay scenes (Keogh et al., 2009). Similarly, younger LGBT people have described their experiences of stereotypical assumptions on the part of their doctors based on the fact that they are homosexual, with a prevailing presumption that they must be using alcohol in a disordered fashion and with health professionals jumping to the conclusion that any health problem they present with must be related to their sexuality. Specific alcohol services and programmes can be regarded as intimidating and 'heterocentric' to people who identify as LGBT (Emslie et al., 2015). People who identify as trans face additional harassment and transphobia across their social lives, and this often leads them to expect (and often experience) the same treatment within health services, leading them to avoid such support even when potentially beneficial (Rogers, 2016).

Facilitative factors in encouraging LGBT young people into alcohol treatment and interventions, therefore, may include the provision of targeted LGBT resources around alcohol use, designed and provided by those who have personal awareness of drinking in gay scenes, and who can counter the stereotypical assumptions that such heterogeneous groups can face in heteronormative healthcare provision. This might usefully involve work to increase LGBT inclusion in mainstream alcohol interventions, with sensitivity to any changes that may need to be made to content and delivery to achieve this inclusion. LGBT young people in particular have shown that they are capable and willing to contribute to the appropriate adaptation of mainstream substance use interventions for LGBT recipients (Goldbach & Holleran Steiker, 2011). Further, providing meaningful LGBT access to these existing alcohol interventions increases the range of services available and is likely to be highly effective given the variability of routes into alcohol use for both LGBT groups and the general population (Newcomb, Heinz, & Mustanski, 2012).

Familial Domestic Abuse, Drinking to Cope and Learned Behaviours

Whilst young people experiencing poverty or membership of an LGBT group are readily identifiable as socially marginalised in a range of contexts, there are also some hidden groups of young people who experience social exclusion alongside alcohol problems. Young people living in families where domestic abuse (or intimate partner violence) is present are often

10 Alcohol Consumption Among Young People in Marginalised Groups   201

overlooked as a marginalised group (perhaps given the perceived temporal nature of the problem), though recent research has started to explore this type of adverse experience (ACE) in relation to the development of alcohol problems. Whilst children who have parents with alcohol problems are between 2 and 14 times more likely to develop alcohol problems themselves (Dube et al., 2001), the addition of domestic violence to this toxic environment has been associated with increased rates of associated harm where young people are more likely to turn to alcohol to cope with related stress (Velleman, Templeton, Reuber, Klein, & Moesgen, 2008).

Domestic abuse (as a wider term than domestic violence) can include emotional, physical and sexual harm perpetrated by an intimate partner, and gendered appraisals of male-on-female violence cite the use of children in perpetrating this harm. Whether threatening to take children away, using them to verbally or physically abuse the mother, or abusing the children physically in order to coercively control the mother, growing up in a family where domestic abuse is present can be developmentally devastating for the offspring (Stark, 2007). The secrecy and stigma surrounding intimate partner abuse (including female-perpetrated violence) can serve to exclude and marginalise involved children and young people from society (especially in education and peer relationships), with health professionals experiencing difficulty in accessing these young people to provide support (Gallagher, 2014).

In a Scottish context, 88% of domestic abuse convicted prisoners were found to have AUDIT scores indicating that they were hazardous or harmful drinkers (Gilchrist, Ireland, Forsyth, Godwin, & Laxton, 2017). International research has linked alcohol use and domestic abuse in two-thirds of cases (though causal patterns are refrained from, lest the abuse be excused by alcohol use), with the consequences for young people subjected to this familial life ranging from significantly poorer psychological adjustment, to adverse social and educational outcomes (Forrester & Harwin, 2006; Kitzmann, Gaylord, Holt, & Kenny, 2003). These consequences of familial domestic abuse can thus be linked with social exclusion and poor coping for young people in later life. Indeed, the high rates of alcohol use among parents in domestic abuse relationships have been linked with transmission of the means by which the offspring learn to cope themselves

(Velleman et al., 2008). Specifically, and across a range of studies, witnessing domestic abuse has been linked with a greater rate of alcohol problems in later life (Tonmyr, Thornton, Draca & Wekerle, 2010).

In considering the means by which this intergenerational transmission of drinking behaviours and associated domestic abuse in relationships occurs, it may be useful to consider schema theory, and the way in which blueprints for adult relationships are modelled in childhood and youth. Children observe their parents' relationship, the strategies that are utilised in resolving conflict and the contexts around using alcohol, and they often assimilate these experiences as cognitions guiding their own behaviour. Research evidence has linked faulty attribution around alcohol use with perpetration of domestic abuse, such that drunkenness has been shown to excuse domestic violence for male perpetrators, but has been used as a means of victim-blaming female sufferers (Gilchrist, Ireland, Forsyth, Laxton, & Godwin, 2014). This exculpatory use of alcohol for men in domestic abusive behaviours (e.g. 'I was drunk, I didn't mean to hit her') could be argued to be implicit in the social learning of male–female relationships for young people in families affected by domestic abuse. Similarly, the inculpatory use of drunkenness against women as victims of domestic abuse (e.g. 'She was drunk – I had a right to hit her') must also impact on the growing child's ideas of relationship dynamics, with young adults being particularly susceptible to social imitation of alcohol drinking behaviours (Robinson et al., 2016).

A problematic aspect of domestic abuse in terms of the developmental progression of young people within the family is that mothers who are victims of such abuse may resist accessing support for their own drinking (often utilised as a coping mechanism) because they fear for the custody of their children (Galvani, 2010). Thus, young people who are raised in the context of domestic violence and related alcohol misuse learn that both the violence and alcohol problems are shameful and must be hidden, creating further barriers for much-needed intervention to address their needs.

This is a new and emerging area of research in terms of marginalised groups of young people and their experiences with alcohol and domestic abuse. Future research work might best explore lived experiences, qualitatively, from the perspective of young people themselves and investigate the effects of alcohol and domestic abuse on young people with non-heterosexual parents. It would also be useful to longitudinally test the effectiveness and appropriateness of available alcohol interventions. The aforementioned Violence Reduction Unit (VRU) has intervened in cases of domestic abuse in Scotland, utilising the holistic public health approach and using hospital admittance as a means of acting upon a 'reachable moment' where victims can access support and build relationships intended to enable and empower them in building new lives free from victimisation. This involves multi-agency preventative work, rehabilitation, and attitudinal change and has crucially been supported by the Scottish Government—interventions may be effective but not feasible without this support at policy level (VRU, 2016). Long-term research work is required to assess the effectiveness and scalability of this VRU approach for young people living with domestic abuse and parental alcohol misuse.

Conclusions

This chapter has shown that there is an emergent body of research literature that explores the particular alcohol-related experiences of various marginalised groups of young people. Whilst alcohol use among young people is not necessarily problematic, alcohol problems among those experiencing social exclusion and stigma have been shown to be related to an exponential risk of associated harms. Recent research has shown that young offenders living in poverty have complex relationships with particular alcohol brands, related to social identity and drinking vessel. LGBT groups have been shown to have had little alternative to drinking 'on the gay scene' until very recently with the advent of SNS and apps, and young people experiencing domestic abuse and parental alcohol problems have been shown to have among the highest levels of problematic alcohol use into adulthood.

In terms of intersectional marginalisation, some young people will be young offenders, LGBT, and have experience of domestic abuse in their parental homes. It may be useful to separate out such groups to understand and attempt to ameliorate specific harms around alcohol, whilst remaining cognisant of the reality that humans are not easily pigeon-holed as one thing or another, in isolation. Instead, useful interventions will aim to target specific group-related needs, whilst balancing treatment readiness and access to further (or indeed more holistic) interventions as required. Some marginalised groups may not need help with their alcohol use, but for those that do, we must (ethically) ensure they are meaningful, appropriate and feasible, as well as being regarded as effective in the research literature.

Where alcohol interventions are required for the groups of marginalised young people discussed here, the possibility of iatrogenic harm (harm inadvertently caused by the intervention itself) must be considered when assuming that majority-effective interventions will work (unaltered) for marginalised groups. Adaption of existing interventions, by the affected groups themselves seems to emerge in the literature as optimal, many of these young people are already socially excluded, and further segregation from the general public may be damaging. Population-level alcohol interventions, such as MUP and VRU, require longitudinal research work to gauge their efficacy.

Finally, with all the progressive intention and research evidence in the world, in the context of a backdrop of social and political austerity, one must consider the extent to which any required interventions are likely to be available. Adapting existing interventions to meet the needs of various excluded groups of young people may be the most feasible approach. Recent English research has tracked the emergence of 'Generation Sensible', where young people are far less likely than their parents to binge drink and develop alcohol problems (Oldham et al., 2018). These findings have been replicated in an international context, with reductions in access to alcohol and parental permissiveness around alcohol use being implicated as causal factors (Livingston, Callinan, Raninen, Pennay, & Dietze, 2017; Pennay, Livingston, & MacLean, 2015). Perhaps then, the problems associated with alcohol consumption among marginalised young people will reduce over time, and in conjunction with shifting social norms and multi-agency, population-level interventions.

References

Ahmed, A., & Rogers, M. (Eds.). (2016). *Working with marginalised groups: From policy to practice*. UK: Palgrave Macmillan.

Alcohol Concern. (2016). *Alcohol in the system report: An examination of alcohol and youth offending in London*. Trust for London. https://www.trustforlondon.org.uk/publications/alcohol-system-examination-alcohol-and-youth-offending-london/.

Babor, T. F., Higgins-Biddle, J. C., Saunders, J. B., & Monteiro, M. G. (2001). *AUDIT: The alcohol use disorders identification test—Guidelines for use in primary care* (2nd ed.). World Health Organisation. http://whqlibdoc.who.int/hq/2001/WHO_MSD_MSB_01.6a.pdf.

Cortes, J., Fletcher, T. L., Latini, D. M., & Kauth, M. R. (2018). Mental health differences between older and younger lesbian, gay, bisexual, and transgender veterans: Evidence of resilience. *Clinical Gerontologist: The Journal of Aging and Mental Health, 42*(2), 162–171.

Crawford, L. A., & Novak, K. B. (2006). Alcohol abuse as a rite of passage: The effect of beliefs about alcohol and the college experience on undergraduates' drinking behaviors. *Journal of Drug Education, 36*(3), 193–212.

Crichton, J. H. M. (2017). Falls in Scottish homicide: Lessons for homicide reduction in mental health patients. *BJ Psych Bulletin, 41*(4), 185–186.

Dube, S. R., Anda, R. F., Felitti, V. J., Croft, J. B., Edwards, V. J., & Giles, W. H. (2001). Growing up with parental alcohol abuse: Exposure to childhood abuse, neglect, and household dysfunction. *Child Abuse and Neglect, 25*(12), 1627–1640.

DSM-V. (2013). *Diagnostic and Statistics Manual v5—Factsheet: Substance-related and addictive disorders*. American Psychological Association (APA). http://www.dsm5.org/documents/substance%20use%20disorder%20fact%20sheet.pdf.

Emslie, C., Lennox, J., & Ireland, L. (2015). The social context of LGBT people's drinking in Scotland. *Scottish Health Action on Alcohol Problems*. http://www.sarn.ed.ac.uk/wp-content/uploads/2015/12/shaap-glass-report-web1.pdf.

Emslie, C., Lennox, J., & Ireland, L. (2017). The role of alcohol in identity construction among LGBT people: A qualitative study. *Sociology of Health & Illness, 39*(8), 1465–1479.

Felitti, V. J., Anda, R. F., Nordenberg, D., Williamson, D. F., Spitz, A. M., Edwards, V., & Marks, J. S. (1998). Relationship of childhood abuse and household dysfunction to many of the leading causes of death in adults: The

Adverse Childhood Experiences (ACE) Study. *American Journal of Preventive Medicine, 14*, 245–258.

Fish, J. N., & Pasley, K. (2015). Sexual (minority) trajectories, mental health, and alcohol use: A longitudinal study of youth as they transition to adulthood. *Journal of Youth and Adolescence, 44*(8), 1508–1527.

Forrester, D., & Harwin, J. (2006). Parental substance misuse and child care social work: Findings from the first stage of a study of 100 families. *Child and Family Social Work, 11*(4), 325–335.

Forsyth, A. J. M., & Davidson, N. (2010). The nature and extent of illegal drug and alcohol-related litter in Scottish social housing community: A photographic investigation. *Addiction Research & Theory, 18*(1), 71–83.

Forsyth, A. J. M., Khan, F., & McKinley, W. (2010). The use of off-trade glass as a weapon in violent assaults by young offenders. *Crime Prevention and Community Safety, 12*(4), 233–245.

Gallagher, C. (2014). Educational psychologists' conceptualisation of domestic violence. *Educational and Child Psychology, 31*(3), 55–63.

Galloway, J., Forsyth, A. J. M., & Shewan, D. (2007). *Young people's street drinking behaviour: Investigating the influence of marketing & subculture.* London: Alcohol Education Research Council.

Galvani, S. (2010). *Grasping the nettle: Alcohol and domestic violence.* Alcohol Concern. https://www.injuryobservatory.net/wp-content/uploads/2012/09/Cross-Tools-2011-Alcohol.pdf.

Gilchrist, E., Ireland, L., Forsyth, A., Laxton, T., & Godwin, J. (2014). *Roles of alcohol in intimate partner abuse* (pp. 1–61). Alcohol Research UK: Alcohol Insights. http://alcoholresearchuk.org/downloads/finalReports/FinalReport_0117.pdf.

Gilchrist, L., Ireland, L., Forsyth, A., Godwin, J., & Laxton, T. (2017). Alcohol use, alcohol-related aggression and intimate partner abuse (IPA): A cross-sectional survey of convicted versus general population men in Scotland. *Drug and Alcohol Review, 36*, 20–23.

Giles, L., & Robinson, M. (2019). *Monitoring and evaluating Scotland's alcohol strategy: Monitoring report 2019.* Edinburgh: NHS Health Scotland.

Goldbach, J. T., & Holleran Steiker, L. K. (2011). An examination of cultural adaptations performed by LGBT-identified youths to a culturally grounded, evidence-based substance abuse intervention. *Journal of Gay & Lesbian Social Services: The Quarterly Journal of Community & Clinical Practice, 23*(2), 188–203.

Hershberg, R. M., & Johnson, S. K. (2019). Critical reflection about socioeconomic inequalities among white young men from poor and working-class backgrounds. *Developmental Psychology, 55*(3), 562–573.

Keogh, P., Reid, D., Bourne, A., Weatherburn, P., Hickson, F., Jessup, K., & Hammond, G. (2009). *Wasted opportunities. Problematic alcohol and drug use among gay men and bisexual men.* London: Sigma Research.

Kitzmann, K. M., Gaylord, N. K., Holt, A. R., & Kenny, E. D. (2003). Child witnesses to domestic violence: A meta-analytic review. *Journal of Consulting and Clinical Psychology, 71*(2), 339–352.

Lanier, P., Maguire-Jack, K., Lombardi, B., Frey, J., & Rose, R. A. (2018). Adverse childhood experiences and child health outcomes: Comparing cumulative risk and latent class approaches. *Maternal and Child Health Journal, 22*(3), 288–297.

Livingston, M., Callinan, S., Raninen, J., Pennay, A., & Dietze, P. M. (2017, July 25). Alcohol consumption trends in Australia: Comparing surveys and sales-based measures. *Drug and Alcohol Review, 37*, S9–S14.

MacAskill, S., Parkes, T., Brooks, O., Graham, L., McAuley, A., & Brown, A. (2011). Assessment of alcohol problems using AUDIT in a prison setting: More than an 'aye or no' question. *BMC Public Health, 11*, 865.

Marshal, M. P., Friedman, M. S., Stall, R., King, K. M., Miles, J., Gold, M. A., … Morse, J. Q. (2008). Sexual orientation and adolescent substance use: A meta-analysis and methodological review. *Addiction, 103*(4), 546–556.

Marshal, M. P., Friedman, M. S., Stall, R., & Thompson, A. L. (2009). Individual trajectories of substance use in lesbian, gay and bisexual youth and heterosexual youth. *Addiction, 104*(6), 974–981.

McKinlay, W., Forsyth, A. J. M., & Khan, F. (2009). *Alcohol and violence among Young Male Offenders in Scotland* (SPS Occasional Paper No. 1/09). Edinburgh: Scottish Prison Service.

McMurran, M., Vincent Egan, V., Cusens, B., Van Den Bree, M., Austin, E., & Charlesworth, P. (2006). The alcohol-related aggression questionnaire. *Addiction Research & Theory, 14*(3), 323–343.

Meyer, I. H. (2013). Prejudice, social stress, and mental health in lesbian, gay, and bisexual populations: Conceptual issues and research evidence. *Psychology of Sexual Orientation and Gender Diversity, 1*, 3–26.

Millar, R. (2018, November 13). *Buckfast sales rise in Scotland post MUP.* The Drinks Business. https://www.thedrinksbusiness.com/2018/11/buckfast-sales-rise-in-scotland-post-mup/.

Morris, M. (2018). "Gay capital" in gay student friendship networks: An intersectional analysis of class, masculinity, and decreased homophobia. *Journal of Social and Personal Relationships, 35*(9), 1183–1204.

Newcomb, M. E., Heinz, A. J., & Mustanski, B. (2012). Examining risk and protective factors for alcohol use in lesbian, gay, bisexual, and transgender youth: A longitudinal multilevel analysis. *Journal of Studies on Alcohol and Drugs, 73*(5), 783–793.

NHS. (2016). *Alcohol support: Binge-drinking.* National Health Service. https://www.nhs.uk/live-well/alcohol-support/binge-drinking-effects/.

Niño, M. D., Cai, T., & Ignatow, G. (2016). Social isolation, drunkenness, and cigarette use among adolescents. *Addictive Behaviors, 53,* 94–100.

Oldham, M., Holmes, J., Whitaker, V., Fairbrother, H. & Curtis, P. (2018). *Youth drinking in decline.* UK: University of Sheffield. https://www.sheffield.ac.uk/polopoly_fs/1.806889!/file/Oldham_Holmes_Youth_drinking_in_decline_FINAL.pdf.

Pennay, A., Livingston, M., & MacLean, S. (2015). Young people are drinking less: It is time to find out why. *Drug and Alcohol Review, 34*(2), 115–118.

Rogers, M. (2016). Trans and gender diversity: Messages for policy and practice. In A. Ahmed & M. Rogers (Eds.), *Working with marginalised groups: From policy to practice* (Chapter 6). UK: Palgrave Macmillan.

Robinson, E., Oldham, M., Sharps, M., Cunliffe, A., Scott, J., Clark, E., & Field, M. (2016). Social imitation of alcohol consumption and ingratiation motives in young adults. *Psychology of Addictive Behaviors, 30*(4), 442–449.

Scottish Government. (2016). *The Scottish index of multiple deprivation* (SIMD16). http://simd.scot/2016/#/simd2016/BTTTFTT/9/-4.0000/55.9000/.

Spear, L. P. (2000). The adolescent brain and age-related behavioral manifestations. *Neuroscience and Biobehavioral Reviews, 24*(4), 417–463.

Spear, L. P., & Varlinskaya, E. I. (2006). Adolescence: Alcohol sensitivity, tolerance, and intake. In M. Galanter (Ed.), *Alcohol problems in adolescents and young adults: Epidemiology, neurobiology, prevention, and treatment* (pp. 143–159, Chapter xxi). New York, NY: Springer.

Stark, E. (2007). *Coercive control: How men entrap women in personal life.* New York: Oxford.

Stewart, C. (Ed.). (2018a). Lesbian, gay, bisexual, and transgender Americans at risk: Problems and solutions: Adults, Generation X, and Generation Y (Vol. 2, Chapter xxxiv, 290pp.). Santa Barbara, CA: Praeger/ABC-CLIO.

Stewart, C. (2018b, November 19). *Navigators start work at University Hospital Crosshouse*. Violence Reduction Unit. http://actiononviolence.org/news-and-blog/navigators-start-work-at-university-hospital-crosshouse.

Stewart, C. (2018c, September 18). *SVRU welcomes formation of VRU in London*. Violence Reduction Unit. http://actiononviolence.org/news-and-blog/svru-welcomes-formation-of-vru-in-london.

Tonmyr, L., Thornton, T., Draca, J., & Wekerle, C. (2010). A review of childhood maltreatment and adolescent substance use relationship. *Current Psychiatry Reviews, 6*(3), 223–234.

UNESCO. (2017). *What do we mean by youth?* United Nations Educational, Scientific and Cultural Organization. http://www.unesco.org/new/en/social-and-human-sciences/themes/youth/youth-definition/.

Van der Zwaluw, C., Scholte, R. H. J., Vermulst, A. A., Buitelaar, J., Verkes, R. J., & Engels, R. C. M. E. (2009). The crown of love: Intimate relations and alcohol use in adolescence. *European Child and Adolescent Psychiatry, 18*(7), 407–417.

Velleman, R., Templeton, L., Reuber, D., Klein, M., & Moesgen, D. (2008). Domestic abuse experienced by young people living in families with alcohol problems: Results from a cross-European study. *Child Abuse Review, 17*(6), 387–409.

VRU. (2016). *Scotland's violence reduction unit: 10 year strategic plan*. http://actiononviolence.org/sites/default/files/10%20YEAR%20PLAN_0.PDF.

Young, R. (2012). Can neds (or chavs) be non-delinquent, educated or even middle class? Contrasting empirical findings with cultural stereotypes. *Sociology, 46*(6), 1140–1160.

Younge, G., & Barr, C. (2017, December 3). How Scotland reduced knife deaths among young people. Beyond the blade: Knife crime. *The Guardian*. https://www.theguardian.com/membership/2017/dec/03/how-scotland-reduced-knife-deaths-among-young-people.

Part III

Recognizing the Breadth of Young Adult Drinking Styles

11

Non-drinkers and Non-drinking: A Review, a Critique and Pathways to Policy

Emma Banister, Dominic Conroy and Maria Piacentini

Non-drinking and non-drinkers have been the focus of growing cultural interest. This is evident in temporary abstinence campaigns (e.g. 'Dry January' in the UK, 'Dry February' in North America and 'Dry July' in Australia) and in growing evidence of the recent polarisation of alcohol consumption in many 'wet cultures'. While the majority of young adults drink, there are increasing numbers of non-drinkers; the UK media label the current generation of young adults 'Generation Sensible' (BBC, 2018). Academic research has witnessed a growth of studies focused on

---

E. Banister (✉)
University of Manchester, Manchester, UK
e-mail: emma.banister@manchester.ac.uk

D. Conroy
School of Psychology, University of East London, London, UK
e-mail: D.Conroy@uel.ac.uk

M. Piacentini
Lancaster University Management School, Lancaster, UK
e-mail: m.piacentini@lancaster.ac.uk

© The Author(s) 2019
D. Conroy and F. Measham (eds.), *Young Adult Drinking Styles*,
https://doi.org/10.1007/978-3-030-28607-1_11

non-drinking, cutting across disciplinary boundaries including sociology, psychology, criminology and marketing. A key theme of this work concerns difficulties with non-drinking in contexts where heavy drinking features prominently (e.g. university student life). Some research starts from a position that learning about non-drinking lives and experiences may help inform moderate alcohol consumption among young adults more broadly. In this chapter, section one summarises the key themes of emergent research relating to non-drinking. We then problematise aspects of the extant non-drinking literature in section two, advocating for research accounts containing greater nuance in understanding and defining young adult drinking styles which acknowledge the wider cultural context within which 'not drinking' may be understood. Finally, in section three, we consider how the evidence base might help refresh alcohol-related health promotion policy and future alcohol research agendas. Our approach is inclusive, ensuring that accounts of non-drinking and non-drinkers researched from diverse disciplinary and methodological starting points are included.

Non-drinking and Non-drinkers: Literature Themes

Much research on non-drinkers has focused on the links between 'evaluations of non-drinkers' and drinking behaviour. Such studies are conducted within a broader context of interest in how perceived peer norms relating to alcohol consumption might influence drinking behaviour. For example, studies working in the Prototype Willingness Model (PWM) tradition have consistently demonstrated that negative evaluations of 'the prototypical non-drinker' predict increased alcohol consumption among students (Gerrard et al., 2002; Rivis, Sheeran, & Armitage, 2006; Zimmermann & Sieverding, 2010). This PWM research provides a useful way of considering how perceptions of particular peers (non-drinkers) might drive personal drinking behaviours. This offers a theoretically distinctive account of 'the influence of non-drinkers' on drinking behaviour but assumes that 'perceptions of the prototypical drinker' can be measured without difficulty. Similar work has seen the construction of an Attitudes Toward

Non-drinkers (RANDS) measure, which has been explored as a predictor of harmful drinking behaviour among young people (Regan & Morrison, 2011, 2013, 2017). Again, non-drinkers are here understood as a homogenously defined, salient 'outgroup' given their non-engagement with alcohol consumption which could be considered normative and acceptable among many young adults. The RANDS scale has usefully linked people's ideas about non-drinkers to drinking behaviour itself. However, the RANDS measure contains divergent items about non-drinking as an imagined behaviour (e.g. 'I would find it very hard to enjoy my social life if I were a non-drinker'), with items about the impact of an individual's non-drinking behaviour on social occasions (e.g. 'An evening with a non-drinker tends to be predictable'). Conflation of these different aspects is important in that while typical 'non-drinkers' (the actors) might be viewed negatively, the decision to abstain from drinking any alcohol (non-drinking as a lifestyle choice) might be viewed ambivalently, yet views of situation-specific non-drinking might be viewed favourably.

Qualitative research has also been conducted to explore perceptions of non-drinkers among young adults. Focus group research findings suggest that the presence of non-drinkers at student parties involving heavy drinking may exert very little influence over their peers' drinking behaviour and were broadly accepted within drinking environments (Brown, Koelsch, & Yufik, 2010). Stereotypes can link 'being a non-drinker' with 'being unsocial' (Fossey, Loretto, & Plant, 1996). These stereotypes were unsettled in interview research with UK university students which revealed contradictory accounts of non-drinkers as both less sociable for not joining in with alcohol-consuming peers, yet in some respects more sociable than alcohol-consuming peers given their non-use of alcohol to feel socially at ease (Conroy & de Visser, 2013). Research on perceptions of non-drinkers has tended to assume that (a) non-drinkers can be unproblematically defined as a homogenous social group and (b) that non-drinkers and non-drinking mean the same thing to different people. A further difficulty, apparent in efforts to quantitatively measure 'views of non-drinkers', is that 'attitudes toward non-drinkers' might involve disparate aspects of non-drinking, for example whether relating to non-drinking as a perceived or undertaken lifestyle decision, to non-drinking as a behaviour (the act of not drinking in a situation) or to 'non-drinkers' as an (imagined/stereotyped) *type* of person.

Research that has focused on how non-drinkers are viewed among their peers has helped stimulate interest in the experience of being a young adult non-drinker, especially in contexts where relatively high levels of alcohol consumption may be normative and expected (e.g. university campus settings). Interest in experiences of non-drinking young adults has occasionally surfaced in research on social norms. For example, survey research has demonstrated that misperceptions about excessive drinking norms among Canadian college students can produce a socially alienating campus experience for non- or light-drinking students (Perkins, 2007). However, most studies concerning non-drinkers' experiences have been qualitative (e.g. Banister, Piacentini, & Grimes, 2019; Conroy & de Visser, 2014, 2015; Jacobs, Conroy, & Parke, 2018; Nairn, Higgins, Thompson, Anderson, & Fu, 2006; Piacentini & Banister, 2009; Robertson & Tustin, 2018). Such research frequently points to the adversity experienced by those students or young people who do not drink alcohol. For example, interviews with first year female UK university students pointed to experiences of social exclusion, stigma and limited opportunities to connect socially as a non-drinker on campus (Jacobs et al., 2018). Relatedly, a study of 18–25-year-old students based in New Zealand revealed that non-drinkers were commonly denigrated as 'cowards' or 'weirdos' for not drinking alcohol (Robertson & Tustin, 2018). One key theme of research has been to develop insights into how non-drinking is strategically managed or accounted for by young adults in situations where peers are consuming alcohol (e.g. Conroy & de Visser, 2014; Piacentini & Banister, 2009; Seaman & Ikegwuonu, 2010). For example, several studies have pointed to the utility of 'passing as a drinker' to resist deviant labelling and avoid peer scrutiny/pressure during social occasions by claiming to be drinking alcohol and/or by being seen in possession of an alcoholic drink (Conroy & de Visser, 2015; Herman-Kinney & Kinney, 2013; Jacobs et al., 2018; Romo, Dinsmore, Connolly, & Davis, 2015). Other research has revealed how neutralisation/counter-neutralisation techniques are employed by both non-drinkers and drinkers to soften effects of norm-violating behaviour (like non- or light-drinking), for example discursively resisting/reframing negative labels associated with being a 'type' of drinker (Piacentini, Chatzidakis, & Banister, 2012).

Some studies point to mundane practicalities of being a non-drinker in the company of other young adults who may be drinking alcohol excessively. One feature includes the phenomenon of acting as the 'carer' for alcohol-impaired friends/peers during social occasions, for example taking on responsibility to ensure that friends were safe and got home safely (Herring, Bayley, & Hurcombe, 2014; Piacentini & Banister, 2009). This caring role could make non-drinkers feel trapped between irritation about friends' excessive alcohol consumption yet also morally bound to help them (Herring et al., 2014).

Several studies underscored the importance for non-drinkers of enlisting support from like-minded others. This is evident in Piacentini and Banister's (2009) interviews which suggested how mutually supportive coping strategies (e.g. seeking support from other non-drinking others) were employed to resist the social stigma of non-drinking, particularly among female interviewees. Evidence underscores the importance of strategic identity management among non-drinkers attending social occasions involving alcohol and reveal how non-drinkers feel pressured to navigate stereotypical impressions of non-drinkers as 'boring' or 'no fun' (Piacentini & Banister, 2009; Seaman & Ikegwuonu, 2010). However, other studies suggest how greater experience with managing such situations can help bolster feelings of choice and empowerment (Conroy & de Visser, 2015; Herring et al., 2014).

Both qualitative and quantitative studies have focused on reasons/motivations for non-drinking and have concentrated on both lifelong and more recent non-drinkers. Longitudinal research has revealed that reasons for non-drinking related to perceived or experienced negative consequences of alcohol consumption were associated with greater alcohol consumption subsequently (Epler, Sher, & Piasecki, 2009).

Research by Huang, DeJong, Schneider, and Towvim (2011) has suggested that non-drinkers endorse more personal reasons for non-drinking (e.g. not wanting the image of a drinker, beliefs about alcohol's effect on behaviour) compared with more pragmatic reasons for non-drinking during a social occasion endorsed by drinkers (e.g. having to drive later, concern about weight gain). Other research has highlighted the complexity and contradictory way in which non-drinking accounts can be presented. For example, de Visser and Smith's (2007) interviews with demographically diverse young men demonstrated that most light-/non-drinking individuals held reasons for and against drinking. Other accounts of non-drinking reflect multi-faceted motivations that needed to be re-affirmed by non-drinkers on a situation-by-situation basis (Conroy & de Visser, 2014, 2015; Herman-Kinney & Kinney, 2013).

Some studies have drawn attention to how reasons for non-drinking are rhetorically invoked to manage scrutiny around non-drinking. For example, a US study of college abstainers revealed how pronounced 'reasons for non-drinking' evolved while at university, progressing from concealment strategies (e.g. using medical disclaimers such as 'I'm diabetic'), to preventive disclosure strategies (e.g. sharing genuine reasons with trustworthy others) to varying success in terms of diverting peer scrutiny (Herman-Kinney & Kinney, 2013). Recent analysis of reasons for non-drinking during social situations among undergraduates who regularly consume alcohol revealed wide-ranging benefits including enhanced self-esteem and productivity, yet also ambivalence to non-drinking in that not drinking might threaten social inclusion when socialising despite potential benefits (Conroy & de Visser, 2018).

In the next section, we critique the non-drinking literature and consider how a more sophisticated and inclusive way of understanding drinking styles might be permitted. Such discussion involves recognition that choice underpins how personal drinking styles are understood and presented to other people and how drinker categories like 'non-drinker' might be invoked, deployed and negotiated in conversations about drinking practices.

Problematising 'Non-drinking'

In this section, we discuss how research on non-drinking might be constructively problematised. We will first contextualise how non-drinking has traditionally been approached in the academic literature. We then draw on Emma and Maria's recent work concerning the sociology of nothing in relation to non-drinking which provides a way of accommodating existing tensions and complexities in understandings and terminology (Banister et al., 2019). The final section turns to Dominic's ongoing work with colleagues Charlotte Morton and Christine Griffin (Bath University) that explores how 'drinker types' can be understood as rhetorical devices involved in drinking practices. A principal theme of this problematising section is the importance of generating accounts of non-drinking which permit greater agency for the non-drinking actor, and for the practice of non-drinking as an activity or lifestyle decision.

The majority of non-drinking research is conducted in Western countries, primarily the UK (Banister et al., 2019; Piacentini et al., 2012; Conroy & de Visser, 2013, 2014, 2015, 2018), Australia (Jaensch, White-head, Prichard, & Hutton, 2018), New Zealand (Nairn et al., 2006; Niland, McCreanor, Lyons, & Griffin, 2017) and the United States (Ross et al., 2015), contexts where drinking alcohol is a predominant cultural norm and excess is normalised (Measham, 2004; Szmigin, Bengry-Howell, Griffin, Hackley, & Mistral, 2011). This focus informs the way in which non-drinking behaviours are understood and described—generally in relation to these predominant alcohol consumption norms. Terminology in the context of researching non-drinkers is notoriously messy. The operational meaning of researchers' preferred term—'non-drinker'—is open to interpretation producing a range of difficulties and ambiguities. Individuals tend to define their behaviour in relation to others (Hogg, 2016). In both Nairn et al. (2006) and Piacentini and Banister (2009), this is manifest through light-drinking individuals perceiving their self-definition as non-drinkers 'in comparative terms relative to the dominant norms within the student culture' (Piacentini & Banister, 2009: 281). Such views also point to other ambiguities around the consumption of alcohol—for example whether eating foods containing alcohol constitutes alcohol consumption.

It is also prudent to acknowledge the heterogeneity of reasons that individuals come to occupy the position of a non-drinker, which also informs the adopted terminology (e.g. abstainer, teetotaller). The work of Conroy and de Visser (2014, 2015) distinguishes between those who do not drink for 'culturally sanctioned reasons' (e.g. religion, health, athleticism) and 'culturally unsanctioned' reasons (e.g. don't like being around people when drunk, dislike alcohol's subjective effects, dislike the taste) as an instrumental way to explore non-drinking experiences (Conroy & de Visser, 2014, 2015). This separation helps compartmentalise what is clearly a heterogeneous group and may also inform the perceived legitimacy of non-drinking behaviours (Piacentini et al., 2012).

A number of researchers exclude individuals who do not drink primarily for religious reasons (e.g. Herring et al., 2014; Seaman & Ikegwuonu, 2010), yet no explicit rationalisation is provided. So while those from religious backgrounds are likely to be a significant proportion of the non-drinking population (Measham, 2008), they have seldom provided the focus for research. Generally, it seems those not drinking for culturally sanctioned reasons are considered less interesting, and it is assumed their behaviour is more easily managed and understood by others. However, we might ask who gets to decide whether something is culturally sanctioned, and does this approach to assigning legitimacy potentially deny the subject agency?

In addition to the reasons behind, or justifications of, consumption choices, there can also be a temporal side to non-drinking. Herring et al. (2014) usefully distinguish between individuals' non-drinking on the basis of how it fits within their broader narrative history. For example, they differentiate between individuals who do not drink as an ongoing lifestyle decision ('consistent'), who emerge as self-identified non-drinkers following gradual decreases ('transitional') and who do not drink in response to a particular experience ('turning point'). Distinctions between lifelong non-drinkers and former drinkers have also been made, for example, abstainers and desistors, respectively (Herman-Kinney & Kinney, 2013). Again, these varied definitions of non-drinking reflect the variety of research questions addressed, but also the considerable scope for confusion and misunderstanding within and between research communities when considering accounts of non-drinking and non-drinkers in alcohol research.

The literature lacks a cohesive all-encompassing means by which to frame developing understandings, one that allows for heterogeneity within the non-drinking population and also the varying cultural contexts within which (non-)consumption takes place, reflecting cultural contexts where drinking alcohol, sometimes excessively, is the norm, as well as countries or more local cultural contexts where drinking alcohol goes against the norm.

The sociology of nothing as recently developed by Scott (2018) helps account for elements of (non-) consumption that are unseen. She positions nothing as 'not just a passively endured condition, but a reflexively managed mode of experience' and alludes to the non-drinker as an exemplar of 'commission', under which a conscious decision is made to not drink (pp. 4–5). While this may be the case for many non-drinkers (e.g. the culturally sanctioned reformed alcoholic in Banister et al., 2019), it does not fully capture the range of non-drinking positions. More specifically, it fails to capture those who are classified as non-drinkers by omission, where the decision not to drink may not be as consciously, or actively, enacted. In an earlier study (Piacentini & Banister, 2006), we reported the case of Lena whose religion prohibits alcohol. Living within her own culture, her non-consumption of alcohol would be considered an act of omission (it is just something that she happens to not do), but now she lives within a new culture (studying in the UK) her non-drinking becomes an act of commission, a more conscious act, something to work at. This gives a flavour of the complexity of what it means to be a non-drinker, demonstrating how people move in and out of omission/commission depending on the cultural context within which their behaviours are enacted.

We now turn to a fuller discussion of how demonstrative acts of commission, and more passive acts of omission, can be applied to the field of alcohol consumption. Scott (2018) uses commission to understand the active accomplishment of doing or being a non-something; it involves conscious disengagement or disidentification—*demonstrably* doing nothing. Applied to the alcohol context, it implies an absolute position around not drinking, with an accompanying committed effort to not drink. This emphasis links with culturally sanctioned or legitimate non-drinking positions, illustrated where non-drinking individuals actively account for their choices (Supski & Lindsay, 2017), adapt to peer scrutiny and judgement (Graber, de Visser, & Abraham, 2016) or reveal active appeals to alternative subject positions, which can bring sporting and academic activities to the forefront (Nairn et al., 2006).

However, while for Muslim and other faith communities, abstention fits with Mullaney's 'never identities' (in Scott, 2018), alcohol also has an 'absent presence'—it is there and present in the community, but not talked about (Valentine, Holloway, & Jayne, 2010), suggesting the need for nuance when ascribing something as culturally (un)sanctioned, and relative positions in terms of what are considered culturally sanctioned reasons for not drinking (Conroy & de Visser, 2014).

These issues are also evoked with reference to temporary abstention programmes such as Dry January in the UK which could be understood as offering culturally sanctioned opportunities for individuals to temporarily not drink alcohol. The positive regulative techniques (Yeomans, 2018), their temporary nature and prolific sponsorship activities (e.g. in aid of alcohol and cancer charities) allow participants to demonstrably do nothing, without attachment to the potential negative identities sometimes attached to longer term sober identities.

Within this context of temporary abstention, Cherrier and Gurrieri (2013) suggest that temporary abstainers are still constituted by others as drinkers, which reduces the associated stigma which is reserved for the more permanent or committed non-drinker or abstainer.

Under active commission, non-drinkers are positioned as demonstrably and symbolically opposed to drinkers. In contrast, not drinking can be considered a performance of omission, a more passive act of happening to not do something. We now explore how this can help to develop a more nuanced understanding of (non-)drinking.

Omission refers to a process of *non-identification*, rather than disidentification; the act hovers below the threshold of awareness, not meaning enough to be seen and consciously rejected. This includes people who just do not identify as a drinker rather than explicitly identifying as a non-drinker. This disengagement with the collective identity of the non-drinker is explored in detail in Banister et al. (2019), but was also hinted at in Conroy and de Visser (2014) who refer to one participant, Michelle, and her reluctance to be defined by her practices around alcohol: 'I don't want to be labelled by what I do and don't do' (p. 7). She challenges the 'restrictive definitional and regulatory practices that "non-drinking" as a social category appeared to be felt to impose' (p. 7).

Omission is understood by Scott as a more passive act, involving less emphasis on identity management; this contrasts with prior non-drinking research, which has focused on managing (Piacentini & Banister, 2009) and coping (Piacentini & Banister, 2006) with being a non-drinker. However, Banister et al. (2019) demonstrate how within the context of alcohol consumption, even under omission, *not being* can be more planful than Scott (2018) envisaged. They present two key identity refusal positions, namely distancing through resistance (contesting the existence of a non-drinker as a something) and distancing through othering (accepting the existence of non-drinkers yet denying similarities to them personally). These differing positions have implications for how omission is performed (including different styles of identity talk) to 'minimize the role and impact of alcohol (non-)consumption in the construction of identity' (p. 14).

Considerations of the terminology and the accompanying complexity drive home the need for better understandings to more fully appreciate the relational dynamics at play in consumption choices. A framework that accounts for the possibility of non-drinking as being both commission and omission allows more heterogeneous considerations of drinking behaviours, for example potentially including light and occasional drinkers under omission and recognising that similar non-drinking positions may be dealt with very differently (e.g. varying identity talk and construction). Such a framework can provide a more sensitive approach to understanding how non-drinking can vary according to cultural and situational contexts, depending on the audience as well as the individual (e.g. Cocker, Piacentini, & Banister, 2018). Drawing on Scott's sociology of nothing permits scholars to more fully appreciate the range of (non) drinking positions adopted and the range of responses, both from the individuals themselves and their peers/audiences. The above discussion establishes the importance of recognising the agency involved in non-drinking positions, towards producing a more balanced and sensitive account of non-drinking, one which more effectively reflects its more diverse forms and presentations. We will now suggest how this agency can be understood in another way by drawing on currently unpublished discursive research (for an account of this research please consult Morton, 2016). This work has revealed evidence of mismatches between lay/self-identified and formal definitions of two drinker categories ('light drinkers' and 'binge drinkers') among university students who self-identified as light- or non-drinkers. As far as we are aware, no formal definition of 'non drinking' is available in the academic literature or in policy documents. We used a definition from Herring et al.

(2014) who define light drinkers as individuals who drink two/one UK units or less depending on whether they are male/female and report not being drunk in the previous two months. Moreover, this work suggests how students, faced with concrete definitions, were rhetorically creative in accounting for how someone might 'earn' a drinker category when contextual information was taken into account.

This is illustrated with reference to interview talk from an 18-year-old who self-identified as a non-drinker yet could be categorised as a light drinker using formal criteria. In this interview, participant definitions for non-drinkers, in relation to historical drunken behaviour, revealed shifts in footing from absolutes (i.e. participant talk emphasising tight definitional requirements for qualifying as a light drinker) to a more permissive formulation that could accommodate drunkenness without closing off the possibility of meaningfully self-identifying as a non-drinker. Another interview with a participant who self-identified as a light drinker illustrated how if an individual *decides that they are* a light drinker (evident where a participant indicates that they view themselves as a light drinker) then they *are*, almost regardless of what and how much that individual drinks. Evidence here sharply contrasts the underpinning assumptions of formal definitions, but enables individuals to socialise within a heavy-drinking culture while still identifying as a light drinker.

These rhetorical devices reveal the multiple possible dimensions involved in how drinker categories such as 'non-drinking' could or should be defined. Illustrative examples were abundant in this data and drew on the amount of alcohol consumed; the frequency of drinking and the frequency of getting drunk; and contrasting motivations underlying drinking behaviour. The effect of this might be two-fold: it provides a framework for justifying limited drinking behaviour to self and others, but it also means that drinking behaviour itself (which would contradict a more credible 'non drinker' identity) can remain congruent given the heavy-drinking culture typically experienced by university students. Here, notions of objectively recognisable 'non-drinkers' seem to evaporate and drinker categories become utilised as rhetorical devices for managing identity within university culture, as a distinct cultural setting.

We turn now to the final section of this chapter where we consider the evidence and discussion above in light of health promotion practice and policy and in relation to future research on non-drinking.

Using Non-drinking Research to Inform Policy, Practice and Future Research

Non-drinking has rarely featured in health promotion policy and strategy designed to promote healthier alcohol consumption in the general population. Efforts to promote more moderate drinking traditionally focus on education about 'sensible drinking' (e.g. Department of Health, 2016). Non-drinking is, however, intermittently included in alcohol policy. For example, the recent Change4Life campaign encouraged taking two 'dry days' without alcohol consumption per week (Charles, 2012) and is present in current recommendations to take 'several drink-free days each week' as part of healthy drinking (NHS, 2016).

Health promotion strategy might usefully problematise and challenge the dominating negative views of non-drinkers and non-drinking. Such strategic activity could point, credibly, to how numerically non-drinkers represent a large and growing group of individuals, and therefore, it is not the marginalised drinking position as currently viewed. Similarly, a dedicated social marketing campaign might challenge the suggestion that non-drinking is typically met with negative responses, instead highlighting how non-drinking may attract social praise and admiration and provide a wider variety of social and lifestyle opportunities than might otherwise be possible. Another way in which health strategy might acknowledge positives of the presence of non-drinkers during social occasions might be to acknowledge their important role at a purely practical level during social occasions involving high levels of alcohol consumption, for example as the 'designated driver'.

Applying non-drinking research to a broader alcohol health promotion agenda might involve appealing to the varied potential advantages of 'dry days'. Appeals could draw on recent research (Conroy & de Visser, 2018) to illuminate potential benefits of social non-drinking (e.g. experiencing substance-free social confidence) but could also inoculate against anticipated drawbacks of social non-drinking (e.g. limited peer bonding opportunities). In appealing to these positives, health promotion strategy might acknowledge social challenges that can be encountered by non-drinkers and offer concrete, evidence-based suggestions for how non-drinking is made easier when socialising. In light of discussion about omission in the second section of this chapter, it seems possible that more people taking 'dry days' might help incorporate non-drinking into the mainstream purely by increasing the visibility of non-drinking as a typical behaviour during social occasions and by the same token diluting the numbers of people being crudely pigeon-holed as 'non-drinkers' or indeed, 'drinkers'.

A related strategy/policy approach might problematise simplistic definitions of drinking behaviour and, particularly, specific 'drinker categories' like 'non-drinker' and 'binge drinker'. This approach, again, chimes with the theoretical emphases of commission and omission described in section two of this chapter. For example, softening the hard boundaries between 'drinker categories' (e.g. 'non-drinkers' vs 'social drinkers') might permit young adults to reflect on non-drinking as something they can practice flexibly and freely during social occasions. Appreciating the distinctions between active and passive approaches to non-drinking may equip non-drinkers with strategies and approaches for how they present themselves in their varying social settings, to ameliorate the negative impacts of their positioning on their identity, and indeed help them to fully engage in their social worlds as a positively managed mode of experience (Scott, 2018).

There is some support for the idea that non-drinking may be a relevant 'ingredient' within alcohol interventions designed to promote lower levels of alcohol consumption in clinical settings. For example, evidence has suggested that encouraging individuals to reflect on the benefits of social non-drinking and its strategic 'management' in social situations may help reduce overall alcohol consumption (Conroy, Sparks, & de Visser, 2015). However, very little is known about how non-drinking might be framed from a health promotion perspective. Furthermore, using 'dry days' as a means of promoting moderate drinking carries risks, what if compensatory high levels of drinking follow dry days (as might be predicted from an 'abstinence violation effect' perspective, Curry, Marlatt, & Gordon, 1987).

Health promotion policy and strategy might make greater use of non-drinking as a tool to promote more moderate alcohol consumption among young adults but in light of the ambiguities and uncertainties surrounding 'non-drinking' as a categorical activity, we note here that there are no clear ways in which dry days could be applied to promote moderate drinking in a straightforward way devoid of risks involving compensatory drinks.

While these means of promoting moderate alcohol consumption may draw on non-drinking, a key emergent theme from the non-drinking evidence base suggests the importance of reimagining, planning and reconfiguring social environments so that alcohol consumption is de-emphasised as a central feature. Success in this area would provide an important means to help normalise non-drinking, challenging binary understandings of socialising options that might demarcate one environment for drinking alcohol and other environments for not drinking alcohol. Simple steps are important to recognise here. For example, making pubs and cafes enjoyable places to be in regardless of whether people are drinking alcohol, including innovative variations of beverages and food (e.g. deserts or food to share). We also note here the particular responsibilities held by institutions such as universities and higher education colleges in this respect. Student unions may need to re-envisage their role and responsibilities. In the UK, the National Union of Students (NUS) has piloted a scheme at two universities to reduce levels of harmful drinking among students by screening for harmful drinking and providing guidance around moderate drinking (NUS Alcohol Impact, 2016). However, the NUS also has a pivotal role to play in terms of promoting suitable spaces for individuals who do not drink alcohol as a lifestyle choice, but also those who routinely drink alcohol yet want to be able to not drink alcohol during certain social occasions without closing down social opportunities and access to friendship circles. Initiatives in line with this have involved a growing number of universities offering alcohol-free halls of residence (including, in the UK, University of Manchester and University of Edinburgh). Initiatives to expand opportunities for drinks-free socialising are also growing, partly in response to the growing national, racial and cultural diversity of UK student populations. For example, Leeds Students Union has introduced pottery and coffee making classes and now 'tags' relevant events as 'alcohol free' in line with increasing demands for alcohol-free social events (Leeds

University Union, 2019). A more imaginative and inclusive approach to social environments for young people will help recognise the (growing) variation in drinking habits and to include non-drinkers within this vision. This kind of approach, we suggest, might help to normalise lighter drinking habits and to inculcate an understanding of 'drinking styles' rather than 'drinker types' in social spaces.

Considering how the non-drinking evidence base might inform alcohol policy leads to reflections on productive future directions. Maintaining the profile of research on non-drinking is important for several reasons. Continuing research emphasis on 'binge drinking' among young adults helps reinforce a simplistic view of how young people drink, for example not showing evidence of new and creative responses including wide-spread evidence of resilience to a heavy-drinking culture. With the increase in numbers of young people not drinking, it is reasonable to assume that their presence in varied social settings may have an impact on the alcohol behaviours of others in their social group (drinkers and non-drinkers). Therefore, it may be interesting to map the effect of this on drinking behaviours. This may involve studying drinkers and non-drinkers from the same social groups to understand the effect of the co-existence of both groups in the same social setting impacts on modes of being within the group. This may involve looking at consumption levels of drinkers; identity associations; social connectedness; and general well-being measures. Much of the emphasis in the commission/omission non-drinking research to date has been on young people, and it may be a useful approach to consider some of the issues of the lived experience of the non-drinker in older age categories, to explore the ways in which not drinking influences their mode of being.

References

Banister, E., Piacentini, M., & Grimes, A. (2017). Identity refusal and the non-drinking self. In K. Diehl & C. Yoon (Eds.), *Advances in Consumer Research Volume 43* (pp: 457–458). Duluth, MN: Association for Consumer Research.

Banister, E., Piacentini, M. G., & Grimes, G. (2019). Identity refusal: Distancing from non-drinking in a drinking culture. *Sociology, 53*, 744–761.

BBC. (2018, July 19). *Generation sensible' in five charts*. https://www.bbc.co.uk/news/44880278.

Brown, A. L., Koelsch, L., & Yufik, T. (2010). The exception to the rule: Non-drinkers at college student parties: 834. *Alcoholism: Clinical & Experimental Research, 34*(6), 219A.

Charles, G. (2012). *Change4Life tackles sensible drinking mission*. Campaign. Retrieved 3 October 2019 from https://www.campaignlive.co.uk/article/change4life-tackles-sensible-drinking-mission/1115582.

Cherrier, H., & Gurrieri, L. (2013). Anti-consumption choices performed in a drinking culture: Normative struggles and repairs. *Journal of Macromarketing, 33*(3), 232–244.

Cocker, H., Piacentini, M., & Banister, E. (2018). Managing dramaturgical dilemmas: Youth drinking and multiple identities. *European Journal of Marketing, 52*(5/6), 1305–1328.

Conroy, D., & de Visser, R. (2013). 'Man up!': Discursive constructions of non-drinkers among UK undergraduates. *Journal of Health Psychology, 18*(11), 1432–1444.

Conroy, D., & de Visser, R. (2014). Being a non-drinking student: An interpretative phenomenological analysis. *Psychology & Health, 29*(5), 536–551.

Conroy, D., & de Visser, R. (2015). The importance of authenticity for student non-drinkers: An interpretative phenomenological analysis. *Journal of Health Psychology, 20*(11), 1483–1493.

Conroy, D., & de Visser, R. O. (2018). Benefits and drawbacks of social non-drinking identified by British university students. *Drug & Alcohol Review, 37*, S89–S97.

Conroy, D., Sparks, P., & de Visser, R. (2015). Efficacy of a non-drinking mental simulation intervention for reducing student alcohol consumption. *British Journal of Health Psychology, 20*(4), 688–707.

Curry, S., Marlatt, G. A., & Gordon, J. R. (1987). Abstinence violation effect: Validation of an attributional construct with smoking cessation. *Journal of Consulting and Clinical Psychology, 55*(2), 145.

Department of Health. (2016). *Alcohol guidelines review*. Report from the Guidelines Development Group to the UK Chief Medical Officers. Retrieved 3 October 2019 from https://assets.publishing.service.gov.uk/government/uploads/system/uploads/attachment_data/file/545739/GDG_report-Jan2016.pdf.

de Visser, R. O., & Smith, J. A. (2007). Alcohol consumption and masculine identity among young men. *Psychology and Health, 22*(5), 595–614.

Epler, A. J., Sher, K. J., & Piasecki, T. M. (2009). Reasons for abstaining or limiting drinking: A developmental perspective. *Psychology of Addictive Behavior, 23*(3), 428–442.

Fossey, E., Loretto, W., & Plant, M. (1996). Alcohol and youth. In L. Harrison (Ed.), *Alcohol problems in the community* (pp. 52–75). London: Routledge.

Gerrard, M., Gibbons, F. X., Reis-Bergan, M., Trudeau, L., Vande Lune, L. S., & Buunk, B. (2002). Inhibitory effects of drinker and nondrinker prototypes on adolescent alcohol consumption. *Health Psychology, 21*(6), 601–609.

Graber, R., de Visser, R., & Abraham, C. (2016). Staying in the 'sweet spot': A resilience-based analysis of the lived experience of low-risk drinking and abstention among British youth. *Psychology & Health, 31*(1), 79–99.

Herman-Kinney, N. J., & Kinney, D. A. (2013). Sober as deviant: The stigma of sobriety and how some college students "stay dry" on a "wet" campus. *Journal of Contemporary Ethnography, 42*(1), 64–103.

Herring, R., Bayley, M., & Hurcombe, R. (2014). 'But no one told me it's okay to not drink': A qualitative study of young people who drink little or no alcohol. *Journal of Substance Use, 19*(1/2), 95–102.

Hogg, M. A. (2016). Social identity theory. In S. Mckeown, R. Haji, & N. Ferguson (Eds.), *Understanding peace and conflict through social identity theory* (pp. 3–17). Cham: Springer.

Huang, J. H., DeJong, W., Schneider, S. K., & Towvim, L. G. (2011). Endorsed reasons for not drinking alcohol: A comparison of college student drinkers and abstainers. *Journal of Behavioral Medicine, 34*(1), 64–73.

Jacobs, L., Conroy, D., & Parke, A. (2018). Negative experiences of non-drinking college students in Great Britain: An interpretative phenomenological analysis. *International Journal of Mental Health & Addiction, 16*(3), 737–750.

Jaensch, J., Whitehead, D., Prichard, I., & Hutton, A. (2018). Exploring young peoples' use of alcohol at outdoor music festivals in Australia. *Journal of Applied Youth Studies, 2*(3), 32–42.

Leeds University Union. (2019). *Union events.* Retrieved 30 April 2019 from https://www.luu.org.uk/union-events/.

Measham, F. (2004). The decline of ecstasy, the rise of 'binge' drinking and the persistence of pleasure. *Probation Journal, 51*(4), 309–326.

Measham, F. (2008). The turning tides of intoxication: Young people's drinking in Britain in the 2000s. *Health Education, 108*(3), 207–222.

Morton, C. (2016). *'Coming out', making sacrifices and the fun of being sober: A thematic analysis of non-drinking and light drinking students' accounts* (Dissertation available).

Nairn, K., Higgins, J., Thompson, B., Anderson, M., & Fu, N. (2006). "It's just like the teenage stereotype, you go out and drink and stuff": Hearing from young people who don't drink. *Journal of Youth Studies, 9*(3), 287–304.

Niland, P., McCreanor, T., Lyons, A. C., & Griffin, C. (2017). Alcohol marketing on social media: Young adults engage with alcohol marketing on facebook. *Addiction Research & Theory, 25*(4), 273–284.

NHS. (2016). *The risks of drinking too much.* Retrieved 4 September 2018 from https://www.nhs.uk/live-well/alcohol-support/the-risks-of-drinking-too-much/#low-risk-drinking-advice.

NUS Alcohol Impact. (2016). *Students and alcohol 2016: Research into students' relationship with alcohol.* Available at http://s3-eu-west-1.amazonaws.com/nusdigital/document/documents/27249/9c439fd3a22644fee56ed771c584303a/NUS_Alcohol_Impact_Students_and_alcohol_2016.pdf.

Perkins, H. (2007). Misperceptions of peer drinking norms in Canada: Another look at the "reign of error" and its consequences among college students. *Addictive Behaviors, 32*(11), 2645–2656.

Piacentini, M. G., & Banister, E. N. (2006). Getting hammered? Students coping with alcohol. *Journal of Consumer Behaviour: An International Research Review, 5*(2), 145–156.

Piacentini, M. G., & Banister, E. N. (2009). Managing anti-consumption in an excessive drinking culture. *Journal of Business Research, 62*(2), 279–288.

Piacentini, M. P., Chatzidakis, A., & Banister, E. N. (2012). Making sense of drinking: the role of techniques of neutralisation and counter-neutralisation in negotiating alcohol consumption. *Sociology of Health & Illness, 34*(6), 841–857.

Regan, D., & Morrison, T. G. (2011). Development and validation of a scale measuring attitudes toward non-drinkers. *Substance Use and Misuse, 46*(5), 580–590.

Regan, D., & Morrison, T. G. (2013). Adolescents' negative attitudes towards non-drinkers: A novel predictor of risky drinking. *Journal of Health Psychology, 18*(11), 1465–1477.

Regan, D., & Morrison, T. G. (2017). Temporal stability and predictive validity of the regan attitudes toward non-drinkers scale. *SAGE Open, 7*(2).

Rivis, A., Sheeran, P., & Armitage, C. J. (2006). Augmenting the theory of planned behaviour with the prototype/willingness model: Predictive validity of actor versus abstainer prototypes for adolescents' health-protective and health-risk intentions. *British Journal of Health Psychology, 11*(3), 483–500.

Robertson, K., & Tustin, K. (2018). Students who limit their drinking, as recommended by national guidelines, are stigmatized, ostracized, or the subject of peer pressure: Limiting consumption is all but prohibited in a culture of intoxication. *Substance Abuse: Research and Treatment, 12,* 1178221818792414.

Romo, L. K., Dinsmore, D. R., Connolly, T. L., & Davis, C. N. (2015). An examination of how professionals who abstain from alcohol communicatively negotiate their non-drinking identity. *Journal of Applied Communication Research, 43*(1), 91–111.

Ross, C. S., Maple, E., Siegel, M., DeJong, W., Naimi, T. S., Padon, A. A., ..., Jernigan, D. H. 2015. The relationship between population-level exposure to alcohol advertising on television and brand-specific consumption among underage youth in the US. *Alcohol and Alcoholism, 50*(3), 358–364.

Scott, S. (2018). A sociology of nothing: Understanding the unmarked. *Sociology, 52*(1), 3–19.

Seaman, P., & Ikegwuonu, T. (2010). *Drinking to belong.* York: Joseph Rowntree Foundation. Retrieved 1 November 2019 from https://www.jrf.org.uk/sites/default/files/jrf/migrated/files/alcohol-young-adults-full.pdf.

Supski, S., & Lindsay, J. (2017). 'There's something wrong with you' how young people choose abstinence in a heavy drinking culture. *Young, 25*(4), 323–338.

Szmigin, I., Bengry-Howell, A., Griffin, C., Hackley, C., & Mistral, W. (2011). Social marketing, individual responsibility and the "culture of intoxication". *European Journal of Marketing, 45*(5), 759–779.

Valentine, G., Holloway, S. L., & Jayne, M. (2010). Contemporary cultures of abstinence and the nighttime economy: Muslim attitudes towards alcohol and the implications for social cohesion. *Environment and Planning, 42*(1), 8–22.

Yeomans, H. (2018). New Year, new you: A qualitative study of dry January, self-formation and positive regulation. *Drugs: Education, Prevention and Policy, 26*(6), 460–468.

Zimmerman, F., & Sieverding, M. (2010). Young adults' social drinking as explained by an augmented theory of planned behaviour: The roles of prototypes, willingness, and gender. *British Journal of Health Psychology, 15,* 561–581.

12

Can't Dance Without Being Drunk? Exploring the Enjoyment and Acceptability of Conscious Clubbing in Young People

Emma Davies, Joanne Smith, Mattias Johansson, Kimberley Hill and Kyle Brown

In this chapter, we focus on the emergence of the conscious clubbing movement and its potential benefits to young adults as a way of spending social time without drinking alcohol. Efforts to promote moderate drinking among young people may be challenging when the environment strongly encourages drinking, but conscious clubbing, which has roots

---

E. Davies (✉)
Oxford Brookes University, Oxford, UK
e-mail: edavies@brookes.ac.uk

J. Smith
Northumbria University, Newcastle upon Tyne, UK

M. Johansson
Örebro University, Örebro, Sweden

K. Hill
University of Northampton, Northampton, UK

K. Brown
Birmingham City University, Birmingham, UK

© The Author(s) 2019
D. Conroy and F. Measham (eds.), *Young Adult Drinking Styles*,
https://doi.org/10.1007/978-3-030-28607-1_12

233

in rave culture and involves dancing without the use of alcohol or other drugs, may offer an alternative. Drawing on literature from the rave scene and the benefits of dancing in a group, we introduce conscious clubbing and how it could bring about meaningful experiences in participants' lives, while at the same time, reducing the consumption of alcohol, and in doing so, we draw on our own recent survey research. This research illuminates challenges in the acceptability of conscious clubbing to some young people, which we discuss alongside suggestions for new directions for research in this area, at the end of the chapter.

The Historical and Cultural Significance of Raves

Anderson and Kavanaugh (2007) highlight how raves "*historically referred to grassroots organized, antiestablishment and unlicensed all-night dance parties, featuring electronically produced dance music (EDM), such as techno, house, trance and drum and bass*", while acknowledging a number of additional distinct characteristics. These include: a unique sense of cultural identity, defined by 1960s–1970 era liberalism, tolerance and unity; noncommercial, "grass-roots" organisation in large unlicensed venues, and identity markers or symbols, including language, style, gestures and clothing. Most significantly, many conceptualise the concomitant use of psychoactive drugs, specifically MDMA, a "flagship" rave drug (Kavanaugh & Anderson, 2008) as its defining element. During this time, patrons were drawn to contexts whereby they could dance, socialise and develop a sense of community togetherness with no alcohol-related aggression, violence or sexual harassment and no alcohol hangover (Goulding, Shankar, & Elliott, 2002).

It is important to note, however, that rave culture and psychoactive drug usage were a product of the historical and cultural context. Specifically, similarly to the 1920s US jazz and 1970s UK punk scenes, raves were considered as alternative, deviant or a form of youth subculture and identity in the late 1980s/early 1990s (Anderson & Kavanaugh, 2007; Measham, 2004). In addition to increases in both access and availability of these psychoactive drugs (Klee, 1998) at the time, the media were also considered to be amplifying public disapproval regarding alcohol consumption (and its potential relationship to public disorders), typified with discourses such as "lager lout" (Measham & Brain, 2005).

Recreational drug use is considered cyclical (Kohn, 1997) and subject to fashions and trends with the decline of alcohol consumption/increase in psychoactive drug consumption changing as time progressed through the so-called decade of dance (1988–1998: Reynolds, 2013). The rave movement appears to have "died", resulting from commercialisation and emancipation of electronic dance music, the primary cultural product of the rave scene, now present in many elements of popular culture (Anderson & Kavanaugh, 2007). Alongside this, fashions in psychoactive drugs moved on, with a subsequent recommodification of alcoholic drinks because of policy changes in licensing, and the production of high strength bottled beers, alcopops and shooters (Measham, 2004). Such mixed drinks and legal stimulants are considered to provide a similar buzz to other substances (Measham, 2008). In addition, changes to drinking spaces, tailored for young people in terms of style and themes, became more popular among young people who were moving towards a culture of intoxication and excess. Again, alcohol consumption had become socially acceptable and synonymous with "a good night out" (Measham & Brain, 2005).

After the mid-2000s (considered by some as "peak booze") drinking patterns began to change, and at the time of writing, it appears young people's drinking is in decline (e.g., Ng Fat, Shelton, & Cable, 2018). However, those that do drink may still consume alcohol in large quantities, often with the intention of getting drunk, and this pattern of drinking is particularly prevalent among university students, many of whom drink at hazardous levels (Davoren, Demant, Shiely, & Perry, 2016). Young people are generally aware of the risks associated with excessive alcohol consumption, but because they see drinking as a pleasurable part of their social lives, they discount information about these risks (Hutton, 2012). Existing health campaigns tend to focus on encouraging individuals to reduce their alcohol consumption, without replacing the lost social pleasures. The ubiquity of alcohol in social occasions means that individuals who chose not to drink can feel stigmatised and evidence has suggested that these individuals may adopt strategies including pretending to drink when socialising with friends (Conroy & de Visser, 2014).

Not only the social pressures, but the environment itself, within public houses, bars and nightclub settings, may impact on an individual's ability to regulate their alcohol consumption within these contexts due to the strong associative cues, which prompt drinking in these places (Qureshi, Monk, & Li, 2015). New approaches to understanding such features of both the social and the physical environment may be more effective than putting the focus on individual behaviour change, by limiting opportunities for risky consumption (Hill, Foxcroft, & Pilling, 2018). Here, qualitative research has illuminated the complex interplay between individual and social contexts including the rhetorical dynamics involved in negotiating drink offers as someone not drinking during a social situation (Conroy & de Visser, 2014; Piacentini, Chatzidakis, & Banister, 2012).

Current health campaigns can also fail to account for varieties in "drinking practices"—the different ways that alcohol is consumed. For example, for students, pre-drinking at home may occur prior to entering a nightclub with friends but may not occur prior to a meal with family. Thus, drinking behaviours belong in broader domains of social practice transmitted through "performances" (Blue, Shove, Carmona, & Kelly, 2016). Elements of student drinking, including the materials (e.g. bars attended), the meanings (e.g. expectations and social pressure) and the competencies (e.g. knowing what and how much to drink) performed over time, contribute to a shared understanding of these social practices (Supski, Lindsay, & Tanner, 2017). These elements are related, each shaping the others and contributing to the transmission of drinking practices to new students when they start (and even before they start) university (Supski et al., 2017). The implication of understanding drinking in this broader way is that rather than solely targeting individuals, health campaigns also need to focus on disrupting these materials, challenging meanings and instilling new competencies. For example, removing alcohol from events could change the bar environment, expectations about events and the type of knowledge needed at such events.

However, currently, options for young people at university who chose not to drink, or who want to reduce their consumption, are limited. Some focus on promoting participation in sports, but team sport players at university are often considered as a high-risk drinking group (Zhou, Heim,

& O'Brien, 2015). In the USA, researchers examined the effectiveness of late-night alcohol-free events at a college, such as films and board games, and found decreased consumption and binge drinking in individuals who attended more frequently over the course of their four years at university (Layland, Calhoun, Russell, & Maggs, 2018). However, students may not wish to be excluded from music and dancing events, simply because they chose not to drink, which is why we focus here on the possibilities of conscious clubbing.

Conscious Clubbing

Perhaps in line with decreases in drinking in some groups of the population, alcohol-free organisations and events have increased in recent years. For example, Club Soda, founded in 2015, is an organisation that encourages mindful drinking and aims to ensure that non-drinking is as socially acceptable as drinking. Additionally, there has been a rise in alcohol-free festivals, such as Buddhafield Festival and alcohol-free events, which focus on dancing and movement (e.g. Wild Chocolate Club). There are also a growing number of online movements, such as "Hello Sunday Morning" and "Soberistas", offering support and an accessible community of other individuals.

Our focus here is on those alcohol-free events that involve music and dancing, often described as 'sober raves' or 'conscious clubbing' events. The term 'conscious clubbing' serves to show that this kind of event is an alternative to clubs and festivals where alcohol and other drugs are commonly used; instead, these events place emphasis on playing music alongside other forms of energising entertainment, such as yoga classes and massage. One example is Morning Gloryville, considered to be one of the pioneering alcohol-free clubbing events, which at the time of writing has operated in 14 different countries (including UK, Spain, Netherlands, Australia and Japan) and has attracted many popular mainstream music artists.

Aspects of the modern-day conscious clubbing phenomena have clear similarities to dance cultures' rave scene of the 1980s, and the "conscious-partying" movement of the 1990s (Beck & Lynch, 2009). Such conscious-partying events included creative opportunities for cultural, political and spiritual transformation, alongside music and dancing in contrast to what its proponents viewed as the over-commercialisation of the dance scene (Beck & Lynch, 2009). They can be viewed as a counter-cultural movement away from current alcohol consumption norms, characterised by alternative beverage selections, with electronic dance music and "underground" grass-roots style organisation, as key staples of many of these events. Conscious clubbing could be a response to strong public health discourses regarding the harmful nature of excessive alcohol consumption, and a reduction in youth drinking (Ng Fat et al., 2018). Research into people's experiences of these events is limited at present; however, the act of dancing comes with many interpersonal and psychological pleasures, which is reason to hypothesise that conscious clubbing can extend positive benefits to those who participate, in addition to added health benefits of reducing drinking.

The Pleasures and Benefits of Dancing and Connecting with Others Through Dance

Throughout history, people have gathered in groups for rituals, festivals, events, and carnivals to listen to music and dance (Christensen, Cela-Conde, & Gomila, 2017). While attending these gatherings, individuals may momentarily "lose" themselves in the collective group experience (Ehrenreich, 2006). The anthropologist Victor Turner called these gatherings communitas (1969) and stressed their importance for human health and well-being. In communitas, people connect, social structures are disbanded temporarily, and through dancing, individuals may experience joy, healing and bonding with others (Salamone, 2004). When the gathering is over, people return to normal life and its social structures, rules and order, but feel revitalised through new experiences of joy, connection and meaning. Researchers like Haidt acknowledged this phenomenon and referred to it as the hive-hypothesis, in which people feel that they lose themselves and reach peak levels of human growth by becoming part of a wider social movement (Haidt, Patrick Seder, & Kesebir, 2008).

Reviews of the literature and empirical studies show that dancing may promote a number of health-related beneficial outcomes including improving mood, self-concept, body image and well-being, and reducing symptoms of anxiety and depression (Connolly, Quin, & Redding, 2011). EDM participants also express deep reasons for engaging in these events, such as identity formation and change, a deeper sense of belonging in this world as well as transcendence and flow experiences (Goulding et al., 2002). Self-expression and identity are further expressed for these individuals in pre-event rituals and associated clothing. As mainstream culture has become increasingly individualised and less focused on communities, tradition and rituals, there are fewer opportunities for people to be connected to others, without some larger and more corporate purpose (Giddens, 1991). Dance music events may offer opportunities for interpersonal connections, and the participant may interact with the special characteristics of the music together with other dancers as part of a pleasurable, inter-subjectively embodied experience (Solberg & Jensenius, 2016).

Dancing and being part of groups at festivals where one may lose oneself into a bigger group are beneficial in many ways for creating a sense of community and belonging (St John, 2006). Dance events such as Morning Gloryville and others share similar characteristics found at festivals, EDM culture events and raves without adding alcohol and other drugs. Dressing up and other festival characteristics are part of preparing for the communita and getting into a suitable mood. They cement the notion of letting go of the structure of society and getting into a temporary state where the participants can have fun, take on temporary new identities, explore and express themselves (Goulding et al., 2002). It was through an exploration of these potential positive benefits, in the context of the presumed absence of alcohol and other drugs that we sought to investigate conscious clubbing. Specifically, we sought to examine: (a) whether acceptability of and attitudes towards conscious clubbing events were associated with alcohol consumption, social connectedness and life satisfaction in addition to, (b) people's rationale for choosing (or not choosing) to attend such events and (c) personal experiences of attending them.

Survey

Method

Using a cross-sectional survey design, UK university students were recruited into an online survey presented in Qualtrics software through research participation schemes and social media. Individuals were incentivised to take part by the opportunity to enter a prize draw to win an iPad. The survey took 15 minutes to complete and received ethical approval from Birmingham City University.

Measures

The Alcohol Use Disorders Identification Test (AUDIT) (Babor, Higgins-Biddle, Saunders, & Monteiro, 2001) was used as a self-report indicator of potentially hazardous consumption levels (10 items; $\alpha = .81$). The revised Social Connectedness Questionnaire (Lee & Robbins, 1995) was incorporated to assess the degree to which individuals feel connected to others in their social environment (8 items; $\alpha = .96$). The Satisfaction with Life Scale (Diener, Emmons, Larsen, & Griffin, 1985) was incorporated to assess beliefs about satisfaction with one's life (5 items; $\alpha = .88$).

As part of the process to assess attitudes towards conscious clubbing events, participants were shown a video of a Morning Gloryville event (https://www.youtube.com/watch?v=OeMScv8er5Y) and were asked their views about it. Attitudes were assessed in a similar manner to previous studies of attitudes towards consumption of alcohol-free drinks and binge drinking (Norman, 2011). The following phrase was used: "I think alcohol events like these seem…" (4 items; $\alpha = .85$). Acceptability of the introduction of conscious clubbing events was assessed using an index adapted from Petrescu, Hollands, Couturier, Ng, and Marteau (2016). The question read: "Your university is going to introduce an alcohol-free social event, like the one in the video, in fresher's week instead of a traditional club night involving alcohol consumption". Acceptability was then assessed on a 7-point scale, using the following two items: "Do you support or oppose this policy?" and "How acceptable do you find this policy?" ($\alpha = .74$).

A number of closed and open answer questions were then presented to explore participants' experiences of conscious clubbing. They were firstly asked whether they have previously attended "an alcohol-free social event that involved music such as a sober rave, conscious clubbing event or similar". Individuals who had attended were further questioned about their reasons for attending, followed by their experiences, both of which involved open-ended responses. Individuals yet to attend a conscious clubbing event were asked whether they have heard of such an event before, with those responding "yes" asked to indicate why they chose not to attend (open-ended response). General demographic data (age, gender, ethnicity) were also measured.

Analytic Approach

Pearson correlation coefficients were calculated to assess the association between AUDIT scores, social connectedness, life satisfaction, acceptability and attitudes towards conscious clubbing. Open-ended questions were analysed using content analysis following the steps outlined by Treadwell (2013). These steps involved defining the unit of analysis as each individual response, and subsequently, a coding scheme was developed using the participants' words as a starting point and this was applied to the data set. ELD initially generated the coding scheme and this was checked and further developed by MJ. All other authors checked and agreed with the final coding scheme. Content analysis was used to identify frequently mentioned topics within the open-ended questions. The most frequently identified codes for each of the three questions are presented below, alongside some illustrative quotes from the participants. First, we present the answers for those participants who had previously attended a conscious clubbing event, and then, we present the answers from those who had not.

Results

The sample included 236 students, the majority of whom were female (82%), current drinkers (87%) and white European ethnicity (70%) with an average age of 19 years. From our sample, 39 individuals (16%) specified that they have previously attended a conscious clubbing event, the majority of whom ($N = 23$) attended between two and five times. Of the 197 who have yet to attend an event, 47 respondents (20%) indicated that they had heard of these events (or similar). Highlights of the whole-sample correlational results (Table 12.1) revealed that individuals who consume more alcohol view conscious clubbing less favourably, while both AUDIT scores and attitudes towards conscious clubbing were unrelated to social connectedness or life satisfaction scores.

Previous Attenders: Reasons for Attending Conscious clubbing Events ($N = 39$)

For individuals who had previously experienced a sober rave, the most commonly coded reasoning for their attendance was related to having fun without alcohol ($N = 14$). Others talked about the negative effects of alcohol on a night out:

Table 12.1 Pearson correlations between AUDIT scores, social connectedness, life satisfaction, attitudes towards conscious clubbing and acceptability of policy to introduce conscious clubbing

	AUDIT	Social con-nectedness	Life satisfaction	Conscious clubbing attitude	Acceptability
AUDIT	1	.02	.05	−.17**	−.13
Social con-nectedness		1	.29**	.05	.08
Life satisfac-tion			1	.11	.14*
Conscious clubbing attitude				1	.81**
Acceptability					1

* $p < .05$, ** $p < .01$

12 Can't Dance Without Being Drunk? Exploring the Enjoyment ...   243

> [I'm] Interested in having fun with friends without making stupid decisions and losing memory. (Man, 20)

The second most common code was about connecting with people ($N = 13$). Some discussed the importance of the social aspects, such as meeting likeminded people, or making new friends, while others talked about making more "genuine" connections than were possible when drinking alcohol:

> Normally I would drink during events like these however it is nice to relax and just socialise sober instead. (Man, 20)

Four participants discussed how they enjoyed the feeling of dancing to music without being drunk, while others talked about attending the events specifically for the music:

> Because for me, alcohol is not essential to have a good time and to dance. Dance music is something I'm passionate about, especially with friends. (Woman, 20)

There was specific mention of not liking to be around drunk people by three participants:

> Because I don't like the way people behave after alcohol consumption. I feel safer if there is no alcohol consumption near me. (Woman, 22)

Other less frequently mentioned reasons were about being an alcoholic, trying something new and feeling safer at such events. The mention of safety chimes with people's experiences at rave events reported to feel welcoming and safe spaces for participants (Goulding et al., 2002).

Previous Attenders: Experiences at Conscious clubbing Events ($N = 39$)

The most common code in relation to people's experiences at events was related to the events being fun and joyful ($N = 16$).

> It was fun, due to not consuming alcohol I was far more aware of what I was doing but as everyone there was the same it meant there was still a carefree environment. (Man, 18)

> In my experience they can be great fun, sometimes you can feel just as energized as if you were drinking but the good times and memories aren't ruined by drunken incidents and hangovers. (Woman, 19)

The above accounts illustrate the fun had during the event, and how the positive experiences are continued the next day, due to a lack of hangover. The second most commonly coded experience was the importance of connecting and being comfortable with people ($N = 6$):

> When I connect to myself, to others and to the music while I'm dancing I feel alive, I feel in my element, I feel to be me. Expressing myself in this way of dancing feels very authentic. (Gender and age not supplied)

People also discussed other positive feelings ($N = 5$), such as "letting loose" in "a carefree environment" and people being happier compared to traditional raves. Other common codes were related to the events being relaxed, friendly, connecting with the self and listening to good music.

The positive experiences reported by those participants who had attended a conscious clubbing event demonstrate some of the potential benefits that could be experienced and highlight that these may be important selling points when trying to encourage young people who have not attended to give it a try. The importance of a positive and energised environment where freedom of expression was welcomed and encouraged seemed central to our participants' experiences. Alongside connecting with other attendees, some expressed the notion of connecting with themselves in an authentic manner, which chimes with other research suggesting that student non-drinkers chose not to drink in order to retain authenticity of the self, and one's higher-order functions (Conroy & de Visser, 2015).

Non-attenders: Reasons for Not Attending Conscious clubbing Events ($N = 49$)

The most commonly coded reason for not attending a conscious clubbing event was related to people saying that they felt it was not for them ($N = 14$). For some, this was because the event was not appealing due to early mornings, or that they were simply not interested. Other participants said that they enjoyed drinking when they went clubbing.

> Not interested in sober events, seems to defeat the purpose. (Man, 20)

These kinds of responses reveal that some people may be resistant to attending a conscious clubbing event, as it breaks the normative assumptions about drinking. The second most commonly coded reason for not attending was that there was no opportunity to do so ($N = 9$).

> I wouldn't of minded going to those events but most good clubs or raves offer alcohol. I just never have a reason not to drink. (Woman, 21)

People also said that they thought the event would not be fun as they could not dance without alcohol ($N = 8$).

> I like to drink and dance because I feel less conscious that way. (Woman, 20)

> In order to dance properly and have a good time I feel like I need to be a bit more outgoing and less self-conscious. Which is why I drink before a night out. (Man, 20)

Other less commonly coded reasons included that friends would not want to attend this type of event.

Survey Discussion

In our study, young people who had positive attitudes towards conscious clubbing had higher levels of acceptability of such events, which, in turn, are related to life satisfaction and connectedness. Young people with high AUDIT scores had negative attitudes towards conscious clubbing, which may suggest that it does not appeal to those who drink more.

Although only small numbers of our participants had previously attended a conscious clubbing event, their reasons for doing so were about having fun without alcohol and connecting with others. However, some non-attenders specifically discussed the lack of alcohol. Of further interest is the perceived need for alcohol in order to be able to dance and not feel self-conscious. For those young people who enjoyed having fun without alcohol, the conscious clubbing experience may be set apart from their experience of drinking and dancing, where alcohol is used to lower one's inhibitions and impose less control on the self, albeit often in a controlled fashion (Measham, 2004). Drinkers often have to monitor their feelings when drinking, balancing the desire to reach their ideal state of intoxication, which allows them to dance and socialise, while staying clear of their "danger zone" (Zajdow & MacLean, 2014). This involves a continuous monitoring of the embodied experience of intoxication, which some drinkers experience as entirely negative, with a fear of loss of control at its heart (Burgess, Cooke, & Davies, 2019). Conscious clubbing events may allow participants to engage with music and with others, without the need to attune to bodily sensations at the same time. Clearly, for some young people, it may be challenging to convince them that this could be a positive experience.

Survey Limitations

Alongside the cross-sectional nature of the study, respondents were predominantly women, of White ethnicity, all were students, and most were drinkers. The video depicted only one type of event, and there are many other variations in existence, and we did not recruit large numbers of participants with previous experience of conscious clubbing events. An issue here could also be that these types of events may attract certain groups of people in their present format, perhaps those who are more health conscious or those who had previously experienced problems with alcohol and are specifically looking for an alternative. Although we do not yet have data about what groups of people attend conscious clubbing events, Vergeer et al. (2018) found that people engaged in similar holistic movement practices in Australia were more likely to be older, female, and had higher levels of education than those who did not participate.

Implications and Future Research

The first implication pertains to the positive benefits that young people reported from attending conscious clubbing events, including the chance to socialise away from drinking environments. This needs exploration in future research with individuals who regularly attend such events to understand the mechanisms by which those positive experiences come about.

A second implication relates to the role of alcohol in enabling young people to participate in dancing. Previous research with young people highlights the role of self-consciousness in drinking, with many specifically discussing their need to drink in more to gain confidence to dance in nightclub settings (Davies & Paltoglou, 2019). This may be in contrast to the lack of self-consciousness associated with dancing within the rave scene and the communitas described earlier, probably because MDMA facilitates dancing without self-consciousness, while at the same time enables the user to feel more connected to others (Olavson, 2004). Further work should attempt to understand the experiences of those young people, like the participants in our study, who are able to feel this connectedness to others without alcohol or other drugs.

The drive for pleasure and bonding with others is a strong motivator and drinking alcohol provides a way to try to satisfy such motives: this often goes unacknowledged in alcohol research. Trying to influence young people to drink less alcohol may not be effective in cultures where alcohol is widely acceptable, as it may be difficult for young people to decide not to drink when everybody else around them is doing it. For example, UK students reported that not drinking had a negative impact on their ability to enjoy nights out and meet new people (National Union of Students, 2016). This chapter suggests an alternative way through this challenge: conscious clubbing uses a powerful natural motivator, the search for pleasure and bonding with other people through music and dancing. Focusing on individual behaviour change puts unnecessary pressure on the individual; however, by changing the environment (materials), their expectations and norms (meanings) and their knowledge about drinking (competencies), young people may be guided to healthier behaviours.

Future research on conscious clubbing is justified when looking at the impacts of other dance-based interventions aimed at young people; for example, they have shown promising positive results on improving mood, well-being and self-concept, and reducing anxiety and depression (Connolly et al., 2011; Lopez-Rodriguez et al., 2017). One avenue for future research could be to recruit heavy drinkers to participate in a conscious clubbing activity in place of one of their usual drinking occasions. It would be interesting to explore whether the process of socialising in a space without alcohol allows young people to see themselves as able to have fun without alcohol outside of that space. Seeing oneself as a non-drinker could theoretically impact on alcohol consumption, as previous research has demonstrated that identification with non-drinker prototypes is associated with reduced alcohol consumption (Davies, 2019).

Conclusions

Conscious clubbing experiences within university settings have the potential to offer more than individual benefits to young people. Adding non-alcoholic social events to university environments offers an opportunity to disrupt the meanings, materials and practices associated with drinking for attendees. This disruption of socially shared meanings involving drinking might be an important way to change the prevalent cultures of heavy drinking at university; however, as our findings attest, it may be challenging to sell the idea of dancing without drinking to some young people.

References

Anderson, T. L., & Kavanaugh, P. R. (2007). A 'rave' review: Conceptual interests and analytical shifts in research on rave culture. *Sociology Compass, 1,* 499–519.

Babor, T., Higgins-Biddle, J. C., Saunders, J. B., & Monteiro, M. G. (2001). *The Alcohol Use Disorders Identification Test, guidelines for use in primary care* (2nd ed.). Geneva: World Health Organization.

Beck, G., & Lynch, G. (2009). 'We are all one, we are all gods': Negotiating spirituality in the conscious partying movement. *Journal of Contemporary Religion, 24*(3), 339–355.

Blue, S., Shove, E., Carmona, C., & Kelly, M. P. (2016). Theories of practice and public health: Understanding (un)healthy practices. *Critical Public Health, 26*(1), 36–50.

Burgess, M., Cooke, R., & Davies, E. L. (2019). My own personal hell: Approaching and exceeding thresholds of too much alcohol. *Psychology & Health*, 1–19. https://www.tandfonline.com/doi/abs/10.1080/08870446.2019.1616087?af=R&journalCode=gpsh20.

Christensen, J. F., Cela-Conde, C. J., & Gomila, A. (2017). Not all about sex: Neural and biobehavioral functions of human dance. *Annals of the New York Academy of Sciences, 1400*(1), 8–32.

Connolly, M. K., Quin, E., & Redding, E. (2011). Dance 4 your life: Exploring the health and well-being implications of a contemporary dance intervention for female adolescents. *Research in Dance Education, 12*(1), 53–66.

Conroy, D., & de Visser, R. (2014). Being a non-drinking student: An interpretative phenomenological analysis. *Psychology & Health, 29*(5), 536–551.

Conroy, D., & de Visser, R. (2015). The importance of authenticity for student non-drinkers: An interpretative phenomenological analysis. *Journal of Health Psychology, 20*(11), 1483–1493.

Davies, E. L. (2019). Similarity to prototypical heavy drinkers and non-drinkers predicts AUDIT-C and risky drinking in young adults: Prospective study. *Psychology & Health*, 403–421.

Davies, E. L., & Paltoglou, A. E. (2019). Public self-consciousness, pre-loading and drinking harms among university students. *Substance Use and Misuse, 54*(5), 747–757.

Davoren, M. P., Demant, J., Shiely, F., & Perry, I. J. (2016). Alcohol consumption among university students in Ireland and the United Kingdom from 2002 to 2014: A systematic review. *BMC Public Health, 16*(1), 173.

250   E. Davies et al.

Diener, E., Emmons, R. A., Larsen, R. J., & Griffin, S. (1985). The satisfaction with life scale. *Journal of Personality Assessment, 49*(1), 71–75.

Ehrenreich, B. (2006). *Dancing in the streets.* New York: Metropolitan.

Giddens, A. (1991). *Modernity and self-identity: Self and society in the late modern age.* Stanford, CA: Stanford University Press.

Goulding, C., Shankar, A., & Elliott, R. (2002). Working weeks, rave weekends: Identity fragmentation and the emergence of new communities. *Consumption Markets & Culture, 5*(4), 261–284.

Haidt, J., Patrick Seder, J., & Kesebir, S. (2008). Hive psychology, happiness, and public policy. *The Journal of Legal Studies, 37*(S2), S133–S156.

Hill, K. M., Foxcroft, D. R., & Pilling, M. (2018). "Everything is telling you to drink": Understanding the functional significance of alcogenic environments for young adult drinkers. *Addiction Research & Theory, 26*(6), 457–464.

Hutton, F. (2012). Harm reduction, students and pleasure: An examination of student responses to a binge drinking campaign. *International Journal of Drug Policy, 23*(3), 229–235.

Kavanaugh, P. R., & Anderson, T. L. (2008). Solidarity and drug use in the electronic dance music scene. *The Sociological Quarterly, 49*(1), 181–208.

Klee, H. (1998). The love of speed: An analysis of the enduring attraction of amphetamine sulphate for British youth. In R. Power (Ed.), *Journal of Drug Issues,* Special Edition, Contemporary issues concerning illicit drug use in the British Isles, *28*(1), 33–55.

Kohn, M. (1997). The chemical generation and its ancestors: Dance crazes and drug panics across eight decades. *International Journal on Drug Policy, 8,* 137–142.

Layland, E. K., Calhoun, B. H., Russell, M. A., & Maggs, J. L. (2018). Is alcohol and other substance use reduced when college students attend alcohol-free programs? Evidence from a measurement burst design before and after legal drinking age. *Prevention Science, 20*(3), 342–352.

Lee, R. M., & Robbins, S. B. (1995). Measuring belongingness: The social connectedness and the social assurance scales. *Journal of Counseling Psychology, 42*(2), 232.

Lopez-Rodriguez, M. M., Baldrich-Rodriguez, I., Ruiz-Muelle, A., Cortes-Rodriguez, A. E., Lopezosa-Estepa, T., & Roman, P. (2017). Effects of biodanza on stress, depression, and sleep quality in university students. *Journal of Alternative and Complementary Medicine, 23*(7), 558–565.

Measham, F. (2004). The decline of ecstasy, the rise of 'binge' drinking and the persistence of pleasure. *Probation Journal, 51*(4), 309–326.

Measham, F. (2008). The turning tides of intoxication: Young people's drinking in Britain in the 2000s. *Health Education, 108*(3), 207–222.

Measham, F., & Brain, K. (2005). "Binge" drinking, British alcohol policy and the new culture of intoxication. *Crime, Media and Culture: An International Journal, 1,* 263–284.

National Union of Students. (2016). Students and alcohol: Research into students' relationship with alcohol. Accessed November 1, 2018.

Ng Fat, L., Shelton, N., & Cable, N. (2018). Investigating the growing trend of nondrinking among young people; analysis of repeated cross-sectional survey of England 2005–2015. *BMC Public Health, 18,* 1090.

Norman, P. (2011). The theory of planned behavior and binge drinking among undergraduate students: Assessing the impact of habit strength. *Addictive Behaviors, 36*(5), 502–507.

Olavson, T. (2004). "Connectedness" and the rave experience: Rave as new religious movement? In St. G. John (Ed.), *Rave Culture and Religion* (pp. 85–106). New York: Routledge.

Petrescu, D. C., Hollands, G. J., Couturier, D.-L., Ng, Y.-L., & Marteau, T. M. (2016). Public acceptability in the UK and USA of nudging to reduce obesity: The example of reducing sugar-sweetened beverages consumption. *PLoS ONE, 11*(6), e0155995.

Piacentini, M. G., Chatzidakis, A., & Banister, E. N. (2012). Making sense of drinking: The role of techniques of neutralisation and counter-neutralisation in negotiating alcohol consumption. *Sociology of Health & Illness, 34*(6), 841–857.

Qureshi, A. W., Monk, R. L., & Li, X. (2015). *Development of context-aware measures of alcohol-related impulsivity.* London: Alcohol Research UK.

Reynolds, S. (2013). *Energy flash: A journey through rave music and dance culture.* London: Faber & Faber.

Salamone, F. A. (2004). *Encyclopedia of religious rites, rituals and festival.* New York: Routledge.

Solberg, R. T., & Jensenius, A. R. (2016). Pleasurable and intersubjectively embodied experiences of electronic dance music. *Empirical Musicology Review, 11,* 301–318.

St John, G. (2006). Electronic dance music culture and religion: An overview. *Culture and Religion, 7*(1), 1–25.

Supski, S., Lindsay, J., & Tanner, C. (2017). University students' drinking as a social practice and the challenge for public health. *Critical Public Health, 27*(2), 228–237.

Treadwell, D. (2013). *Content analysis: Understanding text and image in numbers introducing communication research: Paths of inquiry* (2nd ed.). Thousand Oaks, CA: Sage.

Turner, V. (1969). *The ritual process: Structure and anti-structure.* New York: Aldine De Gruyter.

Vergeer, I., Bennie, J. A., Charity, M. J., van Uffelen, J. G. Z., Harvey, J. T., Biddle, S. J. H., & Eime, R. M. (2018). Participant characteristics of users of holistic movement practices in Australia. *Complementary Therapies in Clinical Practice, 31*, 181–187.

Zajdow, G., & MacLean, S. (2014). "I just drink for that tipsy stage": Young adults and embodied management of alcohol use. *Contemporary Drug Problems, 41*(4), 522–535.

Zhou, J., Heim, D., & O'Brien, K. (2015). Alcohol consumption, athlete identity, and happiness among student sportspeople as a function of sport-type. *Alcohol and Alcoholism, 50*(5), 617–623.

13

Young People and Temporary Alcohol Abstinence During Dry January

Richard de Visser

Introduction

In recent years, organisations in several countries around the world have established campaigns in which people are challenged to give up drinking alcohol for one month. Examples in the UK include Dry January (www.alcoholchange.org.uk/get-involved/campaigns/dry-january), Dryathlon (www.cancerresearchuk.org/get-involved/do-your-own-fundraising/dryathlon), and Go Sober for October (www.gosober.org.uk). Similar programmes run in winter in the southern hemisphere: Dry July in Australia (www.dryjuly.com) has been running since 2008 and in New Zealand (www.dryjuly.co.nz) since 2012. More recently, one-month alcohol abstinence challenges have been established in other countries including Belgium (www.tourneeminerale.be), Canada (www.defi28jours.com), and Hungary (www.kekpont.hu/szaraz-november). In

R. de Visser (✉)
School of Psychology, University of Sussex, Falmer, UK
e-mail: rd48@sussex.ac.uk

© The Author(s) 2019
D. Conroy and F. Measham (eds.), *Young Adult Drinking Styles*,
https://doi.org/10.1007/978-3-030-28607-1_13

Thailand, efforts have been made for many years to promote alcohol abstinence during Buddhist Lent (Jirarattanasopha, Witvorapong, & Hanvoravongchai, 2018). It is notable that these challenges tend to be held outside of summer, when the appeal of drinking may be reduced. The focus on January in Dry January allows it to be tied into a tradition of making new year's resolutions, whereas the francophone focus on February may make the challenge slightly easier to complete because it is three days shorter.

The growth of temporary abstinence challenges has occurred at the same time as the emergence of other efforts to encourage people to drink less such as Hello Sunday Morning (e.g. www.hellosundaymorning.org), which has the stated aim of supporting people to change their relationships with alcohol, whether that means abstaining, taking a break from drinking, or just thinking about how and why they drink and what effect this has on their lives. In other lifestyle domains, Stoptober (www.nhs.uk/oneyou/for-your-body/quit-smoking/stoptober) encourages and support smokers to take a one-month break from tobacco. In the context of diet, Veganuary (www.veganuary.com) encourages and supports people not to consume meat or other animal products for one month, and Meat-Free Mondays (www.meatfreemondays.com) helps people to make longer-lasting changes to their diet by not consuming meat on (at least) one day per week. It has been suggested that the impact of such challenges may not be limited to physical or psychological well-being, but that participation may have more fundamental consequences for individuals' self-concepts (Yeomans, 2018).

Alcohol Change first ran Dry January in 2013 (when the charity was called Alcohol Concern). The stated aim of the organisers is for Dry January to help people to reset their relationship with alcohol. The organisers provide to people who register a range of sources of support, including a website, Facebook pages, a smartphone application, and supportive messages via email and SMS. They have also published a book designed to help people to take on the challenge (Dry January, 2018). The popularity of Dry January is growing: the number of people who register via the website or mobile phone application to do Dry January increased from just over 4000 in 2013 to nearly 60,000 in 2016 (de Visser, Robinson,

Smith, Walmsley, & Cass 2017). Additional evidence indicates that millions of people attempt to have a Dry January without registering via the website (de Visser et al., 2017). In the UK, the phrase "Dry January" has entered the public lexicon, and online and print media include numerous articles every January. Furthermore, anecdotal reports indicate a growth in interest in, and provision of alcohol-free drinks, and even alcohol-free bars during January and throughout the year (www.visitbritain.com/gb/en/6-cool-alcohol-free-bars-britain).

The Benefits of Temporary Abstinence

Alcohol abstinence challenges give people a socially sanctioned opportunity to take a break from drinking alcohol. They provide an opportunity for people to try out the skills they have to resist temptation, pressure, or expectations to drink and to develop these. They also provide people with an opportunity to experience the benefits (and also potential downsides) that may come from taking a break from drinking. These may include gaining an increased sense of control and improved well-being.

Evidence from small-scale studies indicates that completion of a month of alcohol abstinence has physiological benefits such as lower blood cholesterol, lower liver fat, and lower blood sugar levels (Coghlan, 2014; Munsterman et al., 2018). Large-scale survey research has revealed that completion of a month of alcohol abstinence also leads to improvements in physical health and general well-being (de Visser & Nicholls, 2018). Although some have questioned the value of alcohol abstinence campaigns, as part of broader efforts to combat alcohol-related harm, it is apparent that the campaigns do more good than harm (Hamilton & Gilmore, 2016; de Visser, 2016). For example, the concern about people who fail in their efforts to attempt a dry month drinking more due to "abstinence-violation effects" (Curry et al., 1987) is not supported by available data. Surveys of Dry January participants indicate although around 10% do report drinking more after taking part in Dry January, around 40% report drinking less, and 50% report no change in their alcohol consumption (de Visser, Robinson, & Bond, 2016). It is also important to note that these challenges are not designed to be *the* solution for alcohol-related harm, nor the preferred approach for all drinkers. Indeed, it is certainly the case that dependent drinkers should not try to quit drinking without support from appropriately trained health professionals. Instead, Dry January is designed to allow people to take a break from alcohol, to prompt discussions about alcohol, and to help people gain a sense of having better control of their drinking.

Previous studies of Dry January have shown that most participants report completing the challenge and that successful completion of Dry January is accompanied by increased confidence in being able to refuse alcohol as well as lower levels of alcohol intake six months later (de Visser et al., 2016). This research has also revealed that "rebound effects" (i.e. drinking more after a period of abstinence) are uncommon and that they are much less likely than sustained reductions in alcohol intake (de Visser et al., 2016).

Success in abstinence challenges is predicted by characteristics of individual drinkers such as drink refusal self-efficacy (DRSE), which is an individual's self-perceived capacity to refuse alcohol (Young, Oei, & Crook, 1991). People with greater DRSE are more likely to complete abstinence challenges, and participants in Dry January experience increases in DRSE—especially those who complete the challenge (de Visser et al., 2016). This may help to explain apparent reductions in alcohol intake six months after Dry January. It is also possible that drinking motives predict success in Dry January and are influenced by participation in Dry January.

People may engage in fundraising through Dry January—for Alcohol Concern or one of its partner charities. However, past studies of Dry January have revealed that few participants engage in fundraising and that fundraising is not a significant predictor of successful completion of Dry January (de Visser et al., 2016).

In addition to considering individual characteristics, it is important to consider the influence of the social settings in which people undertake Dry January. Non-drinkers and non-drinking are sometimes associated with negative connotations such as being less fun, less sociable, and boring (Conroy & de Visser, 2013, 2014; Piacentini & Banister, 2009; Seaman & Ikegwuonu, 2010; Zimmermann & Sieverding, 2010). These negative perceptions of abstinence may increase the demands on Dry January participants: not only must they manage their own urges and temptation, but they must do so in a context where social pressure and societal expectations construct non-drinking as something unusual that must be justified convincingly. However, the growth of Dry January (de Visser et al., 2017) may mean that temporary abstinence is now not so unusual and is therefore easier to manage.

Social support may help people to complete Dry January. Social support has been shown to be helpful in facilitating health behaviour change in various domains (Bauld, Bell, McCullough, Richardson, & Greaves, 2009; Olander et al., 2013). Past research has revealed that many people do undertake Dry January with their partner, friends, and/or work colleagues (de Visser et al., 2016). However, doing Dry January with others is not a significant predictor of completing the challenge (de Visser et al., 2016). Over the years, the Dry January team has increased the type and amount of support given to participants via the websites, email, app, and social media. It is, therefore, important to determine which elements of this support are valued and effective and how various aspects of support may be enhanced.

There is currently a lack of specific information on young people's engagement with, or experience of, abstinence challenges. However, given that young people's alcohol use is often a cause of concern, it is important to explore their engagement with campaigns designed to encourage more moderate alcohol consumption. Indeed, the initial aim of Alcohol Concern and continuing aim of Alcohol Action is not for people to simply take a month off alcohol in January, but to use Dry January to take a break from alcohol, and to develop the motivation and skills to drink less (or perhaps even to stop drinking) after Dry January.

Young People's Alcohol Use

As noted in other chapters in this volume, young people are frequently found to be more likely than older adults to engage in heavy episodic drinking—often referred to colloquially as "binge drinking" (e.g. de Visser, Rissel, Smith, & Richters, 2006). However, in recent years it has also been noted that the proportion of young people who do not drink alcohol has been increasing (e.g. Australian Institute of Health and Welfare, 2017;

Chen, Yi, & Faden 2015; de Looze et al., 2017; Hibell et al., 2012; Office for National Statistics [ONS], 2017).

The observation that young people drink in different ways than older adults may mean that attempting Dry January presents a different challenge for younger and older drinkers. Young people tend to drink on fewer days per week than older adults, but often drink more on the days when they do drink (ONS, 2017). This means that within January, younger people would have fewer potential drinking days to manage than would older drinkers, and it could increase their chances of successfully completing the challenge. However, there is a lack of quantitative or qualitative information about the similarities and differences in older and younger people's experiences of alcohol abstinence challenges. This chapter presents analyses that were designed to explore similarities and differences in the experience of Dry January between younger participants (those aged 18–25-year-olds) and older adults (those aged 26 years and over). Attention was given to motivation for taking part, likelihood of completion of a dry month, and correlates of successful completion of Dry January, such as use of the support provided by the Dry January team.

A Novel Study of Young People and Dry January

The study described in this chapter employed a prospective longitudinal design similar to that used in my previous studies of Dry January: surveys were conducted at the time the people registered for Dry January (baseline) and in the first week of February (one-month follow-up). Data were collected online using self-completed questionnaires conducted at the time of registration for Dry January (baseline) and at the end of Dry January (one-month follow-up). All people who registered on the Dry January website or via the mobile app were invited to take part via a link to the online survey, which was hosted on a secure server. The home page described the study rationale and methods and outlined consent and data protection procedures. Upon completing the first survey, participants were asked to provide contact details so that they could be sent the URL for the follow-up survey and to be entered into a draw to win £100 (USD125) in store vouchers.

The baseline sample consisted of 7642 drinkers aged 18 years or older who had registered on the Dry January website by 5 January 2016 (535 of whom were aged 18–25). Useable follow-up data at the end of Dry January were provided by 4146 people aged 18–82 (247 of whom were aged 18–25).

People who completed the follow-up were older, had lower AUDIT scores, reported less frequent drunkenness, had greater DRSE in all three domains, and were more likely to have participated in Dry January in the past (details of these analyses are available from the author). However, the large sample size meant that some of these significant differences did not represent large actual differences or effect sizes. All subsequent analyses were conducted using data weighted to adjust for the likelihood of completion of the follow-up questionnaire.

Baseline Questionnaire

Respondents completed the 10-item Alcohol Use Disorders Identification Test (AUDIT: Babor, Higgins-Biddle, Saunders, & Monteiro, 2001). The AUDIT assessed alcohol consumption frequency and volume with reference to usual behaviour (with no time frame specified). Questions on alcohol dependence and alcohol-related problems were framed with reference to the last year and/or the lifetime. Scale scores were summed, with higher scores indicating a greater likelihood of harmful or hazardous drinking. Respondents also reported the number of times in the last month that they got drunk. This was a subjective measure of drunkenness: no definition was given.

Drink refusal self-efficacy was assessed via responses to nine items (Young et al., 1991), using 7-point scales ("*very difficult*"—"*very easy*"). The scale consisted of three three-item subscales, each of which was reliable in this sample: social pressure (e.g. "When my friends are drinking", $\alpha = .82$); emotional relief (e.g. "When I am worried", $\alpha = .91$); and opportunistic drinking (e.g. "When I am watching TV", $\alpha = .85$).

260   R. de Visser

A 10-item scale was used to assess general self-efficacy (GSE: Schwarzer & Jerusalem, 1995). Participants used a 4-point scale ("not at all true"—"exactly true") to respond to statements such as "It is easy for me to stick to my aims and accomplish my goals". The mean scale score was used, with higher scores indicating greater self-efficacy ($\alpha = .91$).

Participants reported whether they had participated in Dry January in previous years. They also indicated whether they had registered for Dry January with any other people.

End-of-Month Follow-Up Questionnaire

The primary outcome measure included in the one-month follow-up questionnaire was whether respondents made it through Dry January without drinking alcohol. Respondents were asked, "On how many days did you drink alcohol during January?": responses of "0" were coded to indicate successful completion of Dry January, and all responses of "1" and above were coded to indicate an unsuccessful attempt at Dry January.

Respondents were also asked: "Did you opt-into receive any Dry January support emails?". Those who did were asked: "Did you read them?". Those who responded "yes" then used a 5-point scale ("occasionally/once"—"every one throughout January") to respond to the question: "How often did you read the email support you received?". These questions were combined to create a variable indicating whether respondents read no support emails, some support emails, or all support emails. Respondents used another 5-point scale to answer the question: "How helpful would you say the email support was in helping you achieve your goal for Dry January?".

Respondents used a 7-point scale ("disagree very strongly"—"agree very strongly") to indicate whether they had experienced benefits in five domains as a result of taking part in Dry January: improved health; lost weight; more energy; improved sleep; and saved money. They also used this scale to indicate whether they had a sense of achievement. Analyses paid attention to mean scores and the proportion agreeing with each statement (i.e. those with score above the mid-point of the 7-point scale).

Respondents described their plans for their drinking after Dry January by indicating which of the following they intended to do: stop drinking alcohol; take a break for a longer period; drink on fewer days per week than I used to before Dry January; cut down on the amount I drink on days that I drink; I am not planning to change how I drank before Dry January; and drink on more days per week than I used to before Dry January.

Results

Of the 4146 respondents who completed both the baseline questionnaire and the one-month follow-up, 247 (6.0%) were aged 18–25. Of these respondents, 81% were female and 19% male. Like the rest of the sample, the vast majority (94%) reported "White British" or "Other white" ethnicity; 2% were Asian, 2% mixed race, and 1% black, and 1% other or not defined.

Background to Taking Part in Dry January

The data in Table 13.1 show that young participants differed from older participants on several key variables known to be related to successful completion of Dry January. Young people were heavier drinkers than older people as indicated by higher AUDIT scores and a greater frequency of drunkenness. Young participants' AUDIT scores ranged from 0 to 31, with a median of 14 and a mean of 14.8. In contrast, older drinker's mean AUDIT scores were significantly lower at 10.2 ($F_{(1,\,4143)} = 103.44$, $p < .01$). Based on their AUDIT scores, 18% of young drinkers were "lower risk" drinkers (scores below 8), 37% were "increasing risk" drinkers (scoring 8–16), 17% were "higher risk" (scoring 16–19), and 28% were "possibly dependent" drinkers (scoring 20+).

Frequency of drunkenness among young drinkers ranged from 0 to 25 days per month, with a median of 5 and a mean of 6.2 days per month: 26% reported getting drunk at least twice per week. In contrast, the mean frequency of drunkenness among older drinkers was significantly lower at 3.9 times per month ($F_{(1,\,4143)} = 38.00$, $p < .01$).

262 R. de Visser

Table 13.1 Reasons for taking part in Dry January

Reason*	Young 18–25 years ($n = 247$)	Older 26–82 years ($n = 3899$)	Difference
To give my body a break from booze	5.14 (2.22)	5.19 (2.25)	$F_{(1, 4143)} = 0.10$, $p = .75$
To save money	5.05 (2.01)	4.22 (1.94)	$F_{(1, 4143)} = 42.67$, $p < .01$
Health reasons	4.99 (2.12)	5.39 (2.12)	$F_{(1, 4143)} = 8.03$, $p < .01$
To prove that I can	4.79 (2.18)	4.90 (2.12)	$F_{(1, 4143)} = 0.51$, $p = .47$
To feel energised	4.74 (2.11)	4.76 (2.15)	$F_{(1, 4143)} = 0.01$, $p = .91$
To sleep better	4.63 (1.96)	4.68 (2.12)	$F_{(1, 4143)} = 0.16$, $p = .69$
To lose weight	4.45 (2.24)	4.79 (2.15)	$F_{(1, 4143)} = 5.56$, $p = .02$
I am concerned about my drinking	3.72 (1.84)	3.88 (1.91)	$F_{(1, 4143)} = 1.61$, $p = .20$
For charity	3.41 (1.65)	3.08 (1.44)	$F_{(1, 4143)} = 12.37$, $p < .01$

*Range $= 1$–7: Higher scores indicate greater importance of the reason

Young participants had significantly lower DRSE in social settings than did older participants ($F_{(1, 4143)} = 20.67$, $p < .01$), but they had significantly greater DRSE in emotional drinking contexts ($F_{(1, 4143)} = 5.48$, $p = .02$) and significantly greater DRSE for opportunistic drinking settings ($F_{(1, 4143)} = 30.14$, $p < .01$). Put another way, they felt less confident about being able to refuse a drink if others were drinking, but they felt more confident about being able to refuse a drink if they were feeling upset or anxious, or if alcohol just happened to be available to them. Young participants also had significantly lower general self-efficacy ($F_{(1, 4143)} = 9.23$, $p < .01$).

Table 13.1 displays participants' reasons for taking part in Dry January. Participants used a 7-point scale ranging from $1 =$ "not at all important" to $7 =$ "very important", with higher scores indicating greater importance given to that reason for taking part. The reasons are displayed in order of decreasing importance for young people. Among young people, the three

13 Young People and Temporary Alcohol Abstinence ... 263

Table 13.2 Context of taking part in Dry January

	Young 18–25 years ($n = 247$) (%)	Older 26–82 years ($n = 3899$) (%)	Difference
Fundraising in Dry January	17.0	9.5	$\chi^2_{(1)} = 14.66$, $p < .01$
Dry January with others?	42.3	42.3	$\chi^2_{(1)} = 0.00$, $p < .99$
Dry January in the past?	17.0	43.3	$\chi^2_{(1)} = 66.02$, $p < .01$
Plans for after Dry January?			$\chi^2_{(3)} = 3.16$, $p = .37$
Stop drinking	8.5	9.0	
Drink less	76.1	71.3	
No change	15.0	19.4	
Drink more	0.4	0.4	

most important reasons were to "To give my body a break from booze", "To save money", and "health reasons". Charity was the least important of the reasons displayed in Table 13.2.

From Table 13.1, it can be seen that not only was the rank order of the importance of the reasons different for younger and older participants, but there were some significant differences in the importance given to the reasons. Young participants were significantly less likely than older people to be taking part for their health or to lose weight. However, they were significantly more likely than older people to be taking part to save money and for charity. Overall, financial reasons were more important for young adults' engagement with Dry January, and health reasons were more important for older adults.

The data in Table 13.2 show that one-sixth of young participants were fundraising through Dry January: a significantly greater proportion than the one-tenth of older participants. As noted in relation to Table 13.2, charity was the least important of young people's reasons for taking part in Dry January. It should be noted, however, that although the overall rating of the importance of charity was only 3.41 for young respondents, it was 4.56 among those who were fundraising.

Table 13.2 also shows that young participants were significantly less likely than older participants to have participated in Dry January in the past. However, there was no significant difference in younger and older participants' plans for their drinking after Dry January: the vast majority intended to drink less than they did prior to Dry January, and one in 11 was intending to use Dry January as the beginning of permanent alcohol abstinence.

The Experience of Taking Part in Dry January

Younger respondents were less likely than older respondents to have made use of the supportive emails provided by Dry January ($\chi^2_{(2)} = 30.98$, $p < .01$). Only 29% of young people read every email, and 30% of young people read none of them, whereas 47% of older people read every email. Furthermore, younger people gave lower ratings of how helpful the content of the emails was for achieving a Dry January ($F_{(1, 4082)} = 11.81$, $p < .01$).

At one-month follow-up, 67% of young participants stayed dry during January: this was significantly greater than the 61% of older participants who did so ($\chi^2_{(1)} = 4.45$, $p = .04$). Among those young participants who did drink after registering for Dry January, 15% reported that they drank on fewer days than usual, and 81% reported that they reduced the amount of alcohol they consumed on the days when they did drink.

Analyses were conducted to identify significant predictors of successful completion of Dry January among young participants. Not drinking during Dry January was predicted by:

- significantly lower AUDIT scores at baseline ($F_{(1, 244)} = 9.63$, $p < .01$),
- a significantly lower frequency of drunkenness at baseline ($F_{(1, 244)} = 19.37$, $p < .01$),
- significantly greater social DRSE ($F_{(1, 244)} = 7.08$, $p < .01$),
- rating the supportive emails as more helpful ($F_{(1, 244)} = 6.93$, $p = .01$), and
- making greater use of the supportive emails ($\chi^2_{(2)} = 10.35$ $p = .01$).

Completion of Dry January was not significantly related to emotional DRSE, opportunistic DRSE, general self-efficacy, past participation in

Dry January, fundraising in Dry January, or participating in Dry January with other people.

Multivariate logistic regression analysis was conducted to determine which variables were significant independent multivariate predictors of successful completion of Dry January. Two significant multivariate predictors were identified: a lower frequency of drunkenness prior to Dry January and reading all supportive emails sent by Dry January (see Table 13.3). These variables correctly classified 71% of younger participants as successful or unsuccessful in their attempt at Dry January ($\chi^2_{(2)} = 27.37$, $p < .01$).

Bivariate analyses revealed that among older participants, there was a different pattern of significant predictors of successful completion of Dry January. Whereas only greater social DRSE predicted young people's successful Dry January, successful completion among older people was predicted by greater social DRSE ($F_{(1, 3896)} = 39.66$, $p < .01$), greater emotional DRSE ($F_{(1, 3896)} = 47.97$, $p < .01$), greater opportunistic DRSE ($F_{(1, 3896)} = 29.84$, $p < .01$), and greater general self-efficacy ($F_{(1, 3896)} = 10.80$, $p < .01$). Another difference was that whereas fundraising did not predict likelihood of success among young people, older participants who were fundraising were more likely to make it to the end of January

Table 13.3 Multivariate predictors of successful completion of Dry January

	Young 18–25 years ($n = 247$) OR (95% CI)	Older 26–82 years ($n = 3899$) OR (95% CI)
Age	–	–
AUDIT score	–	0.97 (0.96–0.98)
Drunk days/month	0.89 (0.85–0.94)	–
DRSE social	–	–
DRSE emotional	–	1.09 (1.05–1.14)
DRSE opportunistic	–	–
General self-efficacy	–	–
Dry January in past?	–	–
Fundraising in Dry January?	–	2.17 (1.69–2.79)
Doing Dry January with anyone?	–	–
Read every email?	2.75 (1.38–5.51)	1.76 (1.54–2.01)

without drinking ($\chi^2_{(1)} = 3.26$, $p < .01$). In the older sub-sample—as in the younger sub-sample—successful completion was not related to age ($F_{(1, 3896)} = 0.85$, $p = .36$), having participated in Dry January in the past ($\chi^2_{(1)} = 1.12$, $p = .29$) or doing Dry January with another person ($\chi^2_{(1)} = 0.83$, $p = .36$). However, it was related to significantly lower AUDIT scores ($F_{(1, 3896)} = 57.30$, $p < .01$) and significantly less frequent drunkenness ($F_{(1, 3896)} = 30.97$, $p < .01$).

Logistic regression revealed that four variables were significant multivariate predictors of whether older adults stayed dry during January (see Table 13.3). These three variables—having a lower AUDIT score at baseline, having greater emotional DRSE, fundraising in Dry January, and reading every supportive email—correctly classified 62% of older participants as successful or unsuccessful in their attempt at Dry January ($\chi^2_{(4)} = 180.95$, $p < .01$).

As noted earlier, participants used a 7-point scale ranging from $1 = $ "Disagree very strongly" to $7 = $ "Agree very strongly" to indicate whether they had experienced benefits in various domains as a result of taking part in Dry January. Young people were most likely to report saving money, and they were significantly more likely to do so than older participants ($F_{(1, 4143)} = 12.05$, $p < .01$). For all other benefits—having a sense of achievement, having more energy, having improved sleep, losing weight, and experiencing better overall health—ratings were comparable for younger and older participants. If scores above the mid-point of four on the 7-point scale are taken to indicate experience of the benefit, then among young people, 82% saved money, 76% had a sense of achievement, 55% had more energy, 54% reported better sleep, 48% reported better health, and 42% lost weight.

Although Dry January is not intended to be a cause of long-term behaviour change, it is interesting to explore whether people do intend to change their behaviour after its completion. Most young participants intended to drink on fewer days per week, but the proportion (62%) was similar to that reported by older participants (66%). Most young participants (63%) intended to consume less alcohol on the days when they did drink, and they were significantly more likely to intend to do so than older participants (49%; $\chi^2_{(1)} = 18.27$, $p < .01$).

For younger participants, their participation in Dry January was most likely to be a one-off experience. In response to the question: "How likely is it that you will participate in Dry January again?", younger participants were significantly less likely than older participants to intend to take part in Dry January again ($F_{(1, 4143)} = 14.13$, $p < .01$).

Discussion

Taken together, the results provided above indicate that the experience of Dry January is somewhat different for young participants than it is for older participants. Young adults enter Dry January with patterns of heavier drinking and more frequent drunkenness and with different profiles of drink refusal self-efficacy. They also enter Dry January for different reasons and with different motivations: they are more likely to take part to save money for themselves, and they are more likely to engage in fundraising through Dry January. Young adults are also less likely to have taken part in Dry January in the past and are less likely to make use of email support provided by Dry January.

With these differences in mind, it is notable that young adults were significantly more likely than older adults to stay dry during January, with their success most strongly predicted by a lower frequency of drunkenness, and making more use of the supportive emails sent by Dry January. This may be because young people tend to drink on fewer days per week than older adults, so they have fewer social drinking events to manage and also feel better able to refuse alcohol in these social contexts (as indicated by the bivariate association between social DRSE and staying dry). It is also possible that Dry January was an easier challenge for younger people because they have less money in the post-Christmas period and therefore go out less and as a result have fewer opportunities to drink and face less pressure to drink. However, it is also likely that older adults (especially those with children) may drink less in January due to having spent money on their family at Christmas and having engaged in festive events during this period. There is a need for comparison with a control group to see if the age differences observed in the data are only found among Dry

January participants or are also observed among younger and older people not involved with Dry January.

An important focus for the Dry January team may be to ensure that their promotional material and the support that they provide to Dry January participants include content that is appealing and relevant to younger drinkers. Saving money was young adults' most prominent reason for taking part in Dry January, and 82% reported that they did save money. It may be important, therefore, to ensure that young people are aware of the "money saved" feature of the Dry January app, which could provide personalised feedback on just how much money they had saved by not drinking during Dry January. However, although young people were less likely than older adults to consider taking part in Dry January again, two-thirds did intend to drink less following Dry January by having fewer drinks on the days when they do drink. There may be value in the Dry January team emphasising the benefits of non-drinking for health, social interactions, and self-concept (Conroy & de Visser, 2018; Yeomans, 2018). Given that engagement with the supportive emails was the only common correlate of success for both older and younger participants, it is important to continue to provide this support and to ensure that age-relevant messages are provided.

One limitation of the study reported here is that there was no longer-term follow-up, so it is not possible to determine whether the short-term effects noted here do carry over into longer-term changes towards healthier drinking. Studies of Dry January participants have shown that around 40% are drinking less 6 months later, with those who successfully complete the challenge most likely to report reductions in alcohol use (de Visser et al., 2016). Furthermore, only around 10% have "rebound effects" that result in them drinking more, with the remaining 50% returning to their previous levels of alcohol consumption. Earlier in this chapter, it was reported that young people were more likely to intend to reduce their daily alcohol intake, so it would be informative to determine whether they are more likely than older drinkers to make such changes these changes.

A further limitation of the study reported here is that there was no comparison group of people not taking part in Dry January. Inclusion of such a group in a longer-term follow-up study would provide answers to several important questions. First, such a study would allow us to determine how similar Dry January participants are to other drinkers in terms of alcohol intake, concern about alcohol intake, and DRSE. The data reported above showed that Dry January participants report a range of drinking styles ranging from fairly light to heavy and harmful (indeed, 28% of young participants were "possibly dependent"). Second, such a study would allow us to determine how changes in drinking among Dry January participants compare to stability or change in drinking in people who do not engage with the campaign. Evaluation of Dry January in 2019 *does* include a parallel general population survey that will provide data to address these and other issues.

In conclusion, the material presented in this chapter shows that young people take part in January for different reasons than older people and experience a different pattern of benefits from taking part. If we wish to encourage more people—and especially more young people—to take part in Dry January—once, or repeatedly—and to use the support available, there may be a need to ensure that recruitment messages reflect their motivations for taking part—particularly saving money—and that support messages are targeted appropriately, so that they can be more likely to experience the short- and longer-term benefits of taking part in an alcohol abstinence challenge. As noted earlier, this chapter is the first report to focus on young people's engagement with, and experiences of, an alcohol abstinence challenge. Given the differences reported here, there is a clear need for more quantitative and qualitative research into young people's experiences of alcohol abstinence challenges such as Dry January.

References

Australian Institute of Health and Welfare. (2017). *National drug strategy household survey 2016: Detailed findings* (Drug Statistics series no. 31. Cat. no. PHE 214). Canberra: AIHW.

Babor, T. F., Higgins-Biddle, J. C., Saunders, J. B., & Monteiro, M. G. (2001). *The Alcohol Use Disorders Identification Test: Guidelines for use in primary care* (2nd ed.). Geneva: World Health Organization.

Bauld, L., Bell, K., McCullough, L., Richardson, L., & Greaves, L. (2009). The effectiveness of NHS smoking cessation services: A systematic review. *Journal of Public Health, 32,* 71–82.

Chen, C. M., Yi, H.-Y., & Faden, V. B. (2015). *Trends in underage drinking in the United States, 1991–2013.* Bethesda, MD: National Institute on Alcohol Abuse and Alcoholism. Viewed on 22 November 2018 at https://pubs.niaaa.nih.gov/publications/surveillance101/Underage13.htm.

Coghlan, A. (2014). Our liver vacation: Is a Dry January really worth it? *New Scientist, 2950:* 6–7. Downloaded 30 June 2014 from http://www.newscientist.com/article/mg22129502.600-our-liver-vacation-is-a-dry-january-really-worth-it.html?full = true#.U7J7jrEylws.

Conroy, D., & de Visser, R. O. (2013). "Man up!": Discursive constructions of non-drinkers among UK undergraduates. *Journal of Health Psychology, 18,* 1432–1444.

Conroy, D., & de Visser, R. O. (2014). Being a non-drinking student: An interpretative phenomenological analysis. *Psychology & Health, 29,* 536–551.

Conroy, D., & de Visser, R. O. (2018). Benefits and drawbacks of social non-drinking identified by British university students. *Drug & Alcohol Review, 37*(Suppl. 1), s89–s97.

Curry, S., Marlatt, G. A., & Gordon, J. R. (1987). Abstinence violation effect: Validation of an attributional construct with smoking cessation. *Journal of Consulting and Clinical Psychology, 55,* 145–149.

de Looze, M. E., van Dorsselaer, S. A. F. M, Monshouwer, K., & Vollebergh, W. A. M. (2017). Trends in adolescent alcohol use in the Netherlands, 1992–2015: Differences across sociodemographic groups and links with strict parental rule-setting. *International Journal of Drug Policy, 50,* 90–101.

de Visser, R. O. (2016). Study shows that Dry January does more good than harm. *British Medical Journal, 352,* i583.

de Visser, R. O., & Nicholls, J. (2018, under review). Temporary abstinence during Dry January: Predictors of success; effects on well-being. *Psychology & Health.*

de Visser, R. O., Rissel, C. E., Smith, A. M. A., & Richters, J. (2006). Sociodemographic correlates of smoking, drinking, injecting drug use, and sexual risk behaviour in a representative sample of Australian young people. *International Journal of Behavioral Medicine, 13,* 153–162.

de Visser, R. O., Robinson, E., & Bond, R. (2016). Voluntary temporary abstinence from alcohol during "Dry January" and subsequent alcohol use. *Health Psychology, 35,* 281–289.

de Visser, R. O., Robinson, E., Smith, T., Walmsley, M., & Cass, G. (2017). The growth of "Dry January": Promoting participation and the benefits of participation. *European Journal of Public Health, 27,* 929–931.

Dry January. (2018). *Try dry: The official guide to a month off booze.* London: Square Peg.

Hamilton, I., & Gilmore, I. (2016). Could campaigns like Dry January do more harm than good? *British Medical Journal, 352,* i143.

Hibell, B., Guttormsson, U., Ahlström, S., Balakireva, O., Bjarnason, T., Kokkevi, A., & Kraus, L. (2012). *The 2011 ESPAD report: Substance use among students in 36 European countries.* Stockholm: Swedish Council for Information on Alcohol and Other Drugs.

Jirarattanasopha, V., Witvorapong, N., & Hanvoravongchai, P. (2018). Impact of Buddhist Lent Dry Campaign on alcohol consumption behaviour: A community level study. *Health and Social Care in the Community, 27,* 863–870.

Munsterman, I. D., Groefsema, M. M., Weijers, G., Klein W. M., Swinkels D. W., Drenth J. P. H., … Tjwa, E. T. T. L. (2018). Biochemical effects on the liver of one month of alcohol abstinence in moderate alcohol consumers. *Alcohol & Alcoholism, 53,* 435–438.

Office for National Statistics. (2017). *Statistics on alcohol, England 2017.* Newport: ONS.

Olander, E. K., Fletcher, H., Williams, S., Atkinson, L., Turner, A., & French, D. P. (2013). What are the most effective techniques in changing obese individuals' physical activity self-efficacy and behaviour: A systematic review and meta-analysis. *International Journal of Behavioral Nutrition & Physical Activity, 10*(29).

Piacentini, M. G., & Banister, E. N. (2009). Managing anti-consumption in an excessive drinking culture. *Journal of Business Research, 62*(2), 279–288.

Schwarzer, R., & Jerusalem, M. (1995). Generalized self-efficacy scale. In J. Weinman, S. Wright, & M. Johnston (Eds.), *Measures in health psychology: A user's portfolio. Causal and control beliefs* (pp. 35–37). Windsor, UK: NFER-Nelson.

Seaman, P., & Ikegwuonu, T. (2010). *Drinking to belong: Understanding young adults' alcohol use within social networks.* York: Joseph Rowntree Foundation.

Yeomans, H. (2018). New year, new you: A qualitative study of Dry January, self-formation and positive regulation. *Drugs: Education, Prevention & Policy, 26*(6), 460–468.

Young, R. M., Oei, T. P., & Crook, G. M. (1991). Development of a drinking self-efficacy questionnaire. *Journal of Psychopathology and Behavioral Assessment, 13*(1), 1–15.

Zimmermann, F., & Sieverding, M. (2010). Young adults' social drinking as explained by an augmented theory of planned behaviour: The roles of prototypes, willingness, and gender. *British Journal of Health Psychology, 15*(3), 561–581.

Part IV

Alcohol Policy Relating to Young Adult Drinking Practices

14

University Alcohol Policy: Findings from Mixed Methods Research and Implications for Students' Drinking Practices

Rose Leontini, Toni Schofield, Julie Hepworth and John Germov

Introduction

Studies have shown that undergraduate university students ('students' henceforth) in Australia and comparable countries are more likely to consume alcohol to hazardous levels than their non-university peers (Hallett

---

R. Leontini (✉)
School of Public Health and Community Medicine, UNSW Sydney, Kensington, NSW, Australia
e-mail: rose.leontini@unsw.edu.au

T. Schofield
School of Health Sciences, Faculty of Medicine and Health, The University of Sydney, Sydney, NSW, Australia

J. Hepworth
MRI-UQ Centre for Health System Reform and Integration, The University of Queensland, Brisbane, QLD, Australia

J. Germov
Faculty of Education and Arts, University of Newcastle, Callaghan, NSW, Australia

© The Author(s) 2019
D. Conroy and F. Measham (eds.), *Young Adult Drinking Styles*,
https://doi.org/10.1007/978-3-030-28607-1_14

et al., 2013; Hutton, 2012). While recent Australian data suggest there has been a modest reduction in youth heavy drinking (Burns et al., 2016), consumption by 18–24-year olds—the group most represented among students—continues to place them at greater risk of harm. The phenomenon of young adults drinking to get drunk has been referred to as a 'culture of intoxication' (Measham & Brain, 2005) and has attracted significant criticism from a variety of political and media commentators (Moore, 2010; Szmigin et al., 2008). Yet, while research shows that numerous sociocultural factors contribute to youth 'binge drinking', the deregulation of the alcohol industry and the liberalisation of alcohol laws over recent years have resulted in easier access to alcohol and normalised excessive consumption among students, as much as in the broader community (Conroy & de Visser, 2013; McCreanor, Moewaka Barnes, Kaiwai, Borell, & Gregory, 2008; Measham & Brain, 2005; Weitzman, Nelson, & Wechsler, 2003).

Internationally, universities and colleges have adopted a variety of policy approaches to students' alcohol use. In one US case, colleges' focus on policy visibility among students was linked to fewer harms from drinking (Wall, BaileyShea, & McIntosh, 2012). Lower rates of consumption were found by another US study among students in colleges where a tougher regulatory approach stemmed the availability of cheap drinks at events (Wechsler & Nelson, 2008). In New Zealand, a multi-pronged approach involving tighter restrictions on alcohol use, a ban on alcohol advertising of university events on- or off-campus, an emphasis on alcohol use and harm minimisation in the students' code of conduct, and a university accord with neighbouring venues saw the incidence of intoxication drop over a ten-year period (Kypri, Maclennan, Cousins, & Connor, 2018). Yet, while these studies have examined the relationship between student drinking, harms and the *visibility* of university policies, none has explored in any detail the role that policy plays in *creating* the social dynamics and practices of drinking environments, and in potentially creating *barriers* to harm minimisation. In this chapter, we report findings from the project *Alcohol Use and Harm Minimisation Among Australian University Students* (AHMS) (Schofield et al., 2009), conducted in Australian universities and residential colleges. The project's original aims were to examine drinking and harm minimisation practices by students and the measures adopted by the participating higher education institutions to minimise alcohol-related harms. In this chapter, however, we focus on the project's findings on the relationship between policy and practice in the context of alcohol use and harm minimisation among university and college students.

Harm Minimisation in Australia

Alcohol leads to many harms with long- and short-term heavy use. Heavy, occasional drinking, particularly relevant to young people, is linked to falls, road accidents, drownings, violence/sexual violence, unplanned/unprotected sex, lost productivity (work and study), vomiting, passing out, acute alcohol poisoning and damage to property (NHMRC, 2009). Australian drug and alcohol policy is overwhelmingly based on harm minimisation. The objective is to minimise alcohol-related harms without prescribing abstinence (Hutton, 2012), the rationale being that alcohol is widely diffused and culturally accepted, with historic, leisure and economic significance and that harm minimisation is aimed at encouraging moderation through self-regulation. This approach presupposes a coordinated effort involving supply reduction, demand reduction and harm reduction (Commonwealth of Australia [Department of Health], 2017).

There are two key national policy documents on alcohol use and harm reduction in Australia: *The National Drug Strategy 2017–2026* (Commonwealth of Australia [Department of Health], 2017), and *The Australian Guidelines to Reduce Health Risks from Drinking Alcohol* (NHMRC, 2009). The Guidelines emphasise the importance of reducing 'cumulative lifetime risk' of alcohol-related disease and injury and advocate limits on daily consumption levels to reduce drink-related harm. A limitation of this approach is that 'risk' is understood as an abstract category unmediated by social differences such as age (Lupton & Tulloch, 2002). A further weakness to alcohol policy is that it is individualistic, presupposing that harms should be 'minimised' by individual drinkers (Zajdow, 2011). Such an individualised approach to both 'problem drinking' and its management fails to capture the complex social dynamics involved in the formation of 'drinking cultures' (Savic, Room, Mugavin, Pennay, & Livingston, 2016), and the role that policy plays in their making.

Despite these limitations, most government and organisational policies on alcohol in Australia adopt the harm minimisation approach. At all levels, harm minimisation emphasises reduction in harms via 'supports and sanctions' (Braithwaite, 2011) ranging from education to punishment. Yet, aside from regulation, the harm minimisation approach appears to have limited success. For example, a systematic review of harm minimisation campaigns from several developed economies found that these do little to influence significant reductions to actual drinking (Burns et al., 2016; Wechsler & Nelson, 2008; Young et al., 2018). One Australian study found that after approximately 22 community-based interventions were implemented over a ten-year period from 2005 to 2015 in four geographic sites in Victoria, there was no impact on the reduction of hospital emergency department presentations (Curtis et al., 2017). Our study, instead, explored the relationship between institutional/organisational alcohol policy, harm minimisation and students' drinking.

Alcohol Use and Harm Minimisation Among Australian University Students Project (AHMS)

Conducted between 2011 and 2014, the AHMS project involved four studies comprising the Alcohol and University Life Survey (AULS, 3010 student participants); analysis of organizational policy documents alongside interviews with management staff; semi-structured interviews with 113 students; and nineteen focus groups with 70 students. The AULS study was conducted from April to October 2011 (Survey in Germov & McGee, 2014 [unpublished]); Evidence of links between harmful alcohol consumption among students and shared accommodation as an environmental risk factor (Wicki, Kuntsche, & Gmel, 2010) informed the research design.

The participating universities were large, public institutions. The residential colleges ('colleges' hereafter) were privately owned but affiliated to the universities. Most colleges and university campuses were situated in lively neighbourhoods with multiple leisure and licensed venues. All the universities and some colleges had their own bars, and in all colleges, students could lawfully purchase, store and consume alcohol in their rooms. Hazardous and harmful drinking patterns were measured using the Alcohol Use Disorders Identification Test (AUDIT, Babor, Higgins-Biddle, Saunders, & Monteiro, 2001). Students were also asked to indicate where they lived while attending university. Recruitment was via email to students at the participating institutions. Participants AUDIT scores ranged from 0 to 36 (from an upper possible score of 40) (readers interested in the survey can contact the survey authors). For the remainder of this chapter, we will focus on presenting the qualitative data from across project activities.

The Role of Policy in Shaping Students' Alcohol Use and Harm Minimisation: Four Major Themes

Lead investigators recruited college staff by direct invitation; for students in the interview and focus group studies an 'opt-in' feature in the survey, announcements, flyers and electronic boards on campuses were used. The semi-structured interviews and the focus groups were conducted with non-college and college students. Drawing on the tradition of interpretative practice, data were examined using thematic analysis (Ezzy, 2002).

Where pertinent, we will refer to published findings from the AHMS project (Hepworth et al., 2016; Hepworth, Schofield, Leontini, & Germov, 2018; Leontini et al., 2015; Leontini, Schofield, Brown, & Hepworth, 2017). However, the chapter's aim is to discuss project aspects using unpublished/unexamined data and to synthesise findings with published project findings. We cannot draw on the empiricist concept of 'methodological triangulation' (Silverman, 2005) given the different epistemological approaches involved (e.g. realist, social constructionist, post-positivist). However, the similarity of findings across independently conducted studies and a close comparative analysis of them (Silverman, 2005) suggest

280   R. Leontini et al.

that *together* the data from all the studies provide compelling evidence for the conclusions we draw in this chapter. The analysis of the data from the four studies yielded four major themes; these are outlined below. For clarity, 'on-campus' refers to events held on university/college grounds; 'off-campus' are all other activities, including private and student societies/clubs events not held on campus grounds. Data reported through direct quotes are labelled using pseudonym and student cohort (C/NC). Principals and management: 'Staff', college # (1–6). No identifiers are used for direct quotes embedded in the main body of the text.

Theme 1: University Students Consumed Alcohol Heavily and/or Frequently, and to Harmful Levels

Students from both college and non-college cohorts engaged in drinking that frequently exceeded the national guidelines on low-risk consumption (see Table 14.1). While there was variation in drinking among *individual* students, alcohol was ubiquitous in college settings and commonplace among non-college students. Students from both cohorts, for example, referred to 'a culture of "*regular, heavy drinkers*"' (Hepworth et al., 2018: 849). Similarly, the harms linked to normative drinking were frequent, including hangovers, missed classes, vomiting, passing out, stumbling, unplanned sex while intoxicated, falls and accidents, and hospitalisation. A small subset of ex-college residents had found the excessive use of alcohol during their residency had affected their studies:

Table 14.1   Patterns of drinking behaviour by living situation

Students' living situation	Drinking frequency 2+ times/week	Drinking frequency 6+ times/week	Typical amount/session 7+ drinks	Harmful drinking (AUDIT score $\geq$ 10)
With partner	34.1	11.6	13.2	24.6
Family home	20.5	13.1	16.8	26.6
College/ residence	36.7	24	22.8	41.3
Shared house	32.1	18.9	20.7	41.3
Live alone	25.7	17	16	37

> *R*: [T]oo much drinking, too much partying, and I needed to study. It was the first semester of the second year and my grades had dropped drastically from a distinction to a pass, and so second semester I said I need to leave, I need to live by myself and just focus on work. So yeah, the partying got too much…Too many people, too many events, no sense of personal space at all … there was no sense of balance. (Mark, NC)

Principals and management from the residential colleges insisted that excessive consumption was only typical of a small number of residents, while the majority of their students drank responsibly. However, the harms they reported suggest heavy drinking was widespread:

> *I*: How extensive is problematic drinking amongst the residents?
> *R*: It is hard to quantify…we do have a damages register and I think it is undeniable that levels of unfair wear and tear or damages are higher when there are large events where alcohol is served. (Staff, C1)

Yet according to students, with few 'dry' events, the 'choice' of whether to drink and to what level was limited. For example, the focus groups revealed that the pressure to drink led some students to '*just choose the easy option*' (Hepworth et al., 2016: 257) and drink. This pressure was acknowledged by some college staff:

> the danger…is partly the peer pressure but partly… students' first week at university is setting a sort of pattern for university life, and very little focus on university… much more focus on partying. (Staff, C2)

While students defended the social events as essential to their integration into college life, they also believed that alcohol made the process *easier*. Thus, they *expected* events to include alcohol, and accordingly, the events were advertised as such. Yet, as the above excerpt by a college manager suggests, the seductive power of these social activities was believed to be outside of management's control and entirely in the hands of students.

Heavy drinking was also reported by *non-college* students who had participated in activities organised by university clubs and societies. While supposedly designed for meeting and bonding with peers, in practice these events turned out to be hours and sometimes days of protracted drinking.

One non-college student, for example, described the weekend camp organised by his faculty club as, '*essentially drinking, there was nothing else… and the Arts student society provided infinite amounts of alcohol for everyone and that was the theme for the weekend*'. Thus, across both cohorts of students, being at university was associated with the heavy and/or frequent use of alcohol.

Theme 2: Students in University Residential Colleges Drink More Heavily and/or More Frequently Than Non-college Students

The survey and the qualitative studies found a correlation between students' residential arrangements and their drinking practices showing that there was considerably more drinking among students in residential colleges. A number of factors were identified as key determinants of this finding. First, there were numerous leisure activities and events held in residential colleges at which alcohol was served. Moreover, alcohol was permitted in most areas of college (lawns, common rooms, students' bedrooms and college bars if held). Drinking at large, 'inter-college' parties was especially heavy and often harmful:

> The biggest night of the year is school boy school girl, they have it twice a year, and they normally get about eight hundred guests… And this one [college] girl climbed over the fence and fell off and smashed her front teeth in, but she was so drunk she continued to go to the party and have drinks… oh a lot of girls do stupid things when they are drunk at college, like you know, hook up with two guys at a time and stuff, and just terrible things. (Lisa, C)

The survey found that a significant number of students in residential colleges drank heavily up to six times per week (Table 14.1), suggesting that this cohort exceeds what is typically the 'occasional' or 'episodic' heavy drinking found among youth in the broader community. Indeed, there was an intensification of alcohol use in colleges resulting in students' drinking exceeding the national guidelines' recommendations in terms of *both* number of drinks per occasion *and* frequency of drinking (NHMRC,

2009). For the students, the drinking games and, in some colleges, 'the hazing' (initiation practices that may involve consuming high levels of alcohol) were quintessential college traditions:

> My very first night was probably the most disgusting night of my life…you meet in the junior common room and…they put all their freshers on their knees on tiled floors for about three hours spraying everyone with cans of beer…and you know, force feeding whoever they can get to do it. (Liam, C)

There was a perception among college students that drinking is *safer* on college grounds than in commercial venues, and in particular on the streets while in transit between locations. The risks were attributed primarily to aggressive strangers, including non-college university students at college parties. But this 'safety' was also linked to convenience. As one participant put it, '*It is a bit of a microcosm here so I kind of tend to stay within the college or the university walls*'. The 'microcosm' rendered the necessity to stay sober redundant given the proximity of their drinking spaces to their own beds.

Second, alcohol in college was cheap and often subsidised by either the colleges or the social clubs. Students took advantage of special offers from bottle shops, entered into deals with suppliers for the larger events and organised ticketed events that included '*all the alcohol you can drink*'. Students also created an 'alcohol economy' (Leontini et al., 2015) whereby the sale of drinks served to finance further events. Thus, students' control over the marketing and sales of alcohol led to promoting alcohol to their peers.

Third, college alcohol policy and management actively contributed to the ubiquity and normalisation of students' heavy alcohol use, *and* to creating significant barriers to students' harm minimisation. On the one hand, the organisational processes involved in the making of students' heavy drinking and the constraints on effective harm minimisation centred on the promotion of responsible and sociable drinking (actively encouraged by colleges). On the other hand, however, the objective of promoting responsible drinking was counteracted by college policy and management liberally fostering opportunities for students to drink regularly as an integral part of college life. As one participant from management put it,

[S]tudents are trusted to be independent and mature and to think for themselves. If a resident wants to hold a private event and wants to have alcohol at that event they are free to do that, they are free to use the common areas to hold an event. (Staff, C3)

Thus, the task of creating responsible drinkers was pursued by management at the same time as they failed to recognise their role in creating barriers for achieving it.

Theme 3: Government Regulation: Impact on Drinking Practices and Harm Minimisation Among Non-college Students

'Harm minimisation' was not an expression adopted by the participants. However, the studies found that non-college students have strategies for *harm reduction* that are largely related to their engagement with the night-time economy. First, students' concerns about safety while drinking led them to taking steps such as drinking in safe venues, refusing unwanted drinks, drinking slowly, counting the number of drinks, having a designated driver, eating while drinking and limiting the number of drinks. The reputation of venues was critical to their selection of drinking locations, with students more likely to choose safety over cheap drinks. For example, venues known to comply with liquor licensing laws and the management of intoxicated and abusive patrons were viewed more favourably than house parties:

The more concerning situation is not in the pubs and clubs but at house parties. I have a friend who was raped at a party, she passed out on the couch and … they were both quite drunk, and…I don't think that would happen so much in clubs. (Jenny, NC)

The presence of bouncers and security guards, surveillance cameras, well-lit surroundings, proximity to public transport, and responsible service of alcohol were indications that a drinking venue would be safe. Cheap drinks were limited to fewer venues around town, and for those who chose the trendy and safer bars, special offers were limited (such as happy hour).

Safe and reliable transport was an issue in large capital cities due to the distance from the venues, the cost of taxis and (often) poor infrastructure. Students enrolled in the regional university rarely participated in campus events (e.g. in university bars) or events held in other towns on account of distance; when they did, they chose to drink less or appoint a non-drinking driver, encouraging them to *support* the choice of non-drinkers not to drink:

> I do have some friends that don't drink or only drink soft drink when they go out, or friends that do drink but are often our designated driver because they don't like to drink, so it is not that they have chosen not to drink it is just they don't choose to drink as much. (Marco, NC)

Second, data from the interview study showed that non-college students' concerns were in relation to anti-social behaviour from intoxicated strangers, including assaults from 'gangs', being drawn into fights to help their friends, and drink spiking and sexual assault. Few reported being victims of these kinds of harms, but most had witnessed them. Thus, among this cohort there was significant consideration given to '*friends [that] will take care of you*' (Hepworth et al., 2018: 852). Furthermore, many non-college students held jobs, which reduced the number of nights they would stay out late or drink heavily. For others, non-academic commitments such as competitive sport or long-term partners led to either spacing out drinking occasions or drinking less during occasions. In essence, regulation and policy that was either directly related to alcohol use (such as drink driving laws) or indirectly (e.g. the occupational code of conduct) led non-college students to planning their drinking occasions.

In spite of these factors playing a role in mitigating harms, students' views on the direct effects of alcohol on their health were varied. Common repercussions of heavy occasional drinking, such as hangovers and vomiting, were not readily acknowledged as 'harms' but rather discomforts to be endured by '*our age group*'. A small subgroup were familiar with government guidelines on low-risk drinking; yet they, like most other participants in this cohort, were sceptical about their relevance to their own drinking:

> *I*: Are you aware of the NHMRC Guidelines [on low risk drinking]?

286   R. Leontini et al.

R: Only in so far are they are the ones that say four drinks…
I: Would you say that you drink more than that or?
R: Oh yeah, crush that!
I: So it would be much more?
R: Yeah easily, um, just thinking, quite often five times that. (Karen, NC)

These views suggest that their knowledge of the Guidelines did not translate into the *intention* to reduce drinking. A few believed that alcohol is something people get used to and attributed their own perceived (low) risk to what they saw as their 'tolerance' to alcohol. Dependency on alcohol was associated with heavy drinking among older people. Kyle, for example, noted that he could consume up to 20 drinks on a single occasion, but thought of addiction as emblematic of someone who has become '*a hermit who just sits around drinking all day*'. An important finding was students' ambivalence towards the concept of 'cumulative lifetime risk of harms' central to the Guidelines. Tom and his girlfriend, for example, drank heavily once or twice a week:

> If I continued the way that I do now as a lifestyle for twenty years I think that I could damage myself quite severely, and definitely the way that [my girlfriend] drinks. But by the same token… it is not an everyday thing. It is not like we knock off or finish a lecture and then go into the uni bar and drink every day. So it isn't that sort of regular alcoholism. (Tom, NC)

Students, in other words, did not reject the concept of cumulative lifetime risk. Instead, they reinterpreted it to argue that, by virtue of being occasional (however heavy), their drinking sessions were *unlikely* to place them at risk of harm.

Theme 4: Students' Knowledge of University and College Alcohol Policy and Implications for Their Drinking and Harm Minimisation

Most participants claimed to never have seen a university or college alcohol policy, though a smaller subgroup could vaguely recollect some rules and expectations. The interview study identified some key differences between cohorts. Among college students, most participants believed that college policy was inexistent or '*no-one knows about it*' given the heavy use of alcohol in college, the many obvious cases of intoxication (including their own), and the '*fact*' that '*everyone here has alcohol*'. Indeed, many believed that management were aware of how much students drank but permitted it anyway. From the students' point of view, this unspoken collusion created the perfect conditions for enjoying alcohol without the pressure of restrictive rules, '*as far as drinking or partying goes – it's an ideal situation*' (Leontini et al., 2015: 178). While a few residents recalled rules around noise or damage to property, when asked to elaborate on the consequences for offenders, most recalled mild penalties or reprimands. In a sense, for college residents drinking and managing its consequences were students' secret business, not a college policy. With colleges' regulatory measures up for interpretation, as students saw it, what constitutes 'responsible drinking' for the residents was limited to the protection of the colleges' reputation. College students were also unaware of policies at their university:

> *I:* Have you seen any residential college policy on alcohol for students that says this is how we expect you to conduct yourself?
> *R:* No not at all, I am guessing there isn't one, I haven't seen one.
> *I:* And have you seen the one for the University?
> *R:* No. (Grace, C)

Staff in colleges were adamant that such documents were given to students upon arrival. But these data suggest that students' certainty was based on their observation and personal experience of widespread drinking in college; thus, whatever meaning management ascribed to policy or regulation, it was lost on their residents.

Among the non-college students in the interview study, none claimed to have seen their university's policy on alcohol use. Some 'guessed' that students could not turn up for class intoxicated, though several reported going to class with hangovers. The majority defended individuals' self-determination and civil liberty when drinking even on campus:

> *I:* Do you think universities, as educational institutions with young people, have a responsibility towards students and staff in terms of safe alcohol consumption?

R: I think as long as no-one is causing any trouble to other people while they are trying to learn or study, then people should be left to their own devices. (Kyle, NC)

However, unlike the college cohort, the non-college students did not assume that an absence of university policy meant management turned a blind eye on intoxication or on the misuse of alcohol. They assumed that harms would be somehow dealt with. Students saw universities as public spaces, and some non-college participants believed that—as such—these institutions should not eschew public regulation of alcohol:

I: Do you think universities and colleges have a responsibility for managing alcohol or the way alcohol is consumed?
R: I think in their capacity as licensed premises they have the same responsibility as other licensed premises which I am not sure they discharge properly.
I: Did you read the news about [drinking] in one of the colleges lately?
R: I did.
I: What do you think of stories like that?
R: I think it is an indictment on the university
I: To do what?
R: That they are essentially not - they have no regard for their own duty of care, they are probably breaking the law and it is unethical.
I: [At] the university there is a policy on alcohol. Have you ever seen it?
R: No. (Dan, NC)

Indeed, for Dan, universities and colleges should focus more on academic engagement than on promoting social activities that (often) include alcohol. The students' comments reflect a broader issue about alcohol use in higher education: neither the universities nor the colleges had made their policies on the use of alcohol visible, let alone known to them. In fact, the policies' focus on reducing harms while protecting students' liberty resulted in students believing their institutions did not have an interest in alcohol regulation. For the colleges in particular, the active support by management of students' freedom to use and market alcohol at their own discretion resulted in students' drinking heavily while remaining ignorant about both policy and harm minimisation.

Discussion and Conclusion

The findings reported in this chapter suggest that university campuses and in particular residential colleges are sites at which drinking cultures and intoxication are normative. According to both students and staff, students—particularly in colleges—were under pressure to drink. This supports similar findings about pressure to drink alcohol among university students who may not wish to drink alcohol regularly, or at all, reported in other research (Conroy & de Visser, 2013; Hallett et al., 2013). Our data from the survey and the qualitative studies with non-college students show that public policy and national guidelines on low-risk drinking played a significant role in shaping *drinking practices*. While these did not always appear to lead to reduction in *actual drinking* (especially the recommendations on low-risk drinking), they did contribute to students' implementation of simple but effective plans that led to harm reduction. On the other hand, students' heavy drinking on campus, or at off-campus events organised by student societies and clubs, was primarily linked to how universities and colleges regulate (or not) the use of alcohol. Importantly, university and college alcohol policy remained invisible to most students and ignored by the few who vaguely recalled 'the rules'. The policy approach to alcohol use in the participating universities and colleges was to adopt 'responsive regulation' (Braithwaite, 2011) whereby students were largely free to drink heavily on campus (for college students) and at events organised by student social clubs and societies off-campus (for both college and non-college students), but could be reprimanded or, according to management, face disciplinary measures if intoxication led to harms to property or other people.

Critically, college alcohol policies and their operationalisation supported, rather than limited, heavy and/or frequent drinking among students, thereby significantly reducing the opportunities for students to develop ways for minimising the harms. Students in colleges drank frequently and often above the government guidelines on low-risk drinking *because they were under two mistaken beliefs*: that heavy drinking in college was 'safe' regardless of their level of intoxication and in spite of their knowledge (anecdotal, witnessed and sometimes experienced) that harms *did* occur; and that there was no policy *regulating* the use of alcohol. Moreover, college students believed that principals turned a blind eye on how students drank, such that minor forms of disciplinary action were the only (potential) consequences for harms that could damage college reputation. Being (mis)guided by these assumptions, college students adopted two approaches to alcohol, both dangerous and (yet) neither entirely unfounded given their impressions of how alcohol was (un)regulated. The first was a fatalistic approach towards alcohol use, even to intoxication. In this sense, they practised what Szmigin et al. (2008) have referred to as 'calculated hedonism', whereby they could drink unreservedly and often, and especially to make the most of cheap or free alcohol. The second was their reliance on other students (or the college itself) to take care of them in the event that their drinking would lead to serious harms. Paradoxically, the goal of college policy to encourage responsible drinking and self-regulation through a regulatory approach that was kept, in a sense, at a distance from the social practices of students, was understood to have led instead to students relinquishing responsibility for their own drinking and safety, and to understandings that management held responsibility for dealing with 'a culture of intoxication' (Measham & Brain, 2005).

The broader political and economic contexts in which universities and colleges operate—the liberalisation of alcohol sales and the deregulation of the night-time economy—further placed these institutions at risk of becoming 'intoxigenic environments' (McCreanor et al., 2008). Within such a landscape, the evident lack of knowledge by students of their respective organisations' policies on alcohol use is, to use a students' expression, *an indictment on the university* to raise awareness of policy, but especially to tighten regulation of alcohol on and around campus, including in privately owned but university affiliated colleges. The students' perspectives were intuitive, but they reflected wider calls among university administrators and academic scholars to reduce consumption and associated risks through thoroughgoing examination of existing organisational policies and of how they pose barriers to harm minimisation (Cremeens et al., 2011; Wall et al., 2012; Wechsler & Nelson, 2008). The call to make university and college alcohol policy more visible, enforceable and tailored to the different cohorts is not new (Wall et al., 2012). However, our own investigation of alcohol policies demonstrates that organizational policies and how they operate can present barriers to harm minimisation. Importantly, there is compelling evidence from the literature and our project that, to reduce harm from alcohol use, there needs to be *a reduction in actual drinking*. A more comprehensive and systematic approach is required, however, for identifying, addressing and redressing these barriers in the higher education context. In the light of our findings and the supporting evidence from the international literature, the key implications for universities and residential college policy are both compelling and interrelated.

Acknowledgements We gratefully acknowledge the funding support from the Australian Research Council (Linkage grant no. LP100100471) and our industry partners, University Colleges Australia, NSW Department of Health and Victorian Department of Health.

References

Babor, T. F., Higgins-Biddle, J. C., Saunders, J. B., & Monteiro, M. G. (2001). *AUDIT: The Alcohol Use Disorders Identification Test: Guidelines for use in primary care* (2nd ed.). Geneva, Switzerland: World Health Organization.

Braithwaite, J. (2011). Essence of responsive regulation: The Fasken lecture. *UBC Law Review, 44*(3), 475–520.

Burns, S., Jancey, J., Crawford, G., Hallett, J., Portsmouth, L., & Longo, J. (2016). A cross sectional evaluation targeting young university students. *BMC Public Health, 16,* 610.

Commonwealth of Australia (Department of Health). (2017). *National Drug Strategy 2017–2026.* https://campaigns.health.gov.au/drughelp/resources/publications/report/national-drug-strategy-2017-2026.

Conroy, D., & de Visser, R. (2013). 'Man up!': Discursive constructions of non-drinkers among UK undergraduates. *Journal of Health Psychology, 18*(11), 1432–1444.

Cremeens, J. L., Usdan, S. L., Umstattd, M. R., Talbott, L. L., Turner, L., & Perko, M. (2011). Challenges and recommendations to enforcement of alcohol policies on college campuses: An administrator's perspective. *Journal of American College Health, 59*(5), 427–430.

Curtis, A., Coomber, K., Droste, N., Hyder, S., Palmer, D., & Miller, P. (2017). Effectiveness of community-based interventions for reducing alcohol-related harm in two metropolitan and two regional sites in Victoria, Australia. *Drug and Alcohol Review, 36*(3), 359–368.

Ezzy, D. (2002). *Qualitative analysis: Practice and innovation.* Crow's Nest, NSW: Allen and Unwin.

Hallett, J., Howat, P., McManus, A., Meng, R., Maycock, B., & Kypri, K. (2013). Academic and personal problems among Australian university students who drink at hazardous levels. A web-based survey. *Health Promotion Journal of Australia, 24*(3), 170–177

Hepworth, J., McVittie, C., Schofield, T., Lindsay, J., Leontini, R., & Germov, J. (2016). 'Just choose the easy option': Students' talk about alcohol use and social influence. *Journal of Youth Studies, 19*(2), 251–268.

Hepworth, J., Schofield, T., Leontini, R., & Germov, J. (2018). Alcohol-related harm minimisation practices among university students: Does the type of residence have an impact? *British Journal of Health Psychology, 23*(4), 843–856.

Hutton, F. (2012). Harm reduction, students and pleasure: An examination of student responses to a binge drinking campaign. *International Journal of Drug Policy, 23,* 229–235.

Kypri, K., Maclennan, B., Cousins, K., & Connor, J. (2018). Hazardous drinking among students over a decade of university policy change: Controlled before and after evaluation. *International Journal of Environmental Research and Public Health, 15*(10), E2137.

Leontini, R., Schofield, T., Brown, R., & Hepworth, J. (2017). "Drinking cultures" in university residential colleges: An Australian case study of the role of alcohol policy, management and organisational processes. *Contemporary Drug Problems, 44*(1), 32–48.

Leontini, R., Schofield, T., Lindsay, J., Brown, R., Hepworth, J., & Germov, J. (2015). "Social stuff" and institutional micro-processes: Alcohol use by students in Australian university residential colleges. *Contemporary Drug Problems, 42*(3), 171–187.

Lupton, D., & Tulloch, J. (2002). 'Risk is part of your life': Risk epistemologies among a group of Australians. *Sociology, 36*(2), 317–334.

McCreanor, T., Moewaka Barnes, H., Kaiwai, H., Borell, S., & Gregory, A. (2008). Creating intoxigenic environments: Marketing alcohol to young people in Aotearoa, New Zealand. *Social Science and Medicine, 67*(6), 938–946.

Measham, F., & Brain, K. (2005). 'Binge' drinking, British alcohol policy and the new culture of intoxication. *Crime, Media, Culture, 1*(3), 262–283.

Moore, D. (2010). Beyond disorder, danger, incompetence and ignorance: Rethinking the youthful subject of alcohol and other drug policy. *Contemporary Drug Problems, 37,* 475–498.

National Health and Medical Research Council (NHMRC). (2009). *Australian guidelines to reduce health risks from drinking*. Canberra: National Health and Medical Research Council. https://www.nhmrc.gov.au/_files_nhmrc/publications/attachments/ds10-alcohol.pdf.

Savic, M., Room, R., Mugavin, J., Pennay, A., & Livingston, M. (2016). Defining 'drinking culture': A critical review of its meaning and connotation in social research on alcohol problems. *Drug Education, Prevention and Policy, 23*(4), 270–282.

Schofield, T., Lindsay, J., Giles, F., Hepworth, J., Germov, J., & Leontini, R. (2009). *Alcohol use and harm minimisation among Australian university students*. ARC Linkage Project LIP100100471.

Silverman, D. (2005). *Doing qualitative research. A practical handbook* (2nd ed.). London: Sage.

Szmigin, I., Griffin, C., Mistral, W., Bengry-Howell, A., Weale, L., & Hackley, C. (2008). Re-framing 'binge drinking' as calculated hedonism: Empirical evidence from the UK. *International Journal of Drug Policy, 19,* 359–366.

Wall, A., BaileyShea, C., & McIntosh, S. (2012). Community college students' alcohol use: Developing context-specific evidence and prevention approaches. *Community College Review, 40,* 25–45.

Wechsler, H., & Nelson, T. (2008). What we have learned from the Harvard School of Public Health college alcohol study: Focusing attention on college student alcohol consumption and the environmental conditions that promote it. *Journal of Studies on Alcohol and Drugs, 69*(4), 481–490.

Weitzman, E. R., Nelson, T. F., & Wechsler, H. (2003). Taking up binge drinking in college: The influences of person, social group, and environment. *Journal of Adolescent Health, 32*(1), 26–35.

Wicki, M., Kuntsche, E., & Gmel, G. (2010). Drinking at European universities? A review of students' alcohol use. *Addictive Behaviours, 34*(11), 913–924.

Young, B., Lewis, S., Katikireddi, S., Bauld, L., Stead, M., Angus, K., … Langley, T. (2018). Effectiveness of mass media campaigns to reduce alcohol consumption and harm: A systematic review. *Alcohol and Alcoholism,* 302–316.

Zajdow, G. (2011). Outsourcing the risks: Alcohol licensing, risk and the making of the night time economy. *Current Issues in Criminal Justice, 23*(1), 73–84.

15

Policies Addressing Alcohol-Related Violence Among Young People: A Gendered Analysis Based on Two Australian States

Aaron Hart and Claire Wilkinson

Understanding Alcohol-Related Violence

Alcohol-related violence associated with young adults' heavy sessional drinking has long been understood as a problem for public policy. The nature of this problem has been theorised in different ways and policies have varied accordingly. Contemporary sociological insights recognise that social problems like the violence associated with young adults (i.e. those aged 18–25 years) drinking do not exist independently of the apparatus used to define and measure them. That is not to say that alcohol-related violence is not a problem, rather it is to say that there are many ways of

---

A. Hart (✉)
School of Social and Political Sciences, University
of Melbourne, Melbourne, VIC, Australia
e-mail: harta2@unimelb.edu.au

C. Wilkinson
Social Policy Research Centre, University of New South Wales, Kensington,
NSW, Australia

© The Author(s) 2019
D. Conroy and F. Measham (eds.), *Young Adult Drinking Styles*,
https://doi.org/10.1007/978-3-030-28607-1_15

understanding it as such, and that each one is shaped by public policies and scientific practices.

Alcohol-related violence has been understood as a problem within cultural groups. MacAndrew and Edgerton (1969) demonstrated that different cultural groups around the world behaved differently when intoxicated. Their insight was that 'drunken comportment' was, at least in part, a cultural practice. Drinking cultures have long been of interest for sociological and anthropological researchers (Kapferer, 1988; Room, 1975). Drinking cultures have been understood and measured from a nationwide perspective (Department of Health, 2018: 7; Ministerial Council on Drug Strategy, 2006: 26), among ethnic groups (Gordon, 1978; Moore, 1990) and in 'social worlds' (Room & Callinan, 2014). Within this mode of study and policy, alcohol-related violence and other problems associated with heavy sessional alcohol use—injury, public disorder and various forms of moral transgression—are understood to be related to group cultures.

A small number of studies have theorised alcohol-related violence as an expression of masculinity within a group drinking culture. While these studies focus on gender rather than sex (Krieger, 2003), some figure masculinity as something stable that individuals may express to greater or lesser degrees (e.g. Miller et al., 2014). Others seek to name and define the specific masculine projects at play within the small minority of male drinkers who are violent (Lindsay, 2012; Tomsen, 2005). While Tomsen (1997) characterised the masculinities involved with alcohol-related violence as 'protest masculinities'—that is, working class and otherwise subordinated—Roberts (2018) has argued that this assignation might be crude, and that the intersections of class and masculinity need to be nuanced with generational and local variations. While there is little consensus on how to theorise masculinities associated with alcohol-related violence, most studies figure their position with reference to Connell's (1995) notion of 'hegemonic masculinities'. Critical studies of alcohol policy have pointed out that this framework for understanding alcohol-related violence rarely gets picked up by government (Manton & Moore, 2016; Moore, Fraser, Keane, Seear, & Valentine, 2017). Instead, policy documents tend to express concern about groups 'at-risk' or 'vulnerable' to 'disproportionate levels of harm' from alcohol: young people; rural and regional populations; people with a mental illness; pregnant women; and

Indigenous and non-Anglophone communities (Department of Health, 2018: 8; Victorian Government, 2008: 11). Men are not mentioned as a group of concern. An Australian policy document (Ministerial Council on Drug Strategy, 2006) includes statistics demonstrating that three quarters of deaths, hospitalisation and injuries from acute and chronic alcohol-related conditions were among men. Nevertheless, male drinking and masculinity are not understood to substantively effect or constitute any of the multiple 'cultures' to which the policy refers. This has the effect of absenting what is evidently a powerful force in drinking cultures from policy initiatives to change them.

At the population level, epidemiology has identified diseases in which alcohol is a causal 'factor' and estimated rates at which alcohol 'causes' death and disability (Rehm et al., 2010). These attributions enable subsequent propositions to be assembled around national healthcare costs (Collins & Lapsley, 2008) and the global burden of disease (Rehm et al., 2009). In these causal propositions, alcohol is figured as a pharmacological agent acting upon bodies in the population. The sex of those bodies may be relevant—in figures associating alcohol with breast cancer, for example—but social processes of gendering are not. In setting out to detect the agency of alcohol as it affects the population, epidemiological research constructs alcohol as having stable and predictable effects (Hart & Moore, 2014). The violence that sometimes occurs during drinking events slips into the list of effects caused by alcohol. In this framing, alcohol, rather than gender, is the *cause* of violence. If alcohol is the cause of violence, then it is reasonable to restrict the availability of alcohol as policy response, and gender is left out of the picture.

'Night-time entertainment precincts' are the focus for another framework for understanding alcohol-related violence. Melbourne's central business district and Sydney's King's Cross are two Australian examples and serve as foci in our analysis below. Some studies have measured the blood alcohol concentration (BAC) levels of young drinkers in night-time entertainment districts (Miller et al., 2014; Quigg, Hughes, & Bellis, 2013). These studies demonstrate a relationship between later hours and greater BAC, and figure high BAC late at night as causing violence. These propositions are expressed in policies to restrict the availability of certain types of alcohol products, or the availability of alcohol during certain hours.

Other responses figure specific individuals who have a propensity to violence, disorder or criminality—rather than alcohol—as the problem. In Aalbourg, Denmark, police can ban specific revellers in a night-time entertainment precinct (Søgaard, 2017). In another variant, the movement of people between venues late at night has been targeted in 'lockout' policies, in which no new patrons may enter a premise after a certain time (Palk, Davey, & Freeman, 2010). Over the past decade, several Australian towns and cities have introduced one or more of these responses simultaneously in response to alcohol-related violence in precincts.

Recent social science theories (see, for example, Bacchi's [2015] the *What is the Problem represented to be?* approach or Law's [2004] discussion of post-representationalist social science) suggest that each of these frameworks bring a selection of the forces to which alcohol-related violence might be attributed to the fore and makes them present and accountable, while other forces are obscured or absented. Understood in this way, social science and social policy are not so much in the business of accurately representing and resolving social problems, but of enacting them in partial, political, and incomplete ways (Latour, 2005). Some alcohol-related practices and entities are deemed to require intervention, while others are left unattended. There are always political choices to be made about which frameworks to use in understanding alcohol-related problems, and how to respond with policy.

The main body of this chapter will focus on two illustrative examples of how violence sometimes associated with young adults' heavy sessional drinking has been addressed in two Australian states. It is hoped that this discussion will provide a productive basis for considering alcohol policy options for researchers and policy makers. We analyse the different policy settings with reference to two questions: How is the problem conceptualised? How does it engage with or elide social power structures, particularly gender? Our analysis focused on policy documents in Victoria, but since New South Wales lacked policy framework documents, we concentrated on the Minister's Second Reading Speech, analyses of media reports, a judicial review and peer-reviewed evaluations of licensing trials in specific precincts. In both cases, we follow the policy claims about what causes alcohol-related violence back to the research literature and discuss some of the epistemological practices that frame the problem in particular ways.

The Policy Context in New South Wales

In New South Wales (NSW), an influential articulation of violence associated with young adults' heavy sessional drinking has been that alcohol acts upon late-night drinkers to make them violent. In research and policies taking up this articulation, perpetrators of violence are not characterised by their sex, gender norms or intolerance of sexual diversity—but by the intoxication of their bodies. This articulation has created the possibility for policies that regulate alcohol's availability in specific late-night precincts. In NSW, these policies have reduced violence, although the specific ways in which they do so have not been demonstrated in the research. Late-night alcohol restrictions have had other effects as well: closing-down night-time environments, restricting nightlife for the majority of drinkers who are not violent and engendering political resistance.

In 2008, the NSW liquor authority introduced a range of licensing restrictions, including 1:30 a.m. lockouts and 3:30 a.m. 'last-drinks' (cessation of sales), on fourteen licensed venues in the main entertainment precinct in Newcastle (Miller, Coomber, Sønderlund, & McKenzie, 2012). The restrictions were introduced in response to police and community complaints about violence, property damage and disorderly behaviour associated with service to the intoxicated in Newcastle's central business district (Jones, Kypri, Moffatt, Borzycki, & Price, 2009). They were also influenced by political contexts, notably an outgoing licensing regulator (Jones et al., 2009). An evaluation conducted 18 months after the restrictions found a substantial decrease in assault from the 3:30 a.m. last-drinks but no impact of the 1:30 a.m. lockouts (Kypri, Jones, McElduff, & Barker, 2011; Kypri, McElduff, & Miller, 2014). While the analysis didn't indicate the gender or number of people implicated in an assault (i.e. one incident could involve multiple perpetrators and/or victims), the authors do present the mean age and gender distributions of persons involved in assaults both before and after the restrictions. This highlights the disproportionate involvement of men in assaults (e.g. men perpetrated 82% of assaults before and after the licensing restrictions; men were victims in 81 and 76% of assault incidents, respectively) (Kypri et al., 2011). The article makes no further mention of gender in analysis or policy recommendations. The subsequent evaluation, five years after the restrictions (Kypri et al., 2014) presents incidence-based analyses only with no person-based data, thus overlooking the disproportionate involvement of men in acute forms of alcohol-related harm. By evaluating the intervention in terms of assaults only, with no data on drinking intensity (e.g. measures of breath alcohol levels at sentinel locations at specified times), it is not possible to attribute the reduction in assaults to a reduction in alcohol consumption. The authors recommend that future evaluations measure the assumed causal pathways of the intervention (i.e. drinking intensity/BAC measurements within the precinct) as well as alternative causal explanations and unintended effects (i.e. reduction in number of people going out at night). The research on the Newcastle interventions, with gender largely absent from the research, became influential to public and political debates about late-night violence elsewhere in NSW.

In January 2014, following the high-profile death of two young men, Thomas Kelly and Daniel Christie in Sydney's Kings Cross, the NSW government introduced a 1.30 a.m. lockout and a 3 a.m. last-drinks in two designated areas in Sydney. The two areas were the Kings Cross entertainment precinct and a newly defined Sydney CBD entertainment precinct, the boundaries of which were defined as part of the 2014 law reform. These 'prescribed precincts'—Kings Cross and Sydney CBD entertainment precinct, which sit within the City of Sydney local government administrative area, were identified as experiencing high levels of alcohol-related violence compared to the State average (New South Wales legislation 'Liquor Amendment Bill 2014', 2014), based on data from the state Bureau of Crime Statistics and Research. Focusing on the problem of alcohol-related violence the government avoided giving any consideration to the use of the space by any particular cultural and social groups and their differential rates of perpetrating violence. The exclusion of Sydney's Star City casino precinct—despite a relatively high number of assaults—and a proposed future casino to be located in the Sydney CBD entertainment precinct were points of public and media contention (Dwyer, Wilkinson, & Room, in press; Lee, 2016). The demarcation of precincts within the city also caused some concern about the potential for displacement of problems to relatively proximal entertainment areas within the City of Sydney (Hughes et al., 2011). Evaluations drew upon police data of non-domestic assault incidence. Evaluations have found similar results to Newcastle: the number of assaults reduced by 26–32% and little evidence of displacement to other areas (Donnelly, Weatherburn, Routledge, Ramsey, & Mahoney, 2016; Menéndez, Weatherburn, Kypri, & Fitzgerald, 2015). Such incidence-based analyses tend to obscure the issue of masculinities in alcohol-related violence as the gender and age as well as the number of persons involved are not visible.

The explicit policy rationale for introducing the 2014 Sydney restrictions was 'alcohol-related violence'. Dwyer et al. (in press) analysed mainstream media coverage on the matter from Thomas Kelly's death. Most reporting defined the problem as one of 'alcohol-related violence' or 'alcohol fueled violence'. Less often the problem was framed in terms of drinking culture, such as 'binge drinking', 'excessive drinking' or 'the culture of drinking and violence', or trading hours and outlet density. A small number of articles referred to a problem with violence in general, not explicitly linked to alcohol, such as problems with violent individuals or violent 'men', 'young men' or 'young people'. Dwyer's analysis also illustrates how the media contributed to and aligned themselves with policy remedies. For example, both major NSW newspapers ran active campaigns calling on government to 'solve' the issue of alcohol-related violence. Liquor licence restrictions were the most prominently reported remedy for the problem, with a substantial number of articles calling for the implementation of the so-called 'Newcastle solution' in the form of lockouts and last-drinks laws. Dwyer et al. (in press) find very few articles reported potential negative impacts of licensing restrictions and none mentioned potential negative impacts on live music venues. This is of note, given the public outcry following Melbourne's trial lockout largely galvanised around negative impacts on live music venues and was a well-established line of argument against lockouts by 2010 (i.e. well before the 2014 Sydney lockout laws) (Cook & Wilkinson, 2018). Media reporting was generally positive immediately following the 2014 reforms, reporting they had achieved their intended effects of reducing assaults. Over time, however, public discontent from sectors of the community grew, culminating in a protest march on 21 February 2016, organised by the community action group Keep Sydney Open. Opponents of the laws highlighted their negative impact on the night-time economy, nightlife culture and diversity, including negative impacts on the live music industry, and minority groups, including LGBTIQ communities active in these precincts (Race, 2016). Race (2016) has suggested that 'certain gender identities' are poorly equipped to handle gender diversity in nightlife precincts, and that 'gender diversity education' might be a more appropriate response to alcohol-related violence.

In February 2016, amidst substantial community backlash, an impending state election and criticism of the state Premier, the NSW Government invited a former High Court judge, Ian Callinan, to independently review the reforms (Callinan, 2016). Callinan's review was based on existing research as well as considerations of public submissions. Callinan determined the restrictions had reduced alcohol-related violence and injury and, in Kings Cross, improved safety and amenity. He concluded the measures were achieving their intended objectives. Callinan did note, however, that he was persuaded by submissions and evidence that the precincts had become less attractive to some visitors and that this had resulted in 'turnovers of licensees and other businesses and reductions in employment opportunities' (p. 10). In particular, Callinan noted that the reforms had 'come at a cost [...] to employment', live entertainment and the vibrancy of the Precincts' (p. 11). Callinan recommended relaxing the licensing restrictions for 'genuine [live] entertainment venues' (p. 149) as part of a two-year trial, noting at the same time, the difficulties inherent in defining genuine live entertainment. Adopting Callinan's recommendation the NSW government extended the lockout and last-drinks time by half an hour for live music venues.

Restricting late-night trading hours has been a form of state intervention largely seen as a justified response to a problem of 'alcohol fuelled violence' in night-time entertainment precincts. Evaluations of licensing reforms in Newcastle and Sydney show significant and sustained reductions in assault rates. These findings closely mirror the findings of international research on the impact of changes to alcohol outlet trading hours, particularly those late at night (Wilkinson, Livingston, & Room, 2016). In NSW, the role of culture or gender in violence has been largely absent in policy debates as have the impacts of policy responses on social and cultural subpopulations.

Particularly vocal opposition has come from sexual minority communities whose members are often targets and rarely perpetrators of night-time violence (Dwyer et al., in press; Tomsen & Markwell, 2009).

The Policy Context in Victoria

In 2008, Victoria began a failed experiment with alcohol licensing restrictions in Melbourne's CBD. Since then, Victorian alcohol policy documents have increased their focus on, and the sophistication of their approach to, drinking cultures. While earlier policies limit their understanding of 'drinking culture' to social groups' relative acceptance of more frequent and intense consumption of alcohol, the most recent policy introduces consideration of the social and gendered norms that govern social practices while drinking. It remains to be seen whether the practical application of these policies achieves culture change among those targeted.

Under the influence of police, doctors and public health bodies, the Victorian Government's (2008) *Alcohol Action Plan 2008–2013: Restoring the Balance* imposed restrictions on late-night venues. The most significant was a temporary, three month 'lockout' from 2 a.m. in the CBD and selected inner-Melbourne municipalities. The 'lockout' policies quickly attracted a public backlash. The most prominent and politically damaging opposition was from the live music industry, for which Melbourne—Victoria's capital city—is famous (Rich, 2014). The trial was compromised when a planning tribunal granted exemptions to over one hundred venues (Harden, 2010; KPMG, 2008). The government withdrew the lockout and struck an accord with the music industry, easing the more onerous restrictions. Critics agreed that the restrictions seemed to fall most heavily on venues that were not the problem. A closer look at the rendering of 'drinking culture' in the 2008 policy shows a simplistic understanding. Although it avoids any abstract or definitional discussion of culture, the document states that one of its 'four key areas' is 'culture—sustaining community awareness to encourage a safe and sensible approach to alcohol' (p. 19). The policy 'actions' included under this heading all focus on education and awareness of the risks posed by alcohol. These actions imply that culture can be changed with rational, evidence-based information, particularly information advocating 'low-risk drinking'. By implication, culture is constituted by the rational knowledge of members of a 'community'; and the desirability of 'drinking culture' turns primarily on the extent to which it encourages or tolerates higher levels of consumption. The norms governing social practices during drinking events, including those associated with gender, are not brought into view within this conceptualisation.

The successor Victorian policy (Department of Health, 2012: 17), entitled *Reducing the Alcohol and Drug Toll: Victoria's Plan 2013–2017*, demonstrates an increasing interest in, and sophistication of approach to 'drinking culture'. This includes 'values, attitudes and other factors' that go beyond consumer awareness of public health information (p. 17). A number of other macrosociological and microsocial entities are enrolled to co-constitute 'drinking cultures'. Among these are 'the [Victorian] community', among whom 24% 'believe it does some people good to get drunk once in a while' (p. 17); 'relatives and friends' comprising 'social networks' through which 'drunkenness' 'can spread through "social contagion"' (p. 17), and 'young people', among whom 'a culture of excessive drinking is contributing to harm'. In developing this theme, it states that: 'evidence shows the importance of influencing not just individuals, but also the shared behaviour and attitudes of groups of interconnected people' (p. 17). The 2012 document thereby goes beyond the 'rational informed consumer' approach to 'drinking culture' taken by its predecessor document, but it has some continuities too. First, the document makes no mention of gender roles, and second, the approach to 'drinking culture' is still limited to norms around the intensity of drinking, rather than the gendered social practices of drinkers during drinking events. In addition to the 2012 policy, the Victorian government has distanced itself from the 2008 policy failure by excluding further consideration of lockouts from licensing regulation (Kairouz, 2016). Victoria has also instituted 24-hour public transport on Fridays and Saturdays, which has been partly articulated as a strategy for reducing late-night violence in entertainment precincts (Li, 2016; Scott et al., 2016). Victorian politicians and media have exploited interstate contrasts (i.e. 'Dear Sydney, drop by for a drink some night. Love, Melbourne' [Coulter, 2016]). Significantly, Victoria's 2012 policy undertakes to 'establish a long-term cultural change program led by VicHealth, a state funded public health agency, to turn around our drinking culture' (p. 18). We now shift our attention towards this programme and its host policy framework.

Victoria's current, primary policy response to alcohol-related violence (VicHealth, 2016) takes a more complex and sociologically informed view of 'drinking culture'. It is framed by a position that 'there is no single drinking culture in Australia'. The policy draws from a literature review concerned with 'drinking cultures' (Savic, Room, Mugavin, Pennay, & Livingston, 2016) commissioned to inform its model of drinking culture. The policy defines drinking culture as: 'the way people drink, including the social norms, attitudes and beliefs around what is and what is not socially acceptable for a group of people before, during and after drinking' (p. 6). This understanding of drinking culture 'encompasses both customs and expectations that encourage increased drinking, as well as social controls and adverse responses to drinking behaviour' (p. 5). There is also an acknowledgement that 'harms from alcohol misuse, such as injury, are experienced more often by men' (p. 6). VicHealth used this framework to call for tenders from community groups to mount subpopulation specific culture change initiatives. A range of programmes have been funded, and at the time of writing, these were still underway. Funded interventions for young people have included a mobile-phone based programme for university students, logging data on individuals' drinks and giving feedback about responsible drinking; a 'story telling booth' and online story sharing service about nightlife for 18–24 year olds in inner Melbourne; theatre, scavenger hunts, social media campaigns and other diversionary activities for regional and peri-urban young people (VicHealth, 2018). While a few of the initiatives addressing older drinkers are gender-specific, none of programmes for young people address gender directly.

While they may avoid a backlash, Victoria's drinking cultures initiatives may also ultimately miss their target. Online videos produced with the 'story telling booth' feature mostly young women and a few young men who could be described as 'hipsters' or 'metrosexuals'. There is little evidence of engagement with young men pursuing the kind of Australian hegemonic, toxic or 'protest' masculinities that are evident in the literature. Like its predecessors, this programme may be in danger of having the greatest effect on groups of people who tend not to be associated with the weight of problems. The evaluations of these programmes will be informed by the policy framework. Hopefully, they will address these important questions.

Engaging with the Epistemological Politics of Alcohol Policy

Drawing on our review of two illustrative examples, we could conclude that different conceptualisations of the violence sometimes associated with young adults' heavy sessional drinking can be viewed as partial, contingent and politically inflected. The cases of Victoria and New South Wales prompt two reflections which might be productive for scholars and policy makers concerned with young people's alcohol use.

First, the divergence between the two cities points towards the political economy of problematisation and the discursive power of social groups to situate their articulation of the problem as the one that becomes operationalised in policy. The dynamics of political resistance to licence restrictions emerged unevenly in the two cities. In both cities, 'live music' emerged as a site of organised resistance and an important cultural practice in need of protection, but only in Melbourne was it strong enough to make 'lock out' policies unworkable. This is understandable, since Melbourne has a significantly more vital music scene than Sydney. However, resistance in Sydney has been mounted by LGBTIQ communities and, with their iconic Mardi Gras and Oxford St nightclubs, these 'scenes' have considerable public profile and enjoy global recognition. Nevertheless, opposition arising from these quarters has not been sufficient to overturn licence restrictions. In both Melbourne and Sydney, the media has played a significant role in defining the problem and in adjudicating on the success of the putative solution, and in Sydney, the media strongly backed the proposition that violence was attributable to high blood alcohol content in young bodies late at night. There can be little doubt that theories about young adults' alcohol-related violence are highly politicised.

A second reflection concerns the role of uncertainty within the methodological design of policy evaluations. Evaluators of the Sydney and Newcastle licence restrictions recommended that future research focus on identifying the causal mechanisms associated with reduced violence. Causation is difficult to determine and rarely definitive within studies of social phenomena (Hart & Moore, 2014). Latour has argued that, within the realm of 'the social', causation is better understood as post hoc simplification of complex and non-linear interactions between social and material forces (Latour, 2005). Race (2014) has argued that policies to regulate alcohol and drug use reconstitute rather than merely effect the target phenomena and that the trajectories of these processes are difficult to anticipate beforehand. If Latour and Race are right, then future investigations of licence restrictions will find it methodologically difficult to determine causation, and the causal mechanisms associating alcohol licensing policy and violence will remain in doubt. Evaluators may have to consider their methodologies and findings in a way that serves to contribute to an informed discussion about good policy without depending on clear evidence about the how specific policies affect alcohol-related violence. This lack of certainty might be especially acute around the efficacy and value of culture change policies. Foucauldian scholars have long registered the power of state to influence the normative parameters of a healthy, productive and 'good' way of life for the populace as a whole; but it is less clear how policies might succeed in influencing the cultural practices of target cohorts, such as young men who perpetrate violence during drinking events. This task is fraught with definitional challenges. The difficulty in theorising the target groups for intervention seems likely to complicate any claims that VicHealth initiatives have resulted in reduced incidence of violence.

With these reflections in mind, we would suggest that it makes little sense for researchers and policy makers to assert the objectivity or impartiality of their theories and methods. Instead, their statements about evidence and causation always intervene within a field of contested claims over the gendered, cultural and economic character of specific places. These interventions can be understood as a kind of epistemological politics. A more overt engagement with the epistemological politics of alcohol policy and research can affect a more capacious, honest and balanced response to the violence sometimes associated with young adult drinking.

References

Bacchi, C. (2015). Problematizations in alcohol policy: WHO's "alcohol problems". *Contemporary Drug Problems, 42*(2), 130–147.

Callinan, I. (2016). *Review of amendments to the Liquor Act 2007 (NSW)*. NSW Department of Justice. Retrieved from http://www.liquorlawreview.justice.nsw.gov.au/Documents/report/LiquorLawReviewReport.pdf.

Collins, D. J., & Lapsley, H. M. (2008). *The costs of tobacco, alcohol and illicit drug abuse to Australian society in 2004/05* [research report]. Available at https://nadk.flinders.edu.au/files/3013/8551/1279/Collins__Lapsley_Report.pdf.

Connell, R. W. (1995). *Masculinities*. Sydney, NSW: Allen & Unwin.

Cook, M., & Wilkinson, C. (2018). How did live music become central to debates on how to regulate the Victorian night-time economy? A qualitative analysis of Victorian newspaper reporting since 2003. *Drugs: Education, Prevention and Policy*, 1–8.

Coulter, M. (2016, 13 February). Dear Sydney, drop by for a drink some night. Love, Melbourne. *The Age*. Retrieved from https://www.theage.com.au/national/victoria/dear-sydney-drop-by-for-a-drink-some-night-love-melbourne-20160212-gms5vd.html.

Department of Health. (2012). *Reducing the alcohol and drug toll: Victoria's plan 2013–2017* [research report]. Available at https://www2.health.vic.gov.au/about/publications/researchandreports/Reducing-the-alcohol-and-drug-toll-Victorias-plan-2013-2017---Strategy.

Department of Health. (2018). *National alcohol strategy 2018–2026: Consultation draft*. Retrieved from https://www.health.gov.au/. Accessed on 18 October 2018.

Donnelly, N., Weatherburn, D., Routledge, K., Ramsey, S., & Mahoney, N. (2016). Did the "lockout law" reforms increase assaults at The Star casino, Pyrmont? *Star, 1*(2).

Dwyer, R., Wilkinson, C., & Room, R. (in press). *Framing the debate in the 2014 NSW liquor licence reforms: A content analysis of NSW newspapers*.

Gordon, A. J. (1978). Summary comments: Ethnicity as a field of study in alcohol research. *Medical Anthropology, 2*(4), 147–152.

Harden, M. (2010). Unique and deplorable: Regulating drinking in Victoria. *Meanjin, 69*(3), 54–61.

Hart, A., & Moore, D. (2014). Alcohol and alcohol effects: Constituting causality in alcohol epidemiology. *Contemporary Drug Problems, 41*(3), 393–416.

Hughes, K., Quigg, Z., Bellis, M. A., van Hasselt, N., Calafat, A., Kosir, M., … Voorham, L. (2011). Drinking behaviours and blood alcohol concentration in four European drinking environments: a cross-sectional study. *BMC Public Health, 11*(1), 918.

Jones, C., Kypri, K., Moffatt, S., Borzycki, C., & Price, B. (2009). *The impact of restricted alcohol availability on alcohol-related violence in Newcastle, NSW.*

Kairouz, M. (2016). *Review of the Liquor Control Reform Act 1998: Terms of reference.* Retrieved from https://engage.vic.gov.au/review-liquor-control-reform-act-1998. Accessed 29 October 2018.

Kapferer, B. (1988). *Legends of people, myths of state.* Washington, DC: Smithsonian Institute Press.

KPMG. (2008). *Evaluation of the temporary late night entry declaration: Final Report.* Retrieved from www.justice.vic.gov.au. Accessed 29 October 2018.

Krieger, N. (2003). Genders, sexes, and health: What are the connections—And why does it matter? *International Journal of Epidemiology, 32*(4), 652–657.

Kypri, K., Jones, C., McElduff, P., & Barker, D. (2011). Effects of restricting pub closing times on night-time assaults in an Australian city. *Addiction, 106*(2), 303–310.

Kypri, K., McElduff, P., & Miller, P. (2014). Restrictions in pub closing times and lockouts in Newcastle, Australia five years on. *Drug and Alcohol Review, 33*(3), 323–326.

Latour, B. (2005). *Reassembling the social: An introduction to actor-network-theory.* Oxford: Oxford University Press.

Law, J. (2004). *After method: Mess in social science research.* New York: Routledge.

Lee, M. (2016). Sydney's lockout laws: For and against. *Current Issues in Criminal Justice, 28,* 117.

Li, N. (2016, May). CBD to remain lockout free. *CBD News,* Issue 20. https://cbdnews.com.au/wp-content/uploads/2016/04/CBD_20.pdf. Accessed on 24 April 2014.

Lindsay, J. (2012). The gendered trouble with alcohol: Young people managing alcohol related violence. *International Journal of Drug Policy, 23*(3), 236–241.

Liquor Amendment Act 2014 No 3. (2014). Available from https://www.legislation.nsw.gov.au/#/view/act/2014/3/full.

MacAndrew, C., & Edgerton, R. B. (1969). *Drunken comportment: A social explanation.* Chicago: Aldine.

Manton, E., & Moore, D. (2016). Gender, intoxication and the developing brain: Problematisations of drinking among young adults in Australian alcohol policy. *International Journal of Drug Policy, 31,* 153–162.

Menéndez, P., Weatherburn, D., Kypri, K., & Fitzgerald, J. (2015). Lockouts and last drinks: The impact of the January 2014 liquor licence reforms on assaults in NSW, Australia. *BOCSAR NSW Crime and Justice Bulletins,* 12.

Miller, P., Coomber, K., Sønderlund, A., & McKenzie, S. (2012). The long-term effect of lockouts on alcohol-related emergency department attendances within Ballarat, Australia. *Drug and Alcohol Review, 31*(4), 370–376.

Miller, P., Pennay, A., Droste, N., Butler, E., Jenkinson, R., Hyder, S., ... Lubman, D. I. (2014). A comparative study of blood alcohol concentrations in Australian night-time entertainment districts. *Drug and Alcohol Review, 33*(4), 338–345.

Miller, P., Wells, S., Hobbs, R., Zinkiewicz, L., Curtis, A., & Graham, K. (2014b). Alcohol, masculinity, honour and male barroom aggression in an Australian sample. *Drug and Alcohol Review, 33*(2), 136–143.

Ministerial Council on Drug Strategy. (2006). *National alcohol strategy 2006–2009: Towards safer drinking cultures.* Available at https://www.indigenousjustice.gov.au/resources/national-alcohol-strategy-2006-2011-towards-safer-drinking-cultures/.

Moore, D. (1990). Drinking, the construction of ethnic identity and social process in a Western Australian youth subculture. *British Journal of Addiction, 85*(10), 1265–1278.

Moore, D., Fraser, S., Keane, H., Seear, K., & Valentine, K. (2017). Missing masculinities: Gendering practices in Australian alcohol research and policy. *Australian Feminist Studies, 32*(93), 309–324.

Palk, G. R. M., Davey, J. D., & Freeman, J. E. (2010). The impact of a lockout policy on levels of alcohol-related incidents in and around licensed premises. *Police Practice and Research, 11*(1), 5–15.

Quigg, Z., Hughes, K., & Bellis, M. A. (2013). Student drinking patterns and blood alcohol concentration on commercially organised pub crawls in the UK. *Addictive Behaviors, 38*(12), 2924–2929.

Race, K. (2014). Complex events: Drug effects and emergent causality. *Contemporary Drug Problems, 41*(3), 301–334.

Race, K. (2016). The sexuality of the night: Violence and transformation. *Current Issues Criminal Justice, 28*(1), 105–110.

Rehm, J., Baliunas, D., Borges, G. L. G., Graham, K., Irving, H., Kehoe, T., ... Taylor, B. (2010). The relation between different dimensions of alcohol consumption and burden of disease: An overview. *Addiction, 105*(5), 817–843.

Rehm, J., Mathers, C., Popova, S., Thavorncharoensap, M., Teerawattananon, Y., & Patra, J. (2009). Global burden of disease and injury and economic cost attributable to alcohol use and alcohol-use disorders. *The Lancet, 373*(9682), 2223–223.

Rich, J. (2014). *Why is alcohol policy difficult? Reflections of a bureaucrat.* Paper presented at the Alcohol Policy Research: Putting together a global evidence base, Melbourne.

Roberts, S. (2018). *Young working class men in transition.* Abingdon, Oxon and New York, NY: Routledge.

Room, R. (1975). Normative perspectives on alcohol use and problems. *Journal of Drug Issues, 5,* 358–368.

Room, R., & Callinan, S. (2014). *How alcohol policies and drinking cultures interact: Concepts and evidence.* Paper presented at the Alcohol Policy Research: Putting together a global evidence base, Melbourne.

Savic, M., Room, R., Mugavin, J., Pennay, A., & Livingston, M. (2016). Defining "drinking culture": A critical review of its meaning and connotation in social research on alcohol problems. *Drugs: Education, Prevention and Policy, 23*(4), 270–282.

Scott, N., Hart, A., Wilson, J., Livingston, M., Moore, D., & Dietze, P. (2016). The effects of extended public transport operating hours and venue lockout policies on drinking-related harms in Melbourne, Australia: Results from Sim-Drink, an agent-based simulation model. *International Journal of Drug Policy, 32,* 44–49.

Søgaard, T. F. (2017). Voices of the banned: Emergent causality and the unforeseen consequences of patron banning policies. *Contemporary Drug Problems, 45*(1), 15–32.

Tomsen, S. (1997). A top night: Social protest, masculinity and the culture of drinking violence. *British Journal of Criminology, 37*(1), 90–102.

Tomsen, S. (2005). 'Boozers and bouncers': Masculine conflict, disengagement and Contemporary governance of drinking-related violence and disorder. *Australian and New Zealand Journal of Criminology, 38*(3), 283–297.

Tomsen, S., & Markwell, K. (2009). Violence, cultural display and the suspension of sexual prejudice. *Sexuality and Culture, 13,* 201–217.

VicHealth. (2016). *VicHealth Alcohol Strategy 2016–19.* Vichealth Health Promotion Foundation, Carlton South, Victoria.

VicHealth. (2018). *Alcohol Culture Change Initiative 2016–2019.* Vichealth Health Promotion Foundation, Carlton South, Victoria.

Victorian Government. (2008). *Victoria's Alcohol Action Plan 2008–2013: Restoring the balance.* South Melbourne.

Wilkinson, C., Livingston, M., & Room, R. (2016). Impacts of changes to trading hours of liquor licences on alcohol-related harm: A systematic review 2005–2015. *Public Health Research & Practice, 26* (4).

16

Making Sense of Alcohol Consumption Among Russian Young Adults in the Context of Post-2009 Policy Initiatives

Vadim Radaev

Introduction

Russia has the fourth-highest per capita alcohol consumption in the world (World Health Organisation, 2016). Russians also tend to engage in a North European style of drinking dominated by strong spirits (Nemtsov, 2011; Popova, Rehm, Patra, & Zatonski, 2007). Increasing concern over excessive alcohol consumption persuaded the Russian government to introduce a new restrictive alcohol policy designed to halve overall alcohol consumption during the 2010s. During this period, alcohol consumption declined overall (Radaev & Kotelnikova, 2016). The impact of alcohol policy has been extensively studied around the world (Chaloupka, Grossman, & Saffer, 2002; Mäkelä, Bloomfield, Gustafsson, Huhtanen, & Room, 2007) and it is important to know the extent to which restrictive measures in Russia affected alcohol consumption, particularly among young adults. Reducing the availability of alcohol has been identified as

---

V. Radaev (✉)
National Research University Higher School of Economics, Moscow, Russia
e-mail: radaev@hse.ru

© The Author(s) 2019
D. Conroy and F. Measham (eds.), *Young Adult Drinking Styles*,
https://doi.org/10.1007/978-3-030-28607-1_16

313

a key factor in decreasing consumption and associated harms. A meta-analysis of 1003 independent effects from 112 studies demonstrated that fiscal measures raising excise and sales taxes normally increase retail prices (Wagenaar, Salois, & Komro, 2009) and since consumer demand for alcohol is price sensitive, increasing retail prices usually reduces legal alcohol sales (Nemtsov, 2015; Neufeld & Rehm, 2013).

Unrecorded alcohol is particularly important given it accounts at least for one-quarter of the total alcohol consumption in Russia (WHO, 2014). Consumption of unrecorded alcohol has been recognised as one of the main contributors to alcohol-attributable premature mortality in Russia (Neufeld & Rehm, 2018). The most dramatic case occurred in the Siberian city of Irkutsk in 2016 when 74 people died and 122 people were poisoned from counterfeit alcohol (bath cosmetics) containing methanol. The impact of restrictive policies on unrecorded/illegal alcohol markets remains unclear. During some periods, illegal alcohol sales could replace legal sales, while, during others, both markets could move in the same direction (Radaev, 2017).

In previous studies of alcohol consumption in Russia, a clear downward trend in consumption during the 2000s and particularly the 2010s was interpreted as an indicator of the success of new government alcohol policy (Neufeld & Rehm, 2013). Restrictions on both the affordability and availability of alcohol may have contributed to this decline together with the impact from two subsequent economic crises. After the first economic crisis of 2008–2009, growth rates in average real disposable income dropped from 10 to 3% before falling for four years during the second economic crisis of 2014–2017. Consumers reduced their alcohol consumption or switched to cheaper alcoholic beverages, including unrecorded alcohol. Understanding how economic strain influences alcohol consumption patterns depends on the country-level context and the specific characteristics of a given economic crisis (de Goeij et al., 2015; Jukkala, Makinen, Ferlander, Vagero, & Kaslitsyna, 2008). However, alcohol may suffer the most during crisis periods, as demonstrated by previous research in Russia (Ekström, Ekström, Potapova, & Shanahan, 2003) and other countries (Barda & Sardianou, 2010; Bor, Basu, Coutts, McKee, & Stuckler, 2013). We should also keep in mind that the downward trend in the consumption of strong spirits started earlier than the enactment of the new policy and the post-2008 economic crises. In particular, vodka consumption has been declining since the mid-1990s, and the consumption of homemade distilled spirits ('samogon', the Russian term for 'moonshine' or illicitly distilled alcohol) has been declining since the 2000s (Denisova, 2010; Radaev, 2015, 2016; Roshchina, 2012). Thus, the downward trend might be affected by other factors, including cultural and generational shifts though these factors are not well understood and would benefit from further exploration.

In this context, the drinking patterns of younger generations require special attention. The decline in young adult drinking in Russia might be accounted for in the context of similar declines observed among other countries, particularly higher-income Anglo-Saxon and Scandinavian countries. In the USA, from 2005 to 2014, reported past-month heavy episodic drinking (HED) among young adults declined from 43 to 39% (Hingson, Zha, & Smyth, 2017). In a longitudinal UK study of drinking patterns, 22% of male individuals born around 1900 abstained from alcohol, reducing to 7% among male individuals born between 1940 and 1969, and then a sharp increase in the number of male individuals born after 1985 who abstain (Meng, Holmes, Hill-McManus, Brennan, & Meier, 2014). In Australia, controlling for age and period effects from 1995 to 2013, alcohol consumption decreased from 89% (individuals born between 1960 and 1979) to 43% (individuals born between 1990 and 1994) indicating more than a twofold decline in consumption volumes (Livingston et al., 2016; Pennay, Livingston, & MacLean, 2015). Similar results have been found for Sweden and some other countries (Raninen, Livingston, & Leifman, 2014). Thus, lower levels of alcohol consumption have been observed among younger generations and this appears to be an international phenomenon. It is important to establish whether recent changes in alcohol consumption in Russia are consistent with these international trends in young adult drinking.

This chapter is structured as follows. I briefly outline the historical background of changes in alcohol consumption in Russia and examine the restrictive measures related to the new governmental alcohol policy. Then, data sources and measures are described. Finally, I use survey data to compare young adults with other age cohorts as an illustration for exploring the extent to which state regulations could affect younger cohorts' drinking patterns.

Russia's Alcohol Policy in Historical Context

The Russian government has made several attempts to reduce alcohol consumption, including anti-alcohol campaigns in 1958 and 1972. However, enforcement of controlling measures has been very limited in its effectiveness. As real disposable income increased, alcohol consumption substantially grew, attaining its peak level in 1980, and this included an increase in popularity of the consumption of strong spirits (Nemtsov, 2011; Popova et al., 2007). At this time, total alcohol consumption (both recorded and unrecorded) reached 13.5 litres of pure alcohol per capita (Nemtsov, 2011; Treml, 1997), with vodka and strong spirits accounting for 6 litres, beer for 1.5 litres, wine for 2 litres, and homemade samogon for 4 litres. Thus, manufactured and homemade strong spirits prevailed, comprising approximately three-quarters of total alcohol consumption. Unrecorded alcohol accounted for 30% of total consumption (Radaev & Kotelnikova, 2016).

This Soviet model of drinking underwent a significant change from the 1980s onward. The first shock was political. Michael Gorbachev's anti-alcohol reform introduced in 1985 significantly increased alcohol prices, restricted alcohol sales, and penalised alcohol-related offences. These measures cut legal alcohol consumption by nearly 60% (Bhattacharya, Gathmann, & Miller, 2012; White, 1996). At the same time, samogon consumption increased by 80%, accounting for nearly two-thirds of total alcohol consumption in 1987. At least one-half of the diminishing recorded alcohol was replaced by an increase in unrecorded alcohol consumption from 4 to 7 litres per capita (Nemtsov, 2011; Vroublevsky & Harwin, 1998). Following the removal of severe restrictions in 1988, sales of legal alcohol (predominantly vodka) started to grow again, while the level of samogon consumption remained the same. Given the local vineyards were largely destroyed, the proportion of strong spirits increased.

The second shock was associated with the radical liberal economic reforms implemented between 1992 and 1994, which abolished the state monopoly on alcohol production and led to the legalisation of private entrepreneurship, the liberalisation of domestic and cross-border trade, an abrupt economic collapse, and weakening state control over markets. These reforms were accompanied by dramatic price increases and a considerable shift in consumer preference to unrecorded alcohol due to the increasing prevalence of cheap domestic and imported spirits, including pure ethanol, and counterfeit alcohol products. Many of these low-quality products were detrimental to human health and are documented as attributable to the doubling of premature mortality from alcohol poisoning, particularly among males (Nemtsov, 2011).

Drinking patterns in the Russian population have also changed over time. The prevalence of vodka as the main beverage type has declined since 1995, particularly among men, corresponding with a ban on TV commercial advertising of vodka that year. The prevalence of samogon consumption increased in the late 1990s and peaked in 2000, before declining steadily in the 2000s and stabilising in the 2010s at the lowest level since the mid-1990s. Thus, homemade spirits have not substituted for the declining consumption of manufactured spirits since 2000 (Radaev, 2015, 2016). Global companies' aggressive advertising and massive investment in the Russian beer industry led to a rise in beer consumption between 1995 and 2001. Beer consumption levelled off at its highest point in 2007 and declined thereafter. Finally, the prevalence of wine decreased from 1994 to 2000, followed by a slight increase in the 2000s (particularly among women) and a decline after a small peak in 2012. These changes have ushered in a new post-Soviet model of drinking in contemporary Russian society characterised by a lower alcohol consumption volume (e.g. 10 litres of pure alcohol per capita) and with less characterised by the consumption of strong spirits which now comprise around half of total alcohol consumption.

New Alcohol Policy

In 2006, a new alcohol policy proposed new tax stamps and a centralised electronic tracking and monitoring system of alcohol (EGAIS) to track the alcohol market and the movement of alcohol in Russia. These reforms were introduced in 2009, when the Federal Service for Alcohol Market Regulation (Rosalkogolregulirovanie) was established to develop and implement new alcohol policies. In December 2009, the Russian government approved a new strategy on national policies (Kontseptsiya, 2009). The official goal was to change drinking patterns, reduce alcohol-related harm, and reduce the volume of alcohol consumption by 55% by 2020. The strategy contained several provisions focusing specifically on adolescents and young adults. Strategy objectives included developing new forms of leisure-time activities for youths and adults to reduce alcohol consumption, as well as implementing pricing and fiscal policies designed to reduce the affordability of alcoholic beverages, particularly for young people. The strategy's proposed policy measures included: educating adolescents and young adults about the harms of high levels of alcohol consumption to encourage healthy lifestyles; and limiting (and even entirely banning) the hidden (i.e. undisclosed) advertising of alcoholic beverages, particularly among adolescents and young adults; and strengthening the administrative liability for selling alcohol to underage customers, with the introduction of criminal liability for repeat non-compliance.

Restrictions of Manufacture and Sales

To implement the new strategy, numerous amendments were introduced to federal legislation. A wide range of new regulations on the manufacture and sale of alcoholic beverages were implemented (Khaltourina & Korotayev, 2015; Nemtsov, 2015; Neufeld & Rehm, 2018). In 2011, a new licensing and registration procedure for alcohol manufacturers was implemented, and the minimal investment capital for alcohol producers and distributors was increased to 80 million roubles (2 million EUR). As a result, approximately 40% of (mainly small) alcohol companies were driven out of the market. In the same year, beer was classified as an alcoholic beverage and became subject to restrictions similar to those on strong spirits, and the federal government banned the sale of alcohol from 11 p.m. to 8 a.m. (some regional authorities extended trading hour restrictions by two to three hours). This measure effectively decreased the retail availability of alcohol by driving several 24-hour stores out of business, many of which had relied on night sales of alcohol as a primary source of income (Kolosnitsina, Khorkina, & Dorzhiev, 2015; Skorobogatov, 2014).

In 2011, the sale of alcohol in medical, educational, sport, and cultural facilities was prohibited and regional authorities could establish exclusion zones of up to 1 km around these alcohol-free locations. In 2013, the sale of alcoholic beverages (including beer) in non-stationary outlets (kiosks) was prohibited. The online trade of any alcoholic beverage was made illegal. In 2012, drinking was forbidden in all public places except for catering services, to prevent gatherings of heavy-drinking individuals. Step-by-step restrictions and eventually a total ban was implemented on the advertising of alcoholic beverages in television, radio, and newspapers. TV commercial advertising of vodka had been prohibited since 1995. In 2004, beer adverts were removed from television in the morning and daytime, with exceptions for soccer games, and alcohol advertising became more stringent (e.g. adverts could no longer include images of underage young people). In 2012, advertisements for beer on television, radio, and in public spaces (e.g. transport) were completely prohibited. In 2013, advertising alcoholic beverages in the press and online was completely prohibited. In 2017, the manufacture and sale of alcoholic beverages (including beer) in plastic packaging in volumes greater than 1.5 L were prohibited, except for export, with further restrictions on plastic packaging planned in the future.

Fiscal Measures and Combating Illegal Alcohol

The steep increase in excise tax rates was an important element of the new alcohol policy, particularly from 2011 to 2014 for strong spirits and 2009–2014 for wine and beer. Overall, excise tax rates implemented from 2009 for eight years experienced a 2.7-fold increase for vodka and strong spirits, a 3.5-fold increase for low-percentage alcohol (under 9%), a 2.6-fold increase for dry and sparkling wine, and a sevenfold increase for beer (see Table 16.1).

The minimum unit price of vodka remained at 32 rubles for 0.5 L from 2000 to 2009 before increasing 2.5 times (from 89 to 220 RBL per 0.5 L

Table 16.1 Excise tax rates on alcoholic beverages, RBL/L 2009–2017, and excise increase by 2009 (%)

	2009	2010	2011	2012 (1)	2012 (2)	2013	2014	2015	2016	2017
Vodka and strong spirits	191	210	231	254	300	400	500	500	500	523
% Increase relative to 2009	100	110	121	133	157	209	262	262	262	274
Sparkling wine	105	14	18	22	22	24	25	25	26	27
% Increase relative to 2009	100	133	171	210	210	229	238	238	248	257
Beer	3	9	10	12	12	15	18	19	20	21
% Increase relative to 2009	100	300	333	400	400	500	600	633	667	700

bottle) from 2010 to 2014. Following a temporary reduction of 16% in 2015, the minimum price was raised again by 11% from 2015 to 2017.

Retail prices and excise rates were correlated at a statistically significant level. As a result, the retail price of vodka increased 2.8-fold, the price of sparkling wine increased 1.9-fold and the price of domestic beer increased 2.3-fold from 2009 to 2017. Given that the real disposable income of the population increased only 3.1% between 2009 and 2017, the economic affordability of alcoholic beverages significantly decreased contributing to a decline in sales (e.g. vodka by 51%, beer by 21%) during this period.

Fiscal measures and multiple restrictions on alcohol availability led to a decline in sales of legal alcohol and created additional incentives for the production and sale of unrecorded alcohol along with other tax-evading behaviours. To strengthen state control and eliminate the illegal alcohol market, the EGAIS was extended from production to the wholesale and retail trade in 2016.

The production and sale of counterfeit alcohol were widespread in the 1990s. In the 2000s, significant changes in state policies regarding counterfeit goods retailers were introduced. In 2002 and 2008, important amendments were added to trademark legislation, including a tightening of liability in Russia's Criminal Code, the Civic Code, and the Code of Administrative Offences. It became legally possible to suspend the activities of infringing merchandising companies and individual entrepreneurs. Equipment and other facilities and materials used or intended for use to commit infringements could be confiscated, and any seized counterfeit goods could be destroyed.

More importantly, the enforcement of legislation protecting intellectual property rights improved considerably. The author collected statistics from several state agencies to assess the effects of new enforcement practices. The number of legal cases initiated against infringing companies increased more than tenfold between 2004 and 2006. Furthermore, arbitration court trials concerning the illegal use of trademarks increased tenfold between 2004 and 2010 and have remained high since this time. The number of criminal sentences for the illegal use of trademarks increased 18-fold between 2004 and 2010. Brand owners started to register and protect their trademarks more actively through available legal mechanisms and, after significant increases in the 2000s and beyond, indicated that both brand owners and state agencies became more alert in relation to the protection of intellectual property rights (see Radaev, 2017 for further details).

Controversies in Russian Alcohol Policy

The new alcohol policy has pursued controversial goals. On the one hand, it was designed to encourage healthy lifestyles and reduce the volume of alcohol consumed by the Russian population. On the other hand, these policy initiatives could be understood to have been implemented primarily to stimulate collection of revenues for the state budget by increasing alcohol sales. Fiscal policy reached a critical point in 2015 when excise tax payments collected from strong spirits declined by 11% and payments from beer and wine declined by 9% despite the fact that tax rates remained largely unchanged. The Russian government perceived this decline in excise tax revenue as a failure of the new alcohol policy and, as a result, some further anticipated restrictive measures were shelved. Instead of further increasing excise taxes on spirits by 32% as planned, excise tax rates were frozen in 2016. Excise taxes were then indexed in 2017 and frozen again until 2019. In 2015, the minimum unit price on a 0.5 L bottle of vodka decreased by 16% from 220 (2.85 EUR) to 185 roubles (2.40 EUR): the first decrease in price since the minimum price was introduced in 1996. Television and radio advertising of domestic wine was allowed again in January 2015. During the three years prior to the FIFA World Cup Russia 2018, advertisements for beer were temporarily reinstated in specific locations (points of sale; television broadcasts of sporting events).

The need to soften alcohol policy was publicly attributed to the expansion of illegal alcohol markets due to the price increase in legal alcohol. However, Russian alcohol policy remains very restrictive raising questions around the relationship between a highly restrictive alcohol policy and alcohol consumption in Russian society. In the remainder of this chapter, I will draw on survey data to explore this relationship in further detail.

Methodological Approach

Survey data were used to examine changes in alcohol consumption by age group in the post-Soviet period. These data were collected from the Russian Longitudinal Monitoring Survey (RLMS-HSE) conducted by the National Research University Higher School of Economics and 'Demoscope', together with Carolina Population Center, University of North Carolina at Chapel Hill and the Institute of Sociology at the Russian Academy of Sciences. The RLMS-HSE is an annual nationally representative panel survey of households and individuals that uses multistage probability sampling with primary sampling units selected from geographically determined strata. The data are representative of all regions and settlement types in Russia. This study used data collected from 258,526 individuals aged 15 or older between 1994 and 2016 (excluding 1997 and 1999, when surveys were not conducted). RLMS-HSE data are available from http://www.hse.ru/org/hse/rlms.

Three main measures of alcohol consumption were utilised. Firstly, percentage of drinkers was measured as the percentage of consumers of any alcoholic beverages during the 30 days preceding the survey. It was also measured separately for each age group and for each main beverage type (vodka, homemade samogon, beer, wine). Secondly, volume of consumed alcohol was measured as the average amount of alcohol consumed per capita during the last 30 days by respondents. For different alcoholic beverages, this volume was recalculated in grams of pure alcohol. Thirdly, excessive drinking was defined as the consumption of 400+ grams of pure alcohol for women and 800+ grams of pure alcohol for men during the last 30 days. This measure was adapted from the Dietary Guidelines of the US Department of Health and Human Services (Dietary Guidelines, 2015; Roshchina, 2012).

Data were available on the percentage of drinkers from 1994 to 2016 and the volume of alcohol consumption from 2006 to 2016. Calculations were made for all respondents aged 15+ and separately for women and men. Population surveys typically underestimate alcohol consumption (Livingston & Callinan, 2015): while numbers of people drinking tends to be more accurate, usually, the volume of alcohol consumed is under-reported. However, it is noted that the 30-day time frame used in this

324   V. Radaev

study may have helped minimise biased (under-) reporting due to recall effects.

The average retail prices of 0.5 litre of vodka and 1 litre of domestic beer (i.e. the main beverage types) were used as proxies for the affordability of alcohol from 2000 to 2016. Price increases over the years reflected the outcomes of fiscal alcohol policy, particularly increases in excise tax rates.

Alcohol Consumption Among Young Adults and Other Age Cohorts

Using RLMS-HSE survey data, the sample is divided into four age groups, including adolescents aged 15–17 (4.8%), young adults (aged 18–30 years, 24.1%), older adults (aged 31–55 years, 42.6%), and senior adults aged 56 years or older (28.5%). In this section, drinking patterns are compared between young adults and other age groups. Then, the effects of fiscal policies on alcohol consumption are considered with a particular emphasis on young adults.

Percentage of Individuals Consuming Alcohol

The percentage of people drinking any alcohol during the last 30 days remained relatively stable between 1994 and 2007 and decreased from 56 to 40% between 2008 and 2016. The percentage of adolescents drinking (who are not legally allowed to drink alcohol) peaked at 30% in 2001 before sharply declining to its lowest level of 5%. Participation rates for young adults and older adults were similar, remaining at 65% until 2007 and declining thereafter. However, drinking participation declined more sharply among young adults (41%) than older adults (50%) by 2016. The percentage of senior adults drinking was stable for most of the observation period and showed a moderate decline, from 40% at the beginning of the period to 32% by the end of the period (Fig. 16.1).

Regarding beverage-specific trends, the most significant decline was observed in the consumption of vodka and strong spirits. The percentage of vodka drinkers decreased from 42 to 16% between 1994 and 2016.

16 Making Sense of Alcohol Consumption Among Russian ...

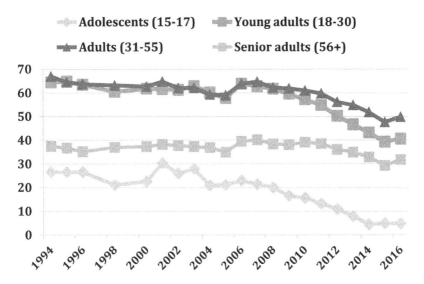

Fig. 16.1 Alcohol consumers for the last 30 days, by age group (%, $n = 258{,}526$)

Under-aged adolescents entirely abstained from drinking vodka by the end of the period. Participation rates in young adults were above the average level in 1994 (46%), followed by the strongest decline compared to other age cohorts by 2016 (8%). The percentage of vodka drinkers also fell in older cohorts: from 52 to 21% among older adults and from 30 to 16% among senior adults.

The percentage of homemade samogon drinkers showed an inverse U-shaped trend with a peak in 2000, with consumption having declined from 10 to 3%. Adolescents entirely abstained from drinking samogon, and there was a decline in samogon consumption among older age groups including, most steeply, among young adults. A similar decline was observed among most groups for the consumption of dry and sparkling wine from 1994 to 2016 (from 19 to 9%). The percentage of drinkers was similar for young adults and older adults, who were more likely to drink wine than senior adults and, particularly, adolescents. Wine was the only alcoholic beverage with a higher level of consumption among women than men in all age groups. The percentage of beer drinkers followed an inverse U-shaped trend with a peak in 2001 and a decrease thereafter. By 2016, the percentage of young adults drinking beer dropped to 30%, similar to that of older adults, and remained much higher than in groups of adolescents and senior adults. Overall, by the end of the period, compared to older age groups, young adults were less likely to drink both manufactured and homemade strong spirits, and under-aged adolescents reported abstaining from drinking strong spirits altogether. With respect to wine and beer, young adults' consumption was similar to that of adults and higher than that of adolescents and senior adults.

Declines in the Volume of Alcohol Consumption and Incidence of Excessive Drinking

The volume of alcohol consumed declined steadily from 2009 in all age groups except senior adults, whose consumption remained relatively stable over time (Fig. 16.2). The volume of self-reported alcohol consumption among adolescents decreased by 45% across the observation period. The volume of alcohol consumed among young adults declined somewhat more steeply than consumption decline among older adults from 2006 to

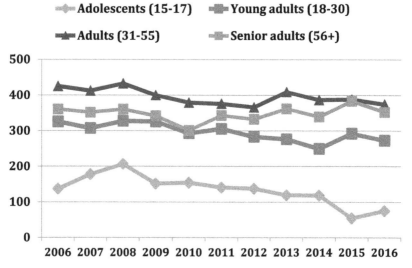

Fig. 16.2 Average volume of alcohol consumption during the last 30 days by age groups (grams of pure alcohol, $n = 80{,}839$)

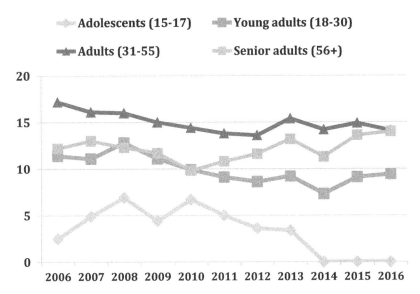

Fig. 16.3 Excessive drinkers by age groups (%, $n = 80{,}839$)

2016 (16% versus 12%). In young adults, it decreased less steeply among young adult women than young adult men (11% versus 21%). Older adults drank above the average level, and senior adults drank slightly above the average level.

Previous studies have shown that a decline in the prevalence of alcohol use during economic recessions may occur in parallel with an increase in the incidence of excessive drinking among young adults (e.g. Bor et al., 2013). In Russia, the incidence of excessive drinking during the last 30 days gradually decreased across all age groups after its peak in 2008 (Fig. 16.3), dropping from 13 to 9% among young adults, from 16 to 14% among older adults, and from 7 to negligible incidence among adolescents.

Effect of Fiscal Measures

The fall both in the numbers of Russian people drinking alcohol and the quantity of alcohol they consumed began in 2009: when Russia's new alcohol policy began to be implemented. To estimate the effect of the fiscal policy measures, the relationship was explored between changes in

328 V. Radaev

the retail prices of major alcoholic beverages and alcohol consumption by age group. Since the increase in retail prices is largely affected by the increase in excise tax rates, it can be used as a proxy for the results of the new alcohol policy. Analyses revealed that the proportion of individuals consuming alcohol was negatively correlated with the retail prices for vodka and domestic beer from 1994 to 2016 in all age groups.

Overall, these findings suggest that fiscal policy measures reducing the affordability of alcohol leading to changes in the number of people who consumed alcohol and the amount of alcohol consumed on occasions when individuals drank. This link between fiscal policy and declines in alcohol consumption was arguably accelerated/facilitated by economic crises starting in 2008 and again in 2014 which led to an eventual decline in real disposable income per capita. Analyses revealed that levels of per capita income among adolescents and young adults were significantly lower than among older adults over all observation periods suggesting that younger cohorts may have been particularly affected by these fiscal measures.

Conclusions

Beginning in 2009, the Russian government imposed multiple restrictions to reduce alcohol consumption and improve drinking patterns. Evidence presented in this chapter has demonstrated how the implementation of these measures was accompanied by a downward trend in alcohol consumption in the 2010s. These reductions varied by drink type and trends and were broadly similar for women and men.

Generational shifts may influence the ongoing decline of alcohol consumption; the younger the age group, the sharper the decline in alcohol consumption. In young adults, the numbers drinking alcohol declined more sharply than the amount of alcohol consumed. The proportion of excessive drinkers among young adults remained the same; however, it was lower than in older age groups.

The significant decline in drinkers and quantities of alcohol consumed started in 2009: the first year of implementation of Russia's new alcohol policy. Using retail prices of major alcoholic beverages types as a proxy for fiscal policy measures, analyses presented in this chapter have provided some evidence that the reduced affordability of alcohol resulted decreased alcohol consumption, particularly among young adults with less money.

In concluding, it is important to acknowledge that it would be fool-hardy to make causal associations between changes in state alcohol policy intervention (particularly restrictions of alcohol manufacture and sales) and changing consumption trends in alcohol consumption. Critically, delineating specific effects of policy on broad drinking patterns requires strict attention to social context, and to ongoing dynamics in the economic and political climate in which changes take place. It is hoped that this chapter has helped to illustrate the importance of disentangling policy initiatives from global or regional economic turbulence as central to efforts to meaningfully interpret declines in drinking at a population level.

Acknowledgements This work was funded by the Program for Basic Research of the National Research University Higher School of Economics. I thank Yana Roshchina for valuable comments.

References

Barda, C., & Sardianou, E. (2010). Analysing consumers' 'activism' in response to rising prices. *International Journal of Consumer Studies, 34,* 133–139.

Bhattacharya, J., Gathmann, C., & Miller, G. (2012). *The Gorbachev anti-alcohol campaign and Russia's mortality crisis* (IZA Discussion Paper 6783).

Bor, J., Basu, S., Coutts, A., McKee, M., & Stuckler, D. (2013). Alcohol use during the great recession of 2008–2009. *Alcohol, 48*(3), 343–348.

Chaloupka, F. J., Grossman, M., & Saffer, H. (2002). The effects of price on alcohol consumption and alcohol-related problems. *Alcohol Research & Health, 26,* 22–34.

de Goeij, M. C. M., Suhrcke, M., Toffolutti, V., van de Mheen, D., Schoenmakers, N. V., & Kunst, A. E. (2015). How economic crises affect alcohol consumption and alcohol-related health problems: A realist systematic review. *Social Science and Medicine, 131,* 131–146.

Denisova, I. (2010). *Potrebleniye alkogolya v Rossii: Vliyaniye na zdorovie i smertnost* [Consumption of alcohol in Russia: Effect on health and mortality] (CEFIR/NES Analytical Reports and Papers 31).

Dietary Guidelines for Americans, 2015–2020. (2015). U.S. Department of Health and Human Services and U.S. Department of Agriculture. Retrieved 2 March 2019 from http://health.gov/dietaryguidelines/2015/guidelines/.

Ekström, K. M., Ekström, M. P., Potapova, M., & Shanahan, H. (2003). Changes in food provision in Russian households experiencing perestroika. *International Journal of Consumer Studies, 27*(4), 294–301.

Hingson, R., Zha, W., & Smyth, D. (2017). Magnitude and trends in heavy episodic drinking, alcohol-impaired driving, and alcohol-related mortality and overdose hospitalizations among emerging adults of college ages 18–24 in the United States, 1998–2014. *Journal of Studies of Alcohol and Drugs, 78*, 540–548.

Jukkala, T., Makinen, I. H., Ferlander, S., Vagero, D., & Kaslitsyna, O. (2008). Economic strain, social relations, gender, and binge drinking in Moscow. *Social Science and Medicine, 66*, 663–674.

Khaltourina, D., & Korotayev, A. (2015). Effects of specific alcohol control policy measures on alcohol-related mortality in Russia from 1998 to 2013. *Alcohol and Alcoholism, 50*, 588–601.

Kolosnitsina, M., Khorkina, N., & Dorzhiev, K. (2015). Vliyaniye tsenovykh mer gosudarstvennoi politiki na potrebleniye spirtnykh napitkov v Rossii [Alcohol pricing policy in Russia: Influence on alcohol consumption]. *Ekonomicheskaya Politika, 10*(5), 171–190.

Kontseptsiya gosudarstvennoy politiki po snizheniyu masshtabov zloupotrebleniya alkogolem I profilaktiki alkogolizma sredi naseleniya Rossiiskoy Federatsii na period do 2020 goda [Strategy paper on national policies to reduce the level of alcohol abuse and on the prevention of alcoholism among the population of the Russian Federation until 2020]. Russian Federation Government, 2009. Retrieved 2 March 2019 from http://fsrar.ru/policy_of_sobriety/koncepcia.

Livingston, M., & Callinan, S. (2015). Under-reporting in alcohol surveys: Whose drinking is under-estimated? *Journal of Studies on Alcohol and Drugs, 76*, 158–164.

Livingston, M., Raninen, J., Slade, T., Swift, W., Lloyd, B., & Dietze, P. (2016). Understanding trends in Australian alcohol consumption—An age–period–cohort model. *Addiction, 111*(9), 1590–1598.

Mäkelä, P., Bloomfield, K., Gustafsson, N. K., Huhtanen, P., & Room, R. (2007). Changes in volume of drinking after changes in alcohol taxes and travellers' allowances: Results from a panel study. *Addiction, 103*, 181–191.

Meng, Y., Holmes, J., Hill-McManus, D., Brennan, A., & Meier, P. S. (2014). Trend analysis and modelling of gender-specific age, period and birth cohort effects on alcohol abstention and consumption level for drinkers in Great

Britain using the General Lifestyle Survey 1984–2009. *Addiction, 109,* 206–215.

Nemtsov, A. (2011). *A contemporary history of alcohol in Russia.* Stockholm, Sweden: Södertörns Högskola.

Nemtsov, A. (2015). Rossijskaja smertnost' v svete potreblenija alkogolja [Russian mortality in light of alcohol consumption]. *Demograficheskoe obozrenie* [Demographic Review], *2,* 113–135.

Neufeld, M., & Rehm, J. (2013). Alcohol consumption and mortality in Russia since 2000: Are there any changes following the alcohol policy changes starting in 2006? *Alcohol and Alcoholism, 48,* 222–230.

Neufeld, M., & Rehm, J. (2018). Effectiveness of policy changes to reduce harm from unrecorded alcohol in Russia between 2005 and now. *International Journal of Drug Policy, 51,* 1–9.

Pennay, A., Livingston, M., & MacLean, S. (2015). Young people are drinking less: It is time to find out why. *Drug and Alcohol Review, 34,* 115–118.

Popova, S., Rehm, J., Patra, J., & Zatonski, W. (2007). Comparing alcohol consumption in Central and Eastern Europe to other European countries. *Alcohol and Alcoholism, 42,* 465–473.

Radaev, V. (2015). Impact of a new alcohol policy on homemade alcohol consumption and sales in Russia. *Alcohol and Alcoholism, 50,* 365–372.

Radaev, V. (2016). Divergent drinking patterns and factors affecting homemade alcohol consumption (the case of Russia). *International Journal of Drug Policy, 34,* 88–95.

Radaev, V. (2017). A crooked mirror: The evolution of illegal alcohol markets in Russia since the late socialist period. In J. Beckert & M. Dewey (Eds.), *The architecture of illegal markets: Towards an economic sociology of illegality in the economy* (pp. 218–241). Oxford, UK: Oxford University Press.

Radaev, V., & Kotelnikova, Z. (2016). Izmeneniye struktury potrebleniya alkogolya v kontekste gosudarstvennoy alkogolnoy politiki v Rossii [Changes in the structure of alcohol consumption in the context of the state alcohol policy in Russia]. *Ekonomicheskaya Politika* [Economic Policy], *5,* 92–117.

Raninen, J., Livingston, M., & Leifman, H. (2014). Declining trends in alcohol consumption among Swedish youth—Does theory of collectivity of drinking cultures apply? *Alcohol and Alcoholism, 49,* 681–686.

Roshchina, Y. (2012). Dinamika i struktura potrebleniya alkogolya v sovermennoy Rossii [Dynamics and structure of alcohol consumption in contemporary Russia]. *Vestnik Rossiiskogo Monitoringa Ekonomicheskogo Polozheniya i Zdorovia Naselenia* [Bulletin of the Russian Longitudinal Monitoring Survey], *2,* 238–257.

Skorobogatov, A. (2014). *The effect of closing hour restrictions on alcohol use and abuse in Russia* (HSE Working Papers 63/EC/2014). Moscow: HSE. Retrieved 2 March 2019 from http://www.hse.ru/data/2014/09/26/1315652159/63EC2014.pdf.

Treml, V. G. (1997). Soviet and Russian statistics on alcohol consumption. In J. L. Bobadilla, C. A. Costello, & F. Mitchell (Eds.), *Premature death in the new independent states* (pp. 220–238). Washington, DC: National Academy Press.

Vroublevsky, A., & Harwin, J. (1998). Russia. In M. Grant (Ed.), *Alcohol and emerging markets: Patterns, problems, and responses* (pp. 203–222). Philadelphia: Brunner and Mazel.

Wagenaar, A. C., Salois, M. J., & Komro, K. A. (2009). Effects of beverage alcohol price and tax levels on drinking: A meta-analysis of 1003 estimates from 112 studies. *Addiction, 104,* 179–190.

White, S. (1996). *Russia goes dry: Alcohol, state and society.* New York: Cambridge University Press.

World Health Organization. (2014). *Global Status Report on Alcohol and Health.* Geneva, Switzerland: WHO.

World Health Organization. (2016). *World health statistics 2016: Monitoring health for the SDGs, Sustainable Development Goals.* Geneva, Switzerland: WHO.

17

Evaluating the Recent 'Integrated Approach' to Alcohol Policy Designed to Promote Moderate Alcohol Consumption Among Dutch Young People

Rob Bovens and Dike van de Mheen

For the last 15 years, alcohol policy in the Netherlands has shifted focus from young adults (and predominantly students) to younger people aged 10–18 years old (mainly university students). A key influence on this was the publication of research in 2004 showing a significant decline in the average age at which children had their first alcoholic drink to 12 years old (Monshouwer, Van Dorsselaer, Gorter, Verdurmen, & Vollebergh, 2004) and a significant increase in 'binge drinking' or, more formally, heavy episodic drinking (HED, defined as consumption of at least 60 grams pure alcohol in a single occasion, World Health Organisation [WHO], 2019) among this age group. Following this, the priority of Dutch alcohol policy shifted to focusing on younger people and young adults (defined for current purposes as approximately 12–17-year-olds and 18–25-year-olds, respectively).

R. Bovens (✉) · D. van de Mheen
Tranzo, Scientific Center for Care and Wellbeing, School of Social and Behavioural Sciences, Tilburg University, Tilburg, The Netherlands
e-mail: R.H.L.M.Bovens@uvt.nl

© The Author(s) 2019
D. Conroy and F. Measham (eds.), *Young Adult Drinking Styles*,
https://doi.org/10.1007/978-3-030-28607-1_17

333

In this chapter, we consider contemporary alcohol consumption in the Netherlands, historical drinking trends and policy change, with a focus on the shift described above to a more integrated approach towards youth and young adult consumption—integrated in the sense that multiple stakeholders and multiple features of policy are involved in efforts to promote moderate drinking among young people and young adults. Drinking trends discussed include an increase in the average age of consuming a first alcoholic drink and a shift in the age at which more serious alcohol problems linked to HED occur from 10–15 years to 16–24 years (Ministry of Health, Wellbeing and Sports, 2018). In a final chapter section, we focus on the alcohol prevention programme that the Dutch government has introduced for the next three years that has focused on problem alcohol use in society. The focus and content of this programme build on the more youth-focused, integrated approach that has characterised the last decade.

Contemporary Alcohol Consumption in the Netherlands

According to a trend report on health conditions in the Netherlands, tobacco, unhealthy diet, inactivity and alcohol use contribute to 18.5% of the disability-adjusted life years (DALYs) of the Dutch population (National Institute for Public Health and Environment, 2018b). Regarding alcohol use, every year about 30,000 patients have been treated for alcohol problems in substance abuse treatment centres ('LADIS Home', z.d.). For example, in 2016, 21,900 patients were treated in emergency rooms for alcohol-related accidents, intoxication or being a victim of violence (Valkenberg & Nijman, 2017). In 2017, 79.5% of people aged eighteen years or older drank alcohol (84.3% males and 74.8% females) (Van Laar & Van Gestel, 2019). In the Global status report on alcohol in 2016, the Netherlands was ranked 32nd of 52 countries with 7.5 litres per capita consumption (WHO, 2018). Data from the seventh round of the European Social Survey showed that the Netherlands was in fourth place of 21 European countries regarding daily drinking and was the country where alcohol was consumed on the largest number of occasions during the course of a week relative to other European countries (Wuyts, Barbier, & Loosveldt, 2016). In the Dutch general adult population in 2017, 9.2% drank above moderate drinking levels (e.g. over 14 units a week for women, over 21 units for men). At this time, there was also growing concern about drinking problems among individuals aged 55 years and older (Van Laar & Van Gestel, 2019). Regarding the frequency of alcohol consumption among young people, we see the same pattern as we see among older adults: in the ESPAD studies, the Netherlands is in fourth position out of 35 countries in terms of how frequently alcohol is used. Regarding HED, the frequency of episodes reported in the general population is average in relative terms in the Netherlands compared to other European countries (The ESPAD Group, 2016). However, when younger people drink, they drink a lot: 71% of young people aged 15–16 years who drink alcohol are classified engaging in HED (Stevens et al., 2018).

Historical Drinking Trends and Policy Change

In 1881, the Alcohol Licensing Act was introduced in the Netherlands (Bovens, 2010). The main goal was to temper the use of spirits in society, with beer consumption a lower-order concern. Liquor stores and bars needed to have a licence from the local government to sell spirits with the number of licences restricted by the national government. The view at that time was that alcohol availability determined the prevalence of alcohol problems. Besides the regulation of licensing, punishments for drunkenness were also introduced (Van der Stel, 1995). The Alcohol Licensing Act of 1904 regulated the licensing of low alcohol beverages (e.g. beer, Tweede Kamer der Staten Generaal, 1997). For the first time, legislation was directed towards the prevention of alcohol consumption among young people as they were forbidden to enter a pub without having someone escort them aged 21 years or older. A national surveillance organisation was established and from 1919 onwards was under the supervision of the National Health Surveillance Organization. The last amendment of the Licensing Act in 1931 increased the number of licences available to sell low alcohol beverages (Tweede Kamer der Staten Generaal, 1997).

After a century of falling levels of alcohol consumption, it quickly increased from 2.6 litres per capita in 1960 to 8.9 litres in 1980 (Van Laar & Van Gestel, 2019), the most rapid increase in the world during this period. At the time, it was felt that the possible reasons for this increase could be found in increased disposable income, decreased alcohol price, new groups drinking within the population, enhanced marketing techniques, as well as catching up with neighbouring countries (Garretsen, 2001). Alcohol use stabilised after 1980 and then after 2000 began to decrease slightly. During this period, Dutch drinking culture gradually changed. Firstly, alcohol consumption while watching sporting events grew as a conventional leisure time activity, which was closely associated with the growth in alcohol industry advertising—particularly beer advertising—at sports and entertainment events. For example, Holland Heineken House has been the location for athletics supporters since the 1992 Olympic Games, demonstrating the closer links between the alcohol industry (Heineken being a leading Dutch beer) and the sporting entertainment industry. Similarly, music events and music halls also have been sponsored by the beer industry. Secondly, alcohol use expanded among youth and also among women, partly illustrated by the introduction of alcopops—a product designed to target female consumers—in the 1990s. Combined with the growth of the event industry (e.g. sporting events, festivals), these changes were associated with a significant increase in alcohol use and HED incidence present among both boys and girls. For example, during this period, alcohol use among 12-year-old boys increased from about 40% to almost 80% and among 12-year-old girls from about 30 to 60% (Van Laar & Van Gestel, 2019).

The age at which young people typically started to drink dropped to 12.2 years for girls and 11.9 years for boys. Another consequence was an increase in hospital admissions due to alcohol intoxication in 2000–2005 among 10–14-year-olds (Fig. 17.1).

Approaches to alcohol prevention programmes in this period reflected the conceptualisation of alcohol problems at that time. Between 1960 and 1990, drink driving became a particular concern in the Netherlands as alcohol-related road traffic accidents increased in line with an increase in the number of cars on the road (Bovens, 2010). Blood tests, breathalyser tests, the strengthening of police surveillance (Bovens & Prinsen,

17 Evaluating the Recent 'Integrated Approach' to Alcohol Policy ...

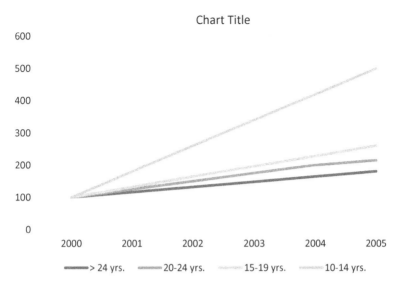

Fig. 17.1 Trends in hospital admissions 2000–2005 due to intoxication by alcohol in the Netherlands (Valkenberg, Van der Lely, & Brugmans, 2007)

1984), mass media campaigns, higher fines and compulsory courses for road traffic offenders were all measures introduced by the government to address the problem of drink driving (Bovens, 1987, 1991). As a result of these preventive measures, the number of alcohol-related fatal accidents dropped significantly after 2000 (I&O Research, 2018). In response to a large increase in per capita consumption of alcohol, the government produced a memorandum 'Alcohol and Society' in 1986 (Tweede Kamer der Staten Generaal, 1986) that led to the Ministry of Welfare, Health and Culture starting mass media campaigns. In 1986, a mass media campaign, 'Booze can break your heart' ('Drank maakt meer kapot dan je lief is'), was launched. This campaign focused initially on heavy drinking by adults, but at the end of the 1990s, the focus shifted to young people. Two specific campaigns started: one for young people aged 14–18 ('Booze: The hangover comes later') and one for university students ('I am Drunk. And who are you?!') (National Institute of Health Promotion and Disease Prevention, 2004). The first campaign focused on young people who frequented the Dutch beaches during summer holidays and the campaign featured peer education sessions by trained students and quiz cards which were aimed in a targeted way at young people likely to engage in HED at beaches and camping sites. When an evaluation suggested that this campaign had been of little effect (De Graaff and Poort, 2004), prevention organisations concluded that a change in strategy was needed and that interventions should focus on the social and physical environment of young people. A student campaign, focused on students when they started university and on student associations, was financed until 2006, and after this point the government refocused from university students and other subgroups to young people (or 'youth') as a broader demographic group.

Besides some modifications of the 1964 Alcohol Licensing and Catering Act (e.g. increasing enforcement of drink driving), there was no national policy to reduce alcohol-related harm through increased regulation and enforcement. Instead, policymakers focused their efforts on mass media campaigns and education programmes in schools. Since the early 1990s, the Healthy School and Drugs programme, offered to 11–17-year-old students, outlined four pillars of effective health promotion: education, screening and early intervention, involving parents and a specific school policy regarding drugs (including alcohol and tobacco) and drug-related behaviour. Despite early evidence of the programme's success (Cuijpers, 2002), more recent studies showed no positive effects on substance use among primary school (De Leeuw, Kleinjan, Lammers, Lokman & Engels, 2014) or secondary school (Malmberg et al., 2015) pupils. Nevertheless, it continued to be the preferred prevention programme in schools.

The Start of an Integrated Approach to Promoting Healthy Drinking Among Younger People: Strategies Aimed at Retailers, Consumers and Government

In recent years, research has accumulated about the harmful effects of alcohol on the developing brain of children and adolescents and of how these risks may be underestimated among both parents and teachers (Tapert & Schweinsburg, 2005; Verdurmen, 2006). Regarding parents, empirical work has demonstrated that Dutch parents believed that offering their children the first drink at home and teaching them to drink were the best ways to educate them to drink in moderation with findings demonstrating that 46% of 12-year-olds were allowed to drink alcohol at home (Monshouwer et al., 2004). By contrast, research suggests that clear rules and delaying the time for when parents permit children to start drinking alcohol are the most effective ways to achieve moderate alcohol use (Van der Vorst, Engels, Meeus, & Deković, 2006). This traditionally laissez-faire attitude towards alcohol in Dutch society is also illustrated by the ease with which minors can purchase alcohol in supermarkets, clubs or pubs: 85% of adolescents under the age of 16 succeeded in buying alcohol (Bieleman, Biesma, Kruize, & Snippe, 2004).

Regarding teachers, there has been growing recognition that education in schools or in settings where young people drink may have little impact on substance use among young people. On 24 March 2005, a letter addressed to the House of Representatives a new policy regarding the youth alcohol use and alcohol-related problems was announced that detailed new legislation, mass media campaigns and collaboration between various stakeholders including alcohol retailers, bar owners, schools and sports clubs (Tweede Kamer der Staten Generaal, 2005). The emphasis of this approach set a particular tone in terms of how norms around how young peoples' alcohol consumption should be viewed with reference to the WHO position on young people's drinking in this appeal. The minister's letter stimulated the start of a huge programme of government initiatives. Firstly, the government started a campaign directed at parents called: 'Prevent alcohol harm to your growing child!' The message was that giving your child an alcoholic drink before their 16th birthday causes harm to the developing brain and increases the likelihood of future alcohol dependence by a factor of four (De Graaf et al., 2008). Parents were offered tips and strategies to successfully educate their children about the dangers inherent in heavy alcohol use and on how to take a moderate approach to alcohol consumption in adult life (De Looze et al., 2014).

Secondly, local governments were required to start regional programmes to prevent alcohol use among children aged younger than 16 years. In these projects, schools, sports clubs, bars and supermarkets could collaborate to avoid offering alcohol to young people aged under 16 years. These recommendations were supported with a government-approved manual that included recommendations about how to set up an effective local programme aimed at young people (Mulder, Bovens, Franken, & Sannen, 2013; National Quality of Nutrition Organization, 2007). In 2005–2012, alcohol prevention programmes were started in more than 200 municipalities (National Institute for Public Health and Environment, 2013).

Thirdly, the supervision of the Dutch National Quality of Nutrition Organization on alcohol retailers was expanded to ensure supermarkets, bars and sports clubs did not sell alcohol to children aged 16 or younger. From 2005 onwards, developments moved quickly. There was a growing awareness about alcohol problems among younger people, and many organisations became involved in initiatives to promote understanding of the risks of starting drinking early among young people. The results, including data generated from monitoring instruments like the HBSC schools surveys (Inchley et al., 2018), along with data concerning hospital admissions due to alcohol-related accidents (Valkenberg & Nijman, 2017), set the public and political agenda to develop a stronger alcohol policy. As an illustration of this, since January 2010, it became forbidden to broadcast alcohol advertisement between 6.00 and 21.00 (Dutch Senate, 2009).

The new Alcohol Licensing Act meant that (1) not only alcohol retailers but also young people aged 16 or under would be punished for possessing alcohol in public places; (2) inspections for violation of rules related to alcohol sales would be conducted by a dedicated team of local supervisors commissioned by the mayor; and (3) municipalities had to establish regulations for alcohol sales by sports clubs and youth clubs.

During the process of changing the law in 2013, it seemed that there was growing support among the public to raise the minimum purchase age for alcohol from 16 to 18 years old. This resulted in a second important amendment to the Alcohol Licensing and Catering Act within a period of just one year. In January 2014, it was forbidden to sell alcohol to minors under 18 and also for minors to possess alcohol in public places. The shift

17 Evaluating the Recent 'Integrated Approach' to Alcohol Policy ... 341

from 16 years to 18 years was accompanied by the introduction of the mass media campaign: 'NIX18' ('Not a drop before 18 years old'). This campaign was supported by the alcohol industry and retailers through a number of compliance activities. For example, supermarkets cashiers were trained and instructed to ask for ID, campaign stickers and signs legally had to appear in licensed bars and off-licence stores, and the new legal minimum purchase age was added to alcohol beverage bottles and alcohol advertisements.

Since the legislative changes, enforcement by local supervisors at a local level has intensified. Enforcement is enhanced by periodical monitoring using so-called mystery shoppers: young people trained to simulate buying alcohol and to supply ID if asked. However, research has suggested that compliance levels with these new regulations have been mixed, with highest compliance levels evident among retailers in off-licence stores and supermarkets and lowest compliance levels with the new minimum purchase age found in sports canteens selling alcohol (Roodbeen, Geurtsen, & Schelleman-Offermans, 2018).

Several regions in the Netherlands started initiatives to encourage periods of sobriety for parents to change their own drinking habits, to provide an example to their children about how a moderate relationship is conducted. Drawing on the success of 'temporary abstinence initiatives' including Ocsober (in Australia) and Dry January (in the UK), the Netherlands introduced IkPas (No Thanks) in 2015, a campaign promoting a period of 30–40 days sobriety at some point during a calendar year (Bovens, Schuitema, & Schmidt, 2017). The IkPas campaign was designed to stimulate and support people to take a break from unhealthy drinking habits. The campaign started as a private initiative with 4595 participants in 2015, supporting by regional Public Health and drug treatment centres, an increasing number of municipalities joined the campaign and it increased to 37,875 participants by 2019. In 2017, the Dutch House of Representatives passed a motion asking the government to finance the campaign resulting in government funding for IkPas since 2018. Participants of the IkPas campaign are variable but are known to include reasonable numbers of heavy drinkers, the elderly, and university students. Evaluations of IkPas since its start are ongoing but promising in terms of promoting more moderate subsequent drinking; for example, in

2018, Dutch participants reported a 36% decrease in weekly alcohol consumption following IkPas participation relative to their pre-participation consumption levels (Bovens, Mathijssen, & van de Mheen, 2018).

In the light of the changes in Dutch alcohol policy and the rise of initiatives like IkPas which suggest some changes in the climate of drinking practices, we will now review recent data concerning alcohol use among young people in the Netherlands. The latest figures suggest a dramatic decline among young people aged 12–16 in drinking practices in terms of annual overall consumption levels and consumption levels for a typical month (please refer to Van Laar and Van Gestel [2019] and Stevens et al. [2018] for further details). Data also suggests that the average age at which young people start to drink alcohol has changed from the 2003 figure (mean starting age = 12 years old) to the 2015 average figure (mean starting age = 13.2 years old). Pinpointing whether and how revisions to Dutch alcohol policy and health promotion strategy during this period are, of course, difficult to establish in a meaningful way. However, recent data from ESPAD (2016) also seem to indicate that HED incidence among 15/16-year-olds remains high—i.e. when young people do drink, there has been evidence that they may drink to excess.

Over the last decade, different factors might be drawn on to explain the expansion of alcohol-specific policies in different health and social care sectors in the Netherlands. These factors include the phenomenon that some young people still regularly engage in HED, a growing problem with alcohol consumption among the Dutch elderly, and an accumulation of evidence implicating alcohol use as a cause of different types of cancer (Wood et al., 2018). These factors have led to alcohol becoming included, in addition to focus on tobacco use and the obesity epidemic, as part of the National Prevention Agreement in November 2018. More than 70 organisations signed this Agreement including NGOs, the sports sector, insurance companies, the National Agency of Municipalities, the alcohol industry, alcohol retailers and the catering industry (Ministry of Health, Wellbeing and Sports, 2018). An overarching goal of the Agreement was to have a healthier population by 2040 through a range of individual and collaborative prevention measures.

Aims of the alcohol component of the National Prevention Agreement included achieving zero alcohol consumption during pregnancy or before the age of eighteen, reduced incidence of HED among adults, and a growing public awareness of the potential health and safety risks posed risked by excessive alcohol consumption. Three key 'best buy' policies were proposed to reduce young adult alcohol consumption: increased prices, making alcohol less widely available and more stringent limitations placed on advertising. Specific features of these proposals included minimising cheap alcohol promotions (e.g. price reductions in supermarkets were not permitted to exceed a 25% reduction of the regular price); arrangements such that legislation over alcohol promotions would be decided at a national rather than regional (municipality) level; and a programme of research designed to explore the feasibility of introducing Minimum Unit Pricing in the Netherlands.

The National Prevention Agreement placed particular emphasis on changes to the availability of alcohol including proposals to promote non-alcoholic beer as an alternative in the sports sector and on college and university grounds. Other proposals included the promotion of other healthy alternatives to alcohol in sports canteens, strengthening controls on 'happy hours' and selling alcohol to minors. The proposals in the Agreement are to be monitored to assess whether goals have been reached.

Recent Developments in Dutch Alcohol Policy Regarding Young Adults

In recent decades, Dutch alcohol policy has focused on young people aged 17 years or younger. This was an understandable and arguably justified initiative given the average age of first alcohol consumption (12 years) at the start of the twenty-first century. There is evidence that the integrated approach taken to Dutch alcohol policy may have been successful, reflected in a reduction in young people aged 12–15 years having consumed a first alcoholic drink and a reduction in the number of individuals in this group who regularly consume alcohol. It is important to contextualise concerns about excessive alcohol consumption among 12–17-year-old young people; the heaviest drinkers in Dutch population are still individuals aged 16–30 years, and university students are a particularly high-risk group for excessive alcohol consumption (Van Laar & Van Gestel, 2019). An ongoing debate between different alcohol harm prevention groups is what measures might be most effective to help promote excessive alcohol consumption in the general population (or in specific subgroups), with some taking the position that macro-level changes (e.g. reducing alcohol availability) are key to addressing harmful drinking practices. Alcohol's significant contribution to the economy and role in entertainment and leisure can place considerable strain on developing and implementing effective measures to curb harmful drinking practices. To note here; such measures may include changing leisure economies leading to new patterns of consumption (e.g. the growing trend across developing countries to eat and drink outside the home) is an important factor to consider in the formulation of effective and sustainable alcohol policies aimed at young people and young adults (Food Service Institute Netherlands, 2018). A growing number of municipalities create new nightlife locations, cafés and bars in an attempt to attract tourists and local residents to spend their time and money in city centres with alcohol playing a key role in attracting customers. Public Health organisations warn that this development will increase the availability of alcohol and is in contradiction with the National Prevention Agreement aim of reducing alcohol availability.

A report published by the National Institute for Public Health and Environment ('RIVM', National Institute for Public Health and Environment, 2018a) considered the possible impact of the Agreement with respect to its tobacco-, obesity- and alcohol-related objectives and concluded that the terms of the Agreement were insufficient to be able to succeed in reaching its defined goals. An important factor here was the difficulty of striking the right balance between industry involvement (necessary to implement key features of the policy) and protecting against industry interests focused around having reasonably liberal legislation in place for the availability, pricing and advertising of alcohol products. By contrast, the RIVM was more positive about tobacco: the tobacco industry was not permitted to take part in Agreement-related consultations and tobacco pricing and availability policies were agreed without major involvement from the tobacco industry. Although the participation of the alcohol industry reduced the opportunity to introduce stricter alcohol controls, a more generous inclusion policy for stakeholders was hoped to commit them to the aims of the final Agreement. Public support for the introduction of stricter alcohol controls has been variable, but despite initial substantial resistance from the general population for the new minimum purchase age of 18, the new law has been implemented without significant controversy from the general public.

We conclude that the change in Dutch alcohol policy in recent years and a focus on reduced consumption may be partly attributable to some Public Health successes, particularly given evidence of increases in the average age at which young people first start to drink alcohol. Part of this success may also be attributable to increases in the minimum purchase age from 16 to 18 years. To conclude, the 2018 National Agreement may have been an important step in addressing alcohol policy and in shifting social norms and conventions around the permissibility of alcohol use among young adults. However, it remains to be seen whether these policy efforts will be met with resistance from the Dutch general public, and whether further measures may be required for wide-scale, sustainable cultural changes in drinking norms and practices among young adults and young people.

References

Bieleman, B., Biesma, S., Kruize, A., & Snippe, J. (2004). *Alcoholverstrekking aan jongeren 2003. Naleving leeftijdsgrenzen 16 en 18 jaar uit de Drank- en Horecawet. Metingen 1999, 2001 en 2003* [Compliance alcohol and licensing act and the legal age]. Groningen and Rotterdam: Intraval.

Bovens, R. (1987). Alcohol program: An educational program for drunken drivers in prison. In M. J. M. Brand-Koolen (Ed.), *Studies on the Dutch prison system* (pp. 151–157). Berkeley, CA: Kugler Publications.

Bovens, R. H. L. M. (1991). *Rijders onder invloed beïnvloed. Onderzoek naar het effect van cursussen alcohol en verkeer* [Driving under the influence of alcohol: Evaluation of alcohol traffic courses. Dissertation]. Groningen: Wolters Noordhoff.

Bovens, R. H. L. M. (2010). *De preventiewerker centraal. Een bijdrage aan de ontwikkeling van de verslavingspreventie* [The focus on the professional in prevention. Oration]. Zwolle: Windesheim.

Bovens, R. H. L. M., Mathijssen, J. J. P., & van de Mheen, H. M. (2018). *Resultaten IkPas-Actie 2018* [PDF]. Tilburg: Tranzo.

Bovens, R. H. L. M., & Prinsen, P. J. (1984). *Extra politie-inzet en rijden onder invloed; verslag van een surveillance-experiment in de gemeente Weert* [Experimental increase of police surveillance in driving under the influence of alcohol]. The Hague: WODC.

Bovens, R. H. L. M., Schuitema, A., & Schmidt, P. M. (2017). IkPas: een definitieve breuk met het verleden? *Verslaving, 13*(4), 208–222.

Cuijpers, P. (2002). Effective ingredients of school-based drug prevention programs: A systematic review. *Addictive Behaviors, 27,* 1009–1023.

De Graaf, I., Bovens, R., Lemmers, L., Naaborgh, L., Schulten, I., & Verdurmen, J. (2008). Beperking alcoholschade bij kinderen en jongeren [Limitation of harm caused by alcohol to children and adolescents]. In A. J. M. Bonnet-Breusers (Ed.), *Praktijkboek Jeugdgezondheidszorg* (pp. Artikel VI 3.3-1 t/m 3.3-26). Maarssen: Elsevier Gezondheidszorg.

De Graaff, D., & Poort, E. (2004). Evaluatie van de Zomercampagne 2003. 'Drank: De kater komt later' [Evaluation study of the summer campaign 2003. 'Booze: the hangover comes later']. Haarlem: ResCon Research and Consultancy.

De Leeuw, R., Kleinjan, M., Lammers, J., Lokman, S., & Engels, R. (2014). De effectiviteit van De Gezonde School en Genotmiddelen voor het basisonderwijs [The effectiveness of the healthy school and substance use]. *Kind en Adolescent, 35*(1), 2–21.

De Looze, M., Vermeulen-Smit, E., Ter Bogt, T. F., Van Dorsselaer, S. A., Verdurmen, J., Schulten, I., ... Vollebergh, W. A. (2014). Trends in alcohol-specific parenting practices and adolescent alcohol use between 2007 and 2011 in the Netherlands. *International Journal of Drug Policy, 25*(1), 133–141.

Dutch Senate. (2009). *Wijziging van de Mediawet 2008 en de Tabakswet ter implementatie van de richtlijn Audiovisuele mediadiensten. Memorie van antwoord* [Change of the Media Legislation 2008]. Dossier 31876, The Hague.

Food Service Institute Netherlands. (2018). FSIN Food500 2018. Ede, FSIN.

Garretsen, H. F. L. (2001). Dutch alcohol policy developments: The last decades and present state of affairs. *Medicine and Law, 20,* 301–311.

I&O Research. (2018). *Rijden onder invloed in Nederland in 2002–2017. Ontwikkeling van het alcoholgebruik van automobilisten in weekendnachten* [Driving while intoxicated in the Netherlands in 2002–2017. Development of the alcohol use among drivers during weekend nights]. The Hague: Ministry of Infrastructure and Environment.

Inchley, J., Currie, D., Vieno, A., Torsheim, T., Ferreira-Borges, C., Weber, M. M., ... Breda, J. (2018). *Adolescent alcohol-related behaviours: Trends and inequalities in the WHO European Region, 2002–2014.* Observations from the Health Behaviour in School-aged Children (HBSC) WHO collaborative cross-national study. Copenhagen: WHO Regional Office for Europe.

Landelijk Alcohol en Drugs Informatie Systeem. Alcohol. Available at https://www.ladis.eu/en.

Malmberg, M., Kleinjan, M., Overbeek, G., Vermulst, A., Lammers, J., Monshouwer, K., … Engels, R. C. M. E. (2015). Substance use outcomes in the Healthy School and Drugs program: Results from a latent growth curve approach. *Addictive Behaviors, 42*, 194–202.

Ministry of Health, Wellbeing and Sports. (2018). *Nationaal Preventie Akkoord: Naar een gezonder Nederland* [National Prevention Agreement: Towards healthier conditions in the Netherlands]. The Hague: Ministry of Health, Wellbeing and Sports.

Monshouwer, K., Van Dorsselaer, S., Gorter, A., Verdurmen, J., & Vollebergh, W. (2004). *Jeugd en riskant gedrag 2003* [Adolescents and risk-taking behaviour 2003]. Utrecht: Trimbos Institute, Netherlands Institute of Mental Health and Addiction.

Mulder, J., Bovens, R., Franken, F., & Sannen, A. (2013). Proces in uitvoering. Een zoektocht naar de operationalisatie van cruciale procesfactoren in de uitvoering van regionale alcoholprojecten [Process in operation: Searching for important criteria to implement regional alcohol programs]. Utrecht: Nederlands Instituut voor Alcoholbeleid (STAP).

National Institute for Public Health and Environment. (2013). *Effectief alcoholbeleid: hoe pakt u dat aan? Aanbevelingen voor alcoholmatiging in de regio* [How to implement effective alcohol policy]. Bilthoven: RIVM.

National Institute for Public Health and Environment. (2018a). *Quickscan mogelijke impact Nationaal Preventieakkoord* [Quickscan possible impact National Prevention Agreement]. Bilthoven: RIVM.

National Institute for Public Health and Environment. (2018b). *Volksgezondheid Toekomstverkenningen 2018* [Orientation on Public Health in the future]. Bilthoven: RIVM.

National Institute of Health Promotion and Disease Prevention. (2004). *Jaarverslag alcoholvoorlichtingscampagne 2003: Drank maakt meer kapot dan je lief is* [Annual Report alcohol education campaign 2003: Alcohol destroys more than you care for]. Woerden, The Netherlands: NIGZ.

National Quality of Nutrition Organization. (2007). *Handleiding lokaal alcoholbeleid: een integrale benadering* [Manual local alcohol policy]. The Hague.

Roodbeen, R., Geurtsen, S., & Schelleman-Offermans, K. (2018). Could you buy me a beer? Measuring secondary supply of alcohol in Dutch on-premise outlets. *Journal of Studies on Alcohol and Drugs, 79*(1), 74–78.

Stevens, G., Van Dorsselaer, S., Boer, M., de Roos, S., Duinhof, E., ter Bogt, T., … de Looze, M. (2018). *HBSC 2017: Gezondheid en welzijn van jongeren in Nederland*. Utrecht: Universiteit Utrecht.

Tapert, S. F., & Schweinsburg, A. D. (2005). The human adolescent brain and alcohol use disorders. *Recent Developments in Alcoholism, 17,* 177–197.

The ESPAD Group. (2016). *ESPAD Report 2015. Results from the European School Survey Project on Alcohol and Other Drugs.* Lisbon, European Monitoring Centre for Drugs and Drug Addiction.

Tweede Kamer der Staten Generaal. (1986). *Alcohol en samenleving. Nota* [House of Representatives. Alcohol and Society. Memorandum]. The Hague, SDu, Tweede Kamer, vergaderjaar 1986–1987, 19 243, nrs. 2–3.

Tweede Kamer der Staten Generaal. (1997). *Wijziging van de Drank- en Horecawet. Memorie van Toelichting* [House of Representatives. Amendment of the Licensing act. Explanatory Memorandum]. The Hague, SDu, Tweede Kamer, vergaderjaar 1997–1998, 25 969, nr. 3.

Tweede Kamer der Staten Generaal. (2005). *Alcoholbeleid. Brief van de minister van Volksgezondheid, Welzijn en Sport, 24 Maart 2005* [House of Representatives. Alcohol Policy. Letter from the Minister of Health, Wellbeing and Sports, 24 March 2005]. The Hague, SDu, Tweede Kamer, vergaderjaar 2005–2006, 27 565, nr. 32.

Valkenberg, H., & Nijman, S. (2017). *Alcoholvergiftigingen en ongevallen met alcohol* [Intoxications and accidents due to alcohol]. Amsterdam: Veiligheid.nl.

Valkenberg, H., Van der Lely, N., & Brugmans, M. (2007). *Alcohol en jongeren: een ongelukkige combinatie* [Alcohol and youngsters: An unfortunate combination). Medisch Contact (online).

Van der Stel, J. C. (1995). *Drinken, Drank en Dronkenschap* [Drink, booze and drunkeness. Dissertation]. Hilversum: Verloren.

Van der Vorst, H., Engels, R., Meeus, W., & Deković, M. (2006). The impact of alcohol-specific rules, parental norms about early drinking and parental alcohol use on adolescents' drinking behavior. *Journal of Child Psychology and Psychiatry, 47*(12), 1299–1306.

Van Laar, M. W., & Van Gestel, B. (2019). *Nationale Drug Monitor 2018* [National Drug Monitor 2018]. The Hague: Scientifical Research and Documentation Center Ministry of Safeness and Justice/Utrecht, Trimbos Institute.

Verdurmen, J. (2006). *Alcoholgebruik en jongeren onder de 16 jaar. Schadelijke effecten en effectiviteit van alcoholinterventies* [Alcohol use and youngster under 16 years. Harmful effects and effectiveness of interventions]. Utrecht: Trimbos Institute, Netherlands Institute of Mental Health and Addiction.

Wood, A. M., Kaptoge, S. K., Butterworth, A. S., Willeit, P., Warnakula, S., Bolton, T., … Bell, S. (2018). Risk thresholds for alcohol consumption: Combined analysis of individual-participant data for 599 912 current drinkers in 83 prospective studies. *The Lancet, 391*(10129), 1513–1523.

World Health Organisation. (2018). *Global status report on alcohol and health 2018.* Geneva: World Health Organization; Licence: CC BY-NC-SA 3.0 IGO.

World Health Organisation. (2019). *Heavy episodic drinking among drinkers.* https://www.who.int/gho/alcohol/consumption_patterns/heavy_episodic_drinkers_text/en/. Accessed 13 June 2019.

Wuyts, C., Barbier, S., & Loosveldt, G. (2016, July 13–15). *Comparison of alcohol consumption in European countries, and some methodological thoughts.* Presented at the 3rd International ESS Conference, Lausanne, Switzerland.

18

Conclusion and Reflections on Future Directions

Dominic Conroy and Fiona Measham

A recurrent theme throughout the production of this book has been a sense of new discourses emerging, along with associated new terminology, that are guiding our understanding of young adult drinking practices. An early starting point in the inception and development of this book—through to communication and discussion with collaborators—was the need to bring together disparate strands of research from different disciplines and different methodological traditions which each were grappling with a sense of change. We hope that this book helps contribute towards steering the trajectory of future research concerning young adult drinking practices but clearly there is much work still to be done.

The production of this book consistently revealed a range of dualisms relevant to the discussion and study of young adult drinking practices. By

---

D. Conroy (✉)
School of Psychology, University of East London, London, UK
e-mail: D.Conroy@uel.ac.uk

F. Measham
Department of Sociology, University of Liverpool, Liverpool, UK
e-mail: f.measham@liverpool.ac.uk

© The Author(s) 2019
D. Conroy and F. Measham (eds.), *Young Adult Drinking Styles*,
https://doi.org/10.1007/978-3-030-28607-1_18

dualisms, we mean the well-established conceptual polarisation of the attitudes and behaviours surrounding young adult drinking practices which can produce coarse, and therefore potentially unhelpful, ways of making sense of these phenomena.

One example of these dualisms concerns drinking practices as rigid/enduring on the one hand and fluid/inconsistent on the other. This dualism is apparent in the context of Marjana Martinic and Arlene Bigirimana's chapter on 'Understanding Life Transitions and Drinking Trajectories in Adulthood' which demonstrated how particular life events and life changes may be linked to drinking modes and practices specific to that time and place in the life course. This dualism was also apparent in the second half of Dominic's chapter with Emma Banister and Maria Piacentini where the conceptual and real-world limitations of employing 'drinking categories' (e.g. 'non-drinker', 'light drinker', 'binge drinker') to guide accurate understanding young adult drinking practices began to be exposed and explored.

Another dualism can be understood in debates around whether and how young adults' drinking practices can be cast in terms of being 'safe versus unsafe' or 'responsible versus irresponsible'. For example, do the declines in alcohol consumption among 16–24-year-old young people discussed throughout this collection provide evidence of a growing commitment to 'safer' consumption levels and a growing level of 'responsibility' among young adults? We might suggest that merely posing the question exposes the political assumptions and potential biases that are tightly embedded in the terminology surrounding notions of safety and responsibility in the context of alcohol and indeed drug consumption of any kind. Notions of 'safe health behaviour' have been critically explored in other areas—notably by Paul Flowers in his studies of 'safe sex' (e.g., Flowers, Smith, Sheeran, & Beail, 1997)—and have revealed the difficulties and dangers involved in restricted definitions of risk and safety regarding particular health behaviours. A third dualism also appears to be important, and this has been touched on in several of the chapters—a dualism concerning the 'pleasurable versus problematic' in young adult drinking and drink-related behaviours.

18 Conclusion and Reflections on Future Directions 353

Clearly, these dualisms only offer one way of making sense of emerging themes in research concerning contemporary young adult drinking practices. Pinning down overarching themes designed to capture a body of work from such a diverse, heterogenous and multidisciplinary group of international researchers and authors may be unhelpful. In reviewing the contributions to this collection and from our own experience as writers and researchers, we simply appeal to colleagues whose fieldwork concerns young adult drinking practices to sustain high levels of criticality, openness and willingness to engage in bold and sophisticated research designs, novel methods for analysing research findings, creative approaches to dissemination, and effective, evidence-based and politically nuanced policy recommendations. In this sense, finding a way to locate research on young adult drinking practices that acknowledges but does not succumb to dualisms feels important in developing a research agenda which is progressive and compassionate to its subject matter.

There are numerous strands present in this collection that alcohol researchers may wish to pursue in future research. Literature on young adults' drinking behaviour in the transition from adolescence to adulthood, highlighted in Martinic and Bigirimana's chapter, is one area that may warrant further research attention. For example, in-depth contemporary studies of initiation into alcohol consumption among young people and how this initial period of drinking (and perhaps non-drinking) practice may blur into later phases of a relationship with alcohol feel valuable. In an area like life transitions, there is clearly scope for more research that adopts longitudinal designs and obviously significant funding commitments are called for here. Such research would be well-positioned to explore how drinking beliefs and practices at one stage of life (e.g. middle adolescence aged 14–17 years) might give way to different modes of drinking in young adulthood (e.g. 18–30-year-olds) when circumstances around education, employment, living status, partner status, peer group norms and complexion may all be prone to radical change.

There is also an emerging and changing policy context relevant to drinking practices among young adults that needs ongoing monitoring and evaluation. Evidence concerning the effects on alcohol consumption and alcohol-related problems with the introduction of minimum unit pricing, restrictions on retail and promotional practices and licensing legislation in several national contexts indicate the extent of policy impact on young adult drinking practices (Angus, Holmes, Pryce, Meier, & Brennan, 2016; Stockwell, Auld, Zhao, & Martin, 2012). Ensuring the impact of policy change on young adult drinking styles in qualitative, quantitative and mixed methods studies will be an important ongoing concern of future research programmes.

The first section of this book included chapters focused on the latest data and discussion concerning changing trends in alcohol consumption and some evidence of decline in consumption levels among young adults. Ongoing research needs not only to chart these changing trends but also to draw us towards a deeper understanding of the range of socio-economic, political and cultural factors at play. Conversely, drinking frequency and quantity of consumption have both increased among senior adults (aged 65 or older in the UK): weekly alcohol consumption has increased from 54% in 2005 to 57% in 2017 and the proportion exceeding minimum recommended levels (4 units of alcohol for men and 3 units for women) on their heaviest drinking day has increased from 16% in 2005 to 20% in 2017 (Office for National Statistics, 2017). Declines in young adult drinking warrant greater scrutiny in this context, not just as a phenomenon in and of itself but we might ask the question 'what can we learn from young adults changed (and changing) drinking practices and how might this be applied to health promotion and risk communications amongst older adults?'.

There is also the interesting possibility of how the current phenomenon of 'drinking less' among youth and young adults around the world might also involve comparative consideration of other potentially 'addictive', dependency-inducing or compulsive practices and behaviours. Specifically, alcohol consumption may have recently been outcompeted by the attractions presented by smartphone technology which gives young adults opportunities for accessible immersion on platforms that offer hybrids of social media communication, video gaming on devices that offer private and immediate sources of entertainment and the emergent possibilities of virtual reality. These declines in young adult consumption have also occurred during a period of emergence and rapid rise in new psychoactive

18 Conclusion and Reflections on Future Directions

substances (NPS), research chemicals whose availability has been facilitated by advances in both the dark and clear web leading to new psychoactive landscapes for future generations (Mounteney et al., 2016).

Whilst there might be displacement between legal and illegal drugs, Chapter 5 by Turner and Measham reminds us to pay close attention to the relationship between legal and illegal drugs including their combined use in situations of atypical and 'extreme' intoxication in contexts such as music festivals. There is a long-standing coupling of alcohol (a depressant) with a range of legal and illegal stimulants, from *Buckfast* (a nineteenth-century wine infused with caffeine made by English monks), *Vin Mariani* (a nineteenth-century French wine infused with cocaine endorsed by the Pope) through to vodka *Red Bull* (a vodka and caffeine energy drink mixer popular with millennials). A further area for future research is to explore atypical, polydrug using and displaced consumption, cultures and contexts. As Turner and Measham's chapter suggests, it may be that holiday time bucks young adult trends towards reduced consumption, with unusually large amounts of alcohol consumed in combination with unusually large amounts of illegal drugs, making polydrug use an atypical distinction of young adult holidays, adding a layer of additional risk at a time of relaxation and potential lowering of usual safeguards. This may be increasingly significant from a health perspective as the contrast between moderation and excess becomes more pronounced within individual lives.

A further key strand of emerging research concerns online drinking identities and social media use involving exposure to alcohol-related content among young adults. This emerging work is well illustrated in Chapters 6 and 7 of this collection where, for example in Chapter 7, Ian Goodwin and Antonia Lyons discussed how the range of social media platforms and opportunities for social media activities exert influences over the real-time dynamics of drinking choices and leisure time activities among young adults. The expansion of the internet and smartphone technology as something that now offers instantaneous immersion in online social networks is something that alcohol researchers must strive to keep abreast of if only to understand the way in which these networks are targeted and utilised by alcohol industry, health promotion and harm reduction organisations. Exploring drinking practices in the context of social media engagement presents, again, significant methodological challenges to produce an account of the dynamic and perhaps reciprocal interplay between 'online' and 'real world' activities and perhaps also how alcohol-related beliefs and narratives are rhetorically employed in these circumstances. Work drawing on the innovative qualitative methods employed by Antonia Lyons and colleagues which have involved integration of data from focus groups, individual interviews alongside online material in work designed to understand the complex dynamics involved in young adults' social networking and drinking practices (see Lyons, Goodwin, McCreanor, & Griffin, 2015 for an account of this research). Thus, changing drinking preferences and practices must be contextualised within broader changes in online as well as real-world consumption and leisure spaces.

As part of the process of producing this book, we have been excited to learn about the work being conducted by our contributors and field colleagues. Through this process, we have learnt about the range of topic areas, relevant theory and methodological approaches employed in the study of changing drinking styles among contemporary young adults in a variety of different national settings. The risk of stereotyping and reaching premature assumptions about 'typical drinking behaviour' among young adults was raised as a concern in the book introduction. Clearly, we cannot refer to the variety of topic areas covered in this book to make general claims about styles of young adult drinking practices in the first quarter of the twenty-first century. That said, there is evidence that young adult drinking is at an exciting juncture: in the growing normative acceptability of not drinking during social occasions and renewed recognition of a responsive relationship between relevant policy and young adult drinking practices warranting a focus on young adults as a discrete group for research attention. Indeed, as hinted at earlier, there might be grounds to believe that lessons might be learnt from young adults and applied to middle-aged and older drinking cohorts to develop more nuanced, reflective and restrained drinking styles.

We hope that you have enjoyed reading this collection and the range of contributions included in the book. We hope that the work included in this collection inspires colleagues to foster new collaborations designed to deliver research projects that offer critical and considered accounts of the varied styles of alcohol practices present among young adults in contemporary cultures.

References

Angus, C., Holmes, J., Pryce, R., Meier, P., & Brennan, A. (2016). *Model-based appraisal of the comparative impact of Minimum Unit Pricing and taxation policies in Scotland.* Sheffield: ScHARR, University of Sheffield.

Flowers, P., Smith, J. A., Sheeran, P., & Beail, N. (1997). Health and romance: Understanding unprotected sex in relationships between gay men. *British Journal of Health Psychology, 2*(1), 73–86.

Lyons, A. C., Goodwin, I., McCreanor, T., & Griffin, C. (2015). Social networking and young adults' drinking practices: Innovative qualitative methods for health behavior research. *Health Psychology, 34*(4), 293.

Mounteney, J., Griffiths, P., Sedefov, R., Noor, A., Vicente, J., & Simon, R. (2016). The drug situation in Europe: An overview of data available on illicit drugs and new psychoactive substances from European monitoring in 2015. *Addiction, 111*(1), 34–48.

Office for National Statistics (2017). *Adult drinking habits in England.* Retrieved on 24 June 2019 from https://www.ons.gov.uk/peoplepopulationandcommunity/healthandsocialcare/drugusealcoholandsmoking/datasets/adultdrinkinghabitsinengland.

Stockwell, T., Auld, M. C., Zhao, J., & Martin, G. (2012). Does minimum pricing reduce alcohol consumption? The experience of a Canadian province. *Addiction, 107*(5), 912–920.

Index

A

Abstinence 5, 24, 37, 48, 126, 162, 213, 226, 256–258, 264, 277, 341

Adolescence 4, 10, 23, 47, 58, 67–69, 77, 157, 353

Advertising 32, 53, 122, 124, 126, 145, 146, 165, 166, 174, 178, 276, 317–319, 322, 336, 343, 344

Aggression 55, 159, 176, 180, 181, 185, 195, 234

Alcohol economy 283

Alcohol identities 116, 118, 119, 124, 195

Alcohol industry 2, 165, 166, 276, 336, 341, 342, 344, 355

Alcohol policy 8, 15, 32, 35, 36, 57, 225, 228, 278, 283, 286, 289, 290, 296, 303, 306, 308, 313, 319, 322, 324, 333, 340, 344

Alcohol-related violence 15, 92, 295–298, 300–302, 305–307

Alcohol Use Disorders Identification Test (AUDIT) measure 37, 194, 201, 240, 242, 246, 279

Atypical intoxication 12, 100, 105, 108, 109

Australian alcohol policy 180, 277, 298

B

Binge drinking 8, 10, 37, 70, 97, 109, 116, 121, 154, 156, 157, 193, 194, 196, 228, 237, 240, 257, 276, 301, 333

Buckfast 194–196, 355

© The Editor(s) (if applicable) and The Author(s), under exclusive license
to Springer Nature Switzerland AG 2019
D. Conroy and F. Measham (eds.), *Young Adult Drinking Styles*,
https://doi.org/10.1007/978-3-030-28607-1

360 Index

C

Class 49, 97, 134, 174, 176, 183, 185, 186, 195, 227, 237, 280, 287, 296
College students 216, 277, 279, 283, 287, 289, 290
Connection 52, 55, 101, 102, 139, 154, 158, 160, 163, 164, 197, 238, 239, 243
Conscious-clubbing 14, 233, 234, 237–248
Cross-national comparisons 22, 41
Culturally sanctioned non-drinkers 219–222
Cumulative lifetime risk 277, 286

D

Dancing 14, 53, 93, 100–102, 105, 234, 237–239, 243, 244, 246–248
Declines in drinking 12, 23, 25–27, 31, 35–37, 40, 41, 47, 48, 50, 59, 69, 72, 235, 328, 329, 352, 354
Discourse 3, 48, 52, 53, 59, 161, 162, 173–184, 186, 235, 238, 351
Discourse analysis 11, 175
Discursive methods 11
Disney 104
Domestic abuse 192, 200–203
Drink 5, 10, 22, 25, 37, 41, 70, 75–77, 97, 98, 116, 121, 122, 137, 144, 146, 156, 158, 159, 163, 177–179, 181–184, 195, 199, 204, 213, 216, 219–221, 224, 227, 228, 235, 236, 243–247, 254, 255, 257, 258, 260, 261, 263, 264, 266–268,

281, 283, 285, 286, 289, 290, 304, 305, 324, 325, 328, 333–336, 338, 339, 342–345, 355
Drink-free challenges 225
Drinking 1–3, 5, 7–15, 22–24, 26–29, 31–41, 50–53, 55–59, 68–78, 88, 92, 97, 98, 109, 115–117, 119–126, 133–138, 141, 142, 144, 147, 156–158, 160–163, 165, 174, 176–186, 191, 192, 195, 197–200, 202, 203, 214–216, 218, 219, 221–228, 233, 235–238, 244–248, 254–258, 260, 262–264, 266–268, 276–278, 280–283, 285–290, 295, 297–300, 303–305, 307, 308, 313, 315, 316, 318, 323–325, 327, 328, 334–337, 339–341, 345, 351–356
Drinking culture 13, 21, 48, 56, 59, 73, 76, 120, 127, 133–136, 140–143, 146, 147, 194, 224, 228, 278, 289, 296, 297, 301, 303–305, 336
Drinking patterns 9, 12, 22, 25, 31, 32, 38, 47, 68–77, 88, 98, 134, 153, 154, 156, 157, 166, 173, 174, 184, 186, 192, 194, 235, 279, 280, 315–318, 324, 328, 329
Drinking practices 5, 6, 8–11, 14, 15, 47, 58, 115, 116, 141, 144, 154, 157–160, 162–165, 175, 181, 182, 186, 218, 219, 236, 282, 284, 289, 342, 344, 351–356

Drinking styles 2, 9, 11, 14, 48, 58, 157, 163, 183, 185, 194, 214, 218, 228, 269, 354, 356
Drinking trajectories 12, 68–70, 72, 73, 76, 77, 184, 352
Drinking transitions 10, 11, 68, 69, 72, 75, 77, 220, 352, 353
Drink refusal self-efficacy (DRSE) 256, 259, 262, 264–267, 269
Drug use 25, 52, 88, 92, 97–99, 102–104, 108, 109, 121, 123, 156, 176, 186, 194, 234, 235, 307
Drunkenness 1, 14, 47, 56, 92, 99, 109, 163, 174, 182, 185, 202, 224, 259, 261, 264–267, 304, 335
Dry January 14, 126, 213, 222, 253–269, 341
Dutch alcohol policy 333, 342, 343, 345

Economic reforms 316
Emerging adulthood 4, 6, 58, 156
Epistemological politics 306, 307
Excluded groups 194, 204

Facebook 55, 116, 118–125, 135–142, 144, 146, 147, 161, 165, 254
Femininity 173, 174, 179, 183
Friendship groups 153, 156–160, 163–165

Friendships 2, 13, 123, 134, 141–143, 153–166, 179, 186, 227

Gay scene 197–200, 203
Gender 12, 15, 24, 49, 51, 70–72, 74, 77, 97, 119, 134, 173, 175–177, 179–181, 183–186, 241, 244, 296–302, 304, 305
Gender roles 73, 77, 304
Generations 48, 49, 51, 52, 54–57, 59, 74, 76, 78, 90, 192, 204, 213, 296, 315, 328, 355
Government alcohol policy 314, 322

Harmful drinking 8, 78, 156, 165, 201, 215, 227, 278–280, 344
Harm minimisation 276–279, 283, 284, 286, 288, 290
Harm reduction 88, 109, 159, 161, 164, 277, 284, 289, 355
Heavy episodic drinking (HED) 23, 28, 29, 31, 35, 71, 257, 315, 333–336, 338, 342, 343
Holiday drinking 88, 97, 355

Ibiza 88, 92–94, 96, 98, 101, 103, 106–108
Identity 4, 6, 10, 12, 13, 47, 52, 53, 56, 59, 60, 69, 107, 116, 118–120, 122–124, 126, 134, 136, 147, 153, 155, 161, 165, 166, 179, 181, 182, 185, 194,

198, 199, 203, 217, 222–224, 226, 228, 234, 239, 302, 355
Identity development 115, 116, 126, 127
IkPas 341, 342
Interventions 8, 22, 78, 116, 125, 127, 164, 166, 192, 196–200, 202–204, 226, 248, 278, 298, 300, 302, 305, 307, 329, 338

L

'Laddish' drinking 180, 182, 185
'Ladette' 178, 183
Lesbian, gay, bisexual and transgender (LGBT) 192, 197–200, 203
Life stage 3, 4, 6, 8–10, 41, 67, 68, 73, 77, 155, 164, 191
Lifestyle 5, 6, 27, 48, 49, 52, 56, 59, 71, 75, 101, 116, 145, 178, 179, 185, 215, 219, 220, 225, 227, 254, 286, 318, 322
Life transitions 12, 67, 68, 71–75, 77, 352, 353

M

Marginalised groups 192, 195, 197, 201–204
Masculinity 73, 74, 159, 173, 174, 180–183, 185, 186, 296, 297, 301, 305
MDMA 96, 102, 104, 234, 247
Mental health 12, 50, 54, 55, 198
Music festivals 12, 88–91, 95, 97, 101, 145, 355

N

National Prevention Agreement 342–344
The Netherlands 15, 237, 333–337, 341–344
NIX18 341
Non-drinkers 2, 11, 14, 123, 158, 163, 213–226, 228, 244, 248, 256, 285, 352
Non-drinking 5, 14, 162, 174, 213–228, 237, 256, 268, 285, 353

O

Occasional drinkers 27, 32, 98, 223, 277, 282, 285

P

Parenthood 10, 12, 58, 67–69, 71–73
Parenting 23, 48, 75, 76
Peer influence 77, 117, 154
Personalised feedback intervention (PFI) 125
Pleasure 41, 59, 87, 88, 90, 94, 96, 99–103, 105, 108, 121, 160, 161, 178, 184, 235, 238, 247, 248
Polydrug use 194, 355
Postfeminism 176, 184
Predrinking 159, 160
Preloading 144, 159
Prototype willingness model (PWM) 214

R

Rationalisation 103, 104, 109, 220

Reciprocal relationships 117
Reducing alcohol consumption 37, 39, 57, 71, 92, 126, 226, 235, 248, 300, 313–318, 328, 329, 336, 342, 352
Respectability 174, 176, 183
Responsive regulation 289
Risk 2, 4, 12, 22, 24, 41, 51, 52, 55, 59, 74, 78, 88, 100, 103–105, 109, 116, 123, 125, 133, 134, 156, 159, 161, 173, 176–180, 183, 192, 197–199, 203, 261, 276, 278, 280, 285, 286, 289, 290, 304, 343, 352, 354–356
Risky drinking 8, 24, 27–30, 32, 36–41, 72, 176
Russia 313–315, 317, 321–323, 327, 328
Russian alcohol policy 15, 315–317, 322, 327, 328

Safe drinking practices 9, 48, 124, 155, 180, 284, 287, 290, 343
Secondary worlds 87–89, 93–96, 99–101, 103, 104, 106, 108, 109
Sociability 12, 52, 55, 101, 102, 108, 157, 158, 161
Social drinking norms 8, 118, 122
Social media ecology 133, 137–142, 144, 146, 147
Social media interactions 69, 115, 135, 137, 174
Social networking sites (SNSs) 13, 115, 116, 118–125, 127, 134–138, 142–144, 147, 199, 203

Social norms 68, 69, 115–118, 122, 125, 126, 139, 174, 199, 204, 216, 305, 345
Social roles 9, 68, 75–78
Sociology 101, 154, 214, 323
Sociology of nothing 219, 221, 223
Story telling 87, 121, 141, 305
Surveys 11, 22–27, 30–32, 34–36, 38, 40, 53, 55, 77, 92, 97, 105, 216, 234, 240, 246, 255, 258, 269, 279, 282, 289, 315, 322–324, 334, 340

Technology 2, 12, 49, 54, 55, 133, 135, 137, 139, 140, 146, 174, 354, 355
Temporary alcohol abstinence 5, 253, 255, 269
Thematic analysis 11, 279
Transition 4, 8, 48–51, 67–69, 72, 75, 76, 78, 91, 106, 118, 153, 156, 198
Trends 2, 9–12, 22–24, 27, 28, 31, 33, 35, 37–40, 54, 57, 59, 74, 235, 314, 315, 324, 325, 328, 329, 334, 335, 337, 344, 354, 355

University students 15, 115–120, 122, 124–127, 158, 162, 214–216, 223, 224, 235, 240, 275, 283, 305, 337, 338, 341, 343

364   Index

V

Violence 15, 51, 105, 159, 180, 181, 185, 192, 194–197, 201, 202, 234, 277, 295–302, 304, 306–308, 334

Y

Young adult 1–15, 22–24, 28, 31–33, 35–41, 47–60, 72, 88, 91–93, 98, 105, 108, 109, 133–135, 137–144, 147, 153–166, 173, 174, 177, 179, 182–186, 202, 213–217, 226–228, 233, 263, 267, 268, 276, 295, 298, 299, 306, 308, 315, 318, 324–329, 333, 334, 343–345, 351–356
Young adult identity 13, 115, 116, 126

Young adult identity 13, 115, 116, 126
Young people 3, 4, 11, 26, 31, 40, 47, 51–53, 58, 69, 88, 90, 93, 95, 103, 104, 116–118, 121, 122, 124, 126, 134, 136, 137, 141–143, 147, 154, 159, 161, 163–165, 176, 191–194, 196–198, 200–204, 215, 216, 228, 233, 235, 244, 246–248, 257, 258, 261–269, 277, 287, 296, 301, 304–306, 318, 319, 334–343, 345, 352, 353
Youth 3, 7, 23, 26, 31, 32, 57, 91, 133, 164, 191, 193, 195, 196, 202, 238, 276, 282, 318, 334, 336, 338–340, 354

CPSIA information can be obtained
at www.ICGtesting.com
Printed in the USA
LVHW052252120121
676313LV00002B/124